Public Opinion, Policy Responses, and Party Politics under the COVID-19 Pandemic

Public Opinion, Policy Responses, and Party Politics under the COVID-19 Pandemic

Examining Taiwan and Its Strategic Neighbors

Edited by
Chia-hung Tsai and Yao-Yuan Yeh

LEXINGTON BOOKS
Lanham • Boulder • New York • London

Published by Lexington Books
An imprint of The Rowman & Littlefield Publishing Group, Inc.
4501 Forbes Boulevard, Suite 200, Lanham, Maryland 20706
www.rowman.com

86-90 Paul Street, London EC2A 4NE

British Library Cataloguing in Publication Information Available

Library of Congress Cataloging-in-Publication Data

Names: Yeh, Yao-Yuan, editor. | Tsai, Chia-hung, 1971– editor.
Title: Public opinion, policy responses, and party politics under the COVID-19 pandemic : examining Taiwan and its strategic neighbors / edited by Yao-Yuan Yeh and Chia-hung Tsai.
Description: Lanham, Maryland : Lexington Books, 2023. | Includes bibliographical references and index. | Summary: "The authors compare the impact of the COVID-19 pandemic on public opinion and the dynamics of party politics in Taiwan, along with some of its strategic neighbors. The book provides profound implications for understanding the interactions between the COVID-19 pandemic and politics for scholars worldwide"— Provided by publisher.
Identifiers: LCCN 2023031879 (print) | LCCN 2023031880 (ebook) | ISBN 9781666940978 (cloth) | ISBN 9781666940985 (epub)
Subjects: LCSH: COVID-19 Pandemic, 2020—-Political aspects—Taiwan. | COVID-19 Pandemic, 2020—Government policy—Taiwan. | Political parties—Taiwan. | Public opinion—Taiwan. | Taiwan—Politics and government—2000–
Classification: LCC RA644.C67 P855 2023 (print) | LCC RA644.C67 (ebook) | DDC 614.5/924144—dc23/eng/20230911
LC record available at https://lccn.loc.gov/2023031879
LC ebook record available at https://lccn.loc.gov/2023031880

To those health professionals who stood on the frontline to combat the COVID-19 pandemic

Contents

Illustrations

Tables

Acknowledgments

We are indebted to many colleagues and organizations who helped to make the book possible. Credits for many of the chapters are due to the online conference "Politics under Pandemic: How COVID-19 Reshapes the Political Landscape in Taiwan and Beyond" on December 17–18, 2021. It was hosted by the Election Study Center and honorably sponsored by the International Doctoral Program in Asia-Pacific Studies and CSS at National Chengchi University, Taiwan, and the East Asia Studies Program at the University of St. Thomas, and the grant support from the Ministry of Education (Taiwan) to the University of St. Thomas. Special thanks to Hui-ling Chen for assisting with the logistics before and after the conference and Stephanie Lu for manuscript formatting and editing.

Introduction

Chia-hung Tsai and Yao-Yuan Yeh

The outbreak of the COVID-19 pandemic silently started in early 2020, and neither individual citizens nor their respective governments had prepared for it. Unlike the last outbreak of a similar coronavirus, SARS, which was less contagious but tended to be more deadly, the COVID-19 virus is much more contagious with a relatively lower chance of causing death. Nevertheless, it is still one of the most dangerous viruses in human history, and so far (February 2022), it has a death toll of more than five million worldwide. Aside from the casualties, the COVID-19 pandemic has also caused a global economic recession due to the need for lockdowns to contain the spread of coronavirus across every country. For example, when the pandemic began spreading in the United States, the unemployment rate rose from 4.4 percent in March 2020 to 14.8 percent in one month.

As one of the many countries suffering the negative impacts of COVID-19, Taiwan was a role model in containing and combating the spread of coronavirus. With the experience gained from SARS and its geographic advantage as an island state, the number of confirmed cases was about one thousand out of 23 million population (0.004 percent) in early May 2021, compared to 33 million cases out of 330 million population (10 percent) in the United States at the same time. However, Taiwan did not completely close the border. The pandemic eventually spun out of control in Taiwan during mid-May 2021, causing the number of cases to grow exponentially, reaching about sixteen thousand cases in September 2021, along with eight hundred deaths. Though the Taiwanese government has regained control and the number of daily new cases has dropped to single digits, the debates over how the government should have dealt with the pandemic and its vaccination policy continue.

Studies of COVID-19 have attracted tremendous attention from academia, governments, and even the general public. However, they tend to focus on the fields of biology, virology, public health, and psychology instead of the politics, policies, and political attitudes related to the pandemic. Of course, it is critical to understand the nature of this virus and seek proper policy remedies to stop the pandemic and help citizens to regain their everyday lives, but how the pandemic has affected the public and their views toward politics are equally important as they will determine political outcomes in the near future. Whether a democratic government could successfully combat the COVID-19 pandemic will certainly be a deterministic factor in explaining its upcoming election outcome. For example, despite a growing market and prosperous economy in the United States prior to the pandemic, the impediments in people's everyday lives and their economic well-being caused by COVID-19 largely contributed to the victory of Joe Biden in defeating the incumbent president Donald Trump in the 2020 U.S. presidential election. Also, as we have witnessed the emergence of vaccine diplomacy initiated by the United States and China, the COVID-19 pandemic dramatically reshapes the political landscape in foreign policy and international relations.

We propose to examine the impact of the COVID-19 pandemic on public opinion and the dynamics of party politics in Taiwan, along with some of its strategic neighbors, for comparison. There are two main reasons for employing Taiwan as the case to study the interaction between the pandemic and politics. First, Taiwan serves as a critical strategic position within growing U.S.-China tensions. Understanding how the pandemic has altered Taiwanese politics and its citizens' political attitudes provides valuable information to policymakers and academic scholars interested in U.S.-China relations and East Asia security. Second, according to the Freedom House, Taiwan is one of the most vibrant democracies in Asia. China claims Taiwan to be part of its territory. In contrast, Taiwan has its own government and has maintained unofficial foreign relations with many countries, including the United States and the European Union. Lying about one hundred miles east of China and using the same language, Taiwan has built up its military against China and has a strong interdependence with China. Therefore, it is interesting to observe how the Taiwanese reacted to the pandemic, which probably started in Wuhan, China.

Third, as Taiwan was one of the few countries that had successfully contained the COVID-19 pandemic at the beginning but lost control after, Taiwan serves as a perfect case to study the impact of the pandemic on public opinion and party politics in three different scenarios: (1) when most countries suffered the pandemic but not Taiwan; (2) when Taiwan suffered the pandemic while many industrial countries were moving toward a relatively better condition through vaccinations; and (3) when Taiwan recovered from the impact of the pandemic while many other countries experienced the delta and omicron variant. In other words, Taiwan provides a methodological advantage for scholars to gauge the influence of the pandemic on public opinion and party politics across different scenarios.

The book is divided into the following sections. First, we include a series of chapters investigating the influence of the COVID-19 pandemic on various political factors concerning public opinion and party politics in Taiwan, including factors contributing to its early success in combating the pandemic, presidential approval ratings, government performance, political trust, partisan opposition, political polarization, and public opinion toward the United States and cross-Strait relations. Second, we include a series of chapters investigating the influence of the COVID-19 pandemic on Taiwan's strategic neighbors for comparison, including China, Japan, Australia, and New Zealand. These chapters will elaborate on the interplay between public opinion, party politics, and the COVID-19 pandemic and how the experiences and observations among these countries can be compared to the case of Taiwan and vice versa. These comparisons provide important perspectives for policymakers to understand the political dynamics among Taiwan and other nations during the pandemic. In addition, these chapters also give trajectories on how the continuing pandemic will change public opinion and party politics among other democracies.

CHAPTER OUTLINE

Part 1. Taiwan under the COVID-19 Pandemic

The first chapter, "Vaccine Policy and Presidential Approval Ratings," examines how, if at all, the vaccine policy and its implementation affected the presidential approval rate. Based on the rational choice calculation, those who most benefited from a policy are more likely to support the policy in particular and the incumbent government in general. Therefore, we hypothesize that other things being equal, people who already received the first jab or are expected to be vaccinated soon are more satisfied with the vaccine priority policy and the presidential performance than people who are set at the lower priority. They tested the hypothesis with a TEDS internet survey conducted in mid-July 2021 when the whole island was still under the high third level of pandemic alarm and high demand for the vaccine. Additionally, they also analyzed a later wave of the survey (that is, telephone interviews conducted in September) to examine whether the hypothesis held during the time that most people took the first jab. The results suggest that the short-term "jab benefit" indeed boosts the support toward the incumbent government.

The second chapter, "Government Performance and Political Trust," engages in growing research that has focused on the role of trust in the government during the COVID-19 crisis. Studies have also shown that the strict measures in combating the pandemic have increased satisfaction with democracy, political support for the government, and vote intention for candidates from the ruling party (Bol et al. 2021). Hence, this chapter questions: Is this the case in Taiwan? Taking data from an internet survey conducted in June 2021, Lin focused on the public's attitudes toward the government's actions on COVID-19 and how those attitudes were associated with trust in the government. Lin examined how trust in the government changed as the pandemic unfolded since 2020 and how threat perceptions shape the public's support of the government. This chapter contributes to a better understanding of public opinion and the role of political trust during the COVID-19 crisis in Taiwan.

National emergencies often prompt a rally-around-the-flag effect in which there is a surge of support for the incumbent government and a lack of criticism from opposition parties. However, if the emergency persists and the initial rally fades, governments are forced to navigate the challenge amid normal, rancorous, partisan politics. In many countries, contentious politics have hindered effective responses to COVID-19. Chapter 3, “The Role of Partisan Opposition,” examines the messy politics Taiwan experienced in the first half of 2021 as it attempted to vaccinate its population. The opposition KMT repeatedly took any available opportunity to question, challenge, and criticize government vaccine policies. Some of these attacks were reasonable, while others were cynical and opportunistic. These attacks created clear partisan patterns in attitudes toward the various vaccines. This was decidedly not a period of opposition deference. Yet vaccination rates in Taiwan have equaled or exceeded those in most other rich democracies. Three crucial factors in this policy success were the fact that the KMT never questioned the desirability of vaccines in general, the spur in public demand for vaccines caused by a sudden outbreak, and the DPP government’s willingness to coopt the KMT’s position by allowing private actors to purchase vaccines on its behalf. Taiwan forged a provaccine consensus because of—not in spite of—its democratic system.

The fourth chapter, “Partisan Cues and Vaccine Hesitancy,” questions why some people do not want a COVID-19 vaccine, even when the number of domestic confirmed cases soared and people were anxious. Despite calling for unification to fight against the pandemic, there is a growing concern that Taiwan is more divided on managing the unprecedented pandemic. Before the unprecedented “lockdown” in place to curb the spread of the pandemic, many people in Taiwan were skeptical about the effect of the AstraZeneca (AZ) vaccine delivered from Japan in March and refused to be vaccinated. While most people were anxious and panicked due to the pandemic, the hesitancy to take a particular brand of the vaccine suggested that the vaccination issue may be politicalized as people view it through the partisan lens. Using panel data collected after the outbreak in Taiwan, this chapter contends that vaccine hesitancy and anxiety are conditional on political preferences. Specifically, the findings imply that people tend to make decisions based on their partisanship, even on the apolitical issue.

Since the outbreak of COVID-19, it has been debated whether democracy is the best political system to fight against COVID-19 has posed a serious threat to global public health. Given that the government must undertake drastic and efficient measures to deal with crises that emerge abruptly, democracy might not be able to respond to the COVID-19 pandemic in a more flexible and timely manner due to the dilemma of weighting public health goals against democratic norms, rights, and freedoms. Because little scholarly attention has been paid to the role of democracy in public health, the fifth chapter, "Political Polarization and Attitudes toward Democracy," aims to understand what factors affect public perceptions of democracy to fight against COVID-19 by focusing on political polarization. Using the data from Taiwan's Election and Democratization Study, 2021 (TEDS2021), this chapter finds that people with higher levels of political polarization are more likely to regard democracy as the best political system to handle COVID-19. The findings broaden our horizons on the consequences of political polarization during the COVID-19 pandemic and imply that political polarization does not necessarily pose a threat to the health of democracy.

In recent years, Taiwan has been at the forefront of the U.S.-China great power competition. In 2021, the United States donated four million vaccines to Taiwan after its first major COVID-19 outbreak. The sixth chapter, "Public Opinion toward U.S. Vaccine Diplomacy," asks how the Taiwanese public view the U.S. vaccine donation drive. Specifically, has the vaccination donation drive been successful in boosting Taiwan's confidence in the United States in the shadow of growing Chinese power? Are there any variations on how the public views the U.S. vaccination donation drive? If so, what are the factors driving how the Taiwanese public assesses this U.S. attempt at resolving the signaling? This chapter examines these questions with an original public opinion dataset from Taiwan. The finding suggests that the Taiwanese public often relies on "bounded rationality"—that is, decision making in which the processes used are rational within the constraints imposed by (a) knowledge limitations, cognitive limitations, and empirical factors arising from the complex, real-life situations in which decisions have to be made—to assess the U.S. vaccine donation drive. The findings contribute to studies of signaling, vaccine diplomacy, and political psychology.

The seventh chapter, "The COVID-19 Pandemic and Cross-Strait Relations," reviews how cross-Strait relations evolved under the COVID-19 pandemic from 2020 to 2021. Chen et al. first discuss various critical events in Taiwan and how the pandemic was employed as an information cue in framing cross-Strait relations, including the Taiwanese government's response to the onset of the COVID-19 pandemic toward China, Chinese information penetration through disinformation tools during the pandemic, and debates over the validity and reliability of COVID-19 vaccines. Furthermore, they investigate whether the COVID-19 pandemic has changed the public perception/assessment of cross-Strait relations and which direction it has brought to the Taiwanese public.

Part 2. Taiwan's Strategic Neighbors under the COVID-19 Pandemic

The COVID-19 pandemic has brought devastating impacts to every country since 2020. Thus far, the pandemic has not reached its end, and various COVID-19 policies have been put forward to counter the spread of the coronavirus and the casualty rates. Scholars also debate whether democracy or autocracy could better cope with the COVID-19 pandemic because numerous examples demonstrate that autocracies may better defend their countries against the pandemic, such as China. Following this trend of arguments, the eighth chapter, "The Effectiveness of the COVID-19 Pandemic Policy in China," discusses how authoritarian governments could better intervene in society by bypassing personal liberties and freedom and allowing more power concentrations in the decision-making process to facilitate quick and fast pandemic responses. Then, we review the COVID-19 policy in China between 2020 and 2021 through a chronological approach and demonstrate how the aforementioned rationales among authoritarian regimes have assisted with better management of the COVID-19 pandemic. Last, we derive the policy implications from observing the case of China and caution against the tradeoff of China's successes in its COVID-19 policy.

The ninth chapter, "Pandemic Policy, Public Opinion, and Election in Japan," examines the case of Japan. The threat of the coronavirus outbreak has transformed lifestyles in East Asian countries as well as Western countries by requiring people to refrain from going out and to wear masks. Restrictions on people's behavior may have sharpened the tradeoff between deterring the spread of infection and maintaining economic activity and may have influenced the formation of people's political attitudes. European countries recorded high numbers of infections and deaths from COVID-19, and health threats boosted public support for the government in the short-term, the so-called the rally-around-the-flag effect. However, Japan's numbers of infections and deaths were much lower than in European countries, and the Japanese public did not react emotionally to the spread of the coronavirus but calmly evaluated the government's policies. The Suga administration started vaccinations four months behind Western countries and held the Olympics without the support of a large majority of the public. These policy failures resulted in the largest number of infections and deaths. However, Prime Minister Suga managed to increase vaccination coverage and contain the spread quickly. Later, Prime Minister Suga resigned due to his lack of popularity, and the Liberal Democratic Party won the 2021 Lower House general election by backing Prime Minister Kishida, who emphasized economic recovery. Analyzing the pre- and postelection surveys shows that Japanese people gave a somewhat positive assessment of the Suga administration's measures against the coronavirus outbreak and supported the Liberal Democratic Party in the hope of Prime Minister Kishida's proposed policy of economic expansion.

The tenth chapter, "Identity Politics and International Relations in Australia," aims to explain this puzzling strategic choice of Australia by looking into the influences of COVID-19 on Australia's domestic politics. When the Donald Trump government released the 2017 National Security Strategy repositioning China as its strategic competitor with a revisionist mind, it ushered in an era of U.S.-China competition for the following years. Along with the unfurling and intensification of the U.S.-China global rivalry, states in East Asia, in particular, face a difficult choice in terms of taking sides. While alliance theories suggest that states stuck in the middle of a great power rivalry tend to avoid making clear security commitments to either side, Australia continuously strengthens its security relations with the United States to balance instead of hedging against China in this U.S.-China rivalry. This chapter argues that COVID-19 has an effect of hardening Australia's new state identity, an order maintainer of the liberal international order (LIO), for Australian policymakers as well as the Australian public in the context of the Great Australian China Debate. Suppose Australia keeps interacting with others based on this new identity. In that case, we may see it takes more and more responsibility for defending its sovereignty and key components of the LIO in the coming years.

The COVID-19 pandemic that began in early 2020 continues to wreak havoc on the world. At the height of the pandemic in 2020, New Zealand was one of the few states that was able to keep the pandemic at bay with relatively low infection and death rates. The exemplary nature of New Zealand's pandemic management propelled its young prime minister, Jacinda Ardern, to global political fame and led to a convincing electoral victory in the October 2020 general election. Indeed, since New Zealand adopted the MMP in 1996, no political party has ever won over 50 percent of the legislative seats in an election, and coalition governments have become the norm. Yet the Ardern-led Labour Party managed to be the first party to win an outright majority. The eleventh chapter, "Leadership, Public Opinion, and Party Politics in New Zealand," examines the convergence of adept handling of the COVID-19 pandemic, the role of public opinion, and the political leadership of Ardern and her cabinet members in political change in New Zealand during these uncertain times.

REFERENCE

Bol, Damien, Marco Giani, Andre Blais, and Peter John Loewen. 2021. "The Effect of COVID-19 Lockdowns on Political Support: Some Good News for Democracy?" *European Journal of Political Research* 60 (2): 497–505.

1

Vaccine Policy and Presidential Approval Ratings

Eric Chen-hua Yu and Chi Huang

INTRODUCTION

The COVID-19 pandemic has changed not only ways of daily lives but also patterns of governance around the world. Since the vaccines became available in late 2020, they offered new hope for relieving us from the pandemic. As the demand for vaccines increases, the supply fails to catch up. When the new wave of pandemic hit the world in 2021, vaccination went beyond routine health policy and emerged as an urgent political issue as allocation of scarce resources.

Compared with other Asian democracies such as Japan and India during the early period of the pandemic, Taiwan's COVID-19 infection and death rates were relatively mild. Yet when the sudden outbreak of the pandemic occurred in mid-May 2021, the government was blamed for not actively procuring vaccines from international pharmaceutical companies. Relying heavily on donations of 2.5 million doses of Moderna from the United States and 3.1 million doses of AZ from Japan in June, the government set the priority order of vaccination for the island's twenty-five million population. Since then, Taiwan has received more donations of vaccines not only from other countries but also from collective purchases made by the founder of Foxconn Terry Kuo, Taiwan Semiconductor Manufacturing Co. (TSMC), and the Buddhist Compassion Relief Tzu Chi Foundation. Along with the urgent supply of Taiwan's local vaccine

Medigen as well as the arrival of previous international purchases, the supply of the vaccine had become sufficient by the end of 2021.

As vaccination has become the primary issue since the hard hit of the pandemic in Taiwan in May 2021, this analysis investigates the extent to which the vaccine policy and its implementation affects the presidential approval rating. It is intuitive that people who benefit from a policy are more likely to support the policy in particular and the incumbent government in general. Thus, we hypothesize that, other things being equal, people who already received the first jab of the vaccine or are expected to be vaccinated soon are more satisfied with not only the vaccine priority policy but also the presidential performance than people who are set at the lower priority. We test our hypothesis by using two waves of survey data collected in mid-July and mid-September 2021, respectively. The first wave of the survey was conducted when the whole island was still under the high third level of pandemic alarm and the demand for vaccines was extremely high. The second wave of the survey was conducted under the second level of pandemic alarm as the supply of vaccines was no longer an issue. The rest of this article is organized as follows: section II reviews the literature that explains the surge and decline of public support toward leaders during crisis. Section III introduces our data and statistical models as well as analysis of the first wave of survey data. Section IV explains the empirical findings of the second wave of the survey data and section V concludes.

PUBLIC SUPPORT TOWARD LEADERS DURING CRISIS

During the outbreak of the COVID-19 pandemic, scholars in public opinion have paid considerable attention on the so-called rally-around-the-flag effect—that is, public opinion becomes more favorable toward political leaders in times of crises (Yam et al. 2020; Esaisson et al. 2021; Johansson, Hopmann, and Shehata 2021; Wang and Cheng 2021). Indeed, in the beginning of the pandemic in early 2020, for example, Taiwan's President Tsai Ing-wen's public approval rating enjoyed a considerable surge of more than 20 percentage points (Wang and Cheng 2021). Yet such a short-term surge did not remain for too long as her approval rating has gradually declined even though the numbers of diagnoses and the death toll of COVID-19 have remained relatively low in Taiwan compared to other countries until May 2021.

Scholars have identified two major theoretical perspectives to explain why there is a boost in approval rating related to a crisis (Hetherington and Nelson 2003)—the patriotism perspective and opinion leader perspective (Hetherington and Nelson 2003; Johansson, Hopmann, and Shehata 2021). Based on social-identity theory (Tajfel 1982), the patriotism perspective suggests that crises trigger support for symbols associated with the in-group, such as the president. Given the uncertainty and insecure feeling brought up by crises, people are more willing to follow their leaders (Doty, Peterson, and Winter 1991). Another relevant social-psychological mechanism posits that negative emotions, such as anger and anxiety, can also become drivers of rally effects (Lambert, Schott, and Scherer 2011).

The opinion leader perspective suggests that the rally effect mainly reflects an unusual perception of the general public toward political leaders during crises. Particularly in the beginning of a crisis, politicians tend to put aside the existing ideological differences and communicate with the general public with a positive tone. Then leaders may gain more support simply because they receive more attention without harsh criticisms (Baker and Oneal 2001). Additionally, people may use other cues than partisan differences to evaluate government performance, such as crisis management (Boin et al. 2017).

As the rally-around-the-flag effect can be regarded as a short-term opinion change in most cases, it is important to explain both its occurrence and duration. Hetherington and Nelson (2003) argue that the patriotism perspective provides a better explanation why the effect occurs in the first place while the opinion leader perspective helps explain its duration. Johansson, Hopmann, and Shehata (2021) further elaborate the argument and develop a three-phase framework to explain the surge and decline of public support toward leaders during crises by using panel data collected during the outbreak of the COVID-19 pandemic in Sweden. Specifically, they argue that at the beginning of the pandemic, the rally effect occurs and leads to a steep increase in public support for political leaders (Yam et al. 2020). During that first phase, the pandemic is highly salient but not politicized. In other words, people do not use the original predispositions to evaluate the government's actual performances. In line with the patriotism perspective, the urgency of the pandemic triggers the social-psychological reasoning behind the surge of the support for leaders.

As the degree of urgency of the pandemic gradually declines, news media and opposition politicians start to criticize the wrongdoing and mismanagement of the government during crises. Although the pandemic remains a salient issue, the discussions about its impacts as well as how to deal with it tend to become politicized. Thus, in this second phase, along with a salient but politicized crisis, the ordinary partisan confrontations gradually kick in and public support for leaders starts declining. The opinion leader perspective, highlighted by communications between politicians and the general public, helps explain the demise of the rally effect. In the third phase, when the pandemic turns to be less urgent and begins to decline in saliency in the public debate, routine politics simply comes back as the public support for leaders again are mainly explained by ordinary partisan or ideological differences (Dalton 2019).

In Taiwan, figure 1.1 confirms the existence of the rally effect during the outbreak of the pandemic in early 2020. The quarterly poll data collected by Taiwan's Election and Democratization Studies (that is, TEDS

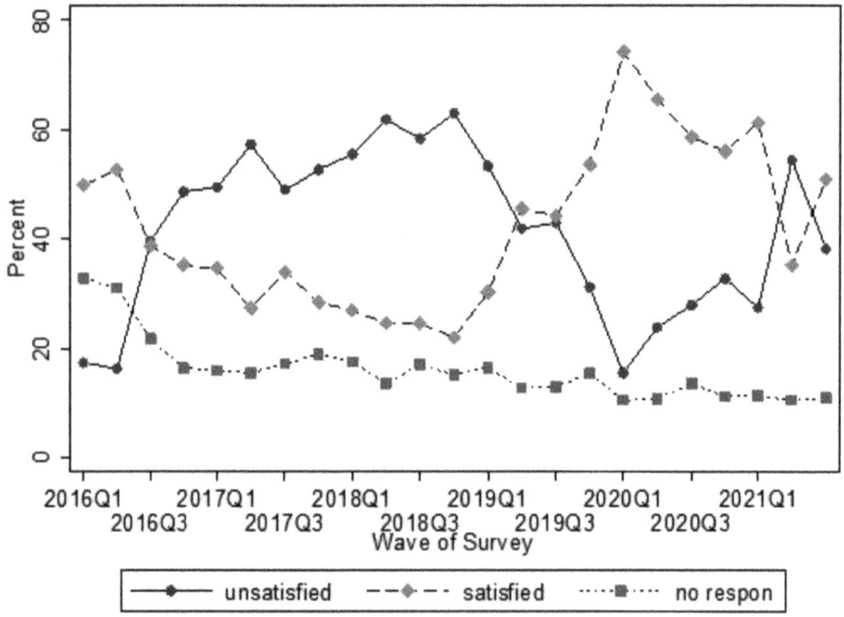

Figure 1.1. President Tsai Ing-wen's Approval Rating, 2016 to 2021
Source: Taiwan's Election and Democratization Studies (TEDS2016-2021_PA series).

Presidential Approval Rating series: TEDS2016-2021_PA series) show that President Tsai Ing-wen's approval rating (that is, percent of satisfaction) indeed increased dramatically from 54.5 percent in the fourth quarter of 2019 (that is, survey conducted in December 2019) to 74.1 percent in the first quarter of 2020 (that is survey conducted in March 2020).[1] Yet because President Tsai was just reelected in mid-January 2020, the high approval rating may also contribute to a certain level of bandwagon effect rather than the rally effect. Figure 1.1 also shows that since the second quarter of 2020, President Tsai's approval rating has dropped in the following three consecutive quarters. In the fourth quarter of 2020, the level of satisfaction with President Tsai's performance reached the point similar to that of the fourth quarter of 2019 (that is, 56 percent versus 54 percent). The small increase in the first quarter of 2021 may reflect the government's success in curbing the spread of the COVID-19 virus as the number of diagnoses had just increased from about eight hundred to one thousand cases during the time. Not to mention that the total death toll related to COVID-19 remained single digits until early March 2021.[2] In short, Tsai's approval rating dropped since early 2020 but stayed high around 60 percent until the real outbreak of the pandemic in Taiwan in May 2021. Given that the pandemic maintained its saliency but less urgent in late 2020 and early 2021, the support for President Tsai seemed to be in the second phase of the previously mentioned framework with respect to the rally effect.

In late 2020, although the vaccine became obtainable in some countries, Taiwan had a very limited quantity of vaccine only available for medical professionals in early 2021. Taiwan's early success of curbing the spread of COVID-19 mainly depended on its strict border control and quarantine regulations. Yet while the number of diagnoses increased dramatically from about one thousand to above eight thousand cases in May 2021, the government was heavily blamed for not actively procuring vaccines in advance. In figure 1.1, the level of satisfaction with President Tsai's performance dropped to about 35 percent in a pseudo-probability sample web survey that took place in the second quarter of 2021 (that is, actually conducted in mid-July at the point that the confirmed diagnoses was about fifteen thousand).[3] Although this number may not be fully comparable to other data points that were obtained via probability sample telephone surveys, it is reasonable to suspect that

President Tsai's approval rating took a hard hit by the sudden outbreak of COVID-19 in May 2021. And not until late June, ordinary people had scarce opportunity to be vaccinated in Taiwan.

Based on another web-based survey conducted by the Election Study Center at National Chengchi University in late May and early July 2021, the demand of vaccines was extremely high during that time.[4] Figure 1.2 indicates that on a 0–10 demand scale, nearly 60 percent of the respondents scored 8 to 10, and more than 75 percent of the respondents score above 6.[5] That is, right after the outbreak of COVID-19 in Taiwan in May 2021, a great majority of Taiwan's general public was willing to take vaccine. Krosnick (1990, 60) defined issue salience as "the degree to which a person is passionately concerned about and personally invested in an attitude." As vaccines were in high demand, the shortage of vaccines surely became a salient issue in Taiwan. Previous empirical studies demonstrated that the ups and downs of a president's approval rating may highly depend on his/her performance on salient issues (Krosnick 1990; Edwards, Mitchell, and Welch 1995; Gronke and Newman 2003; Dennison 2019). The lack of

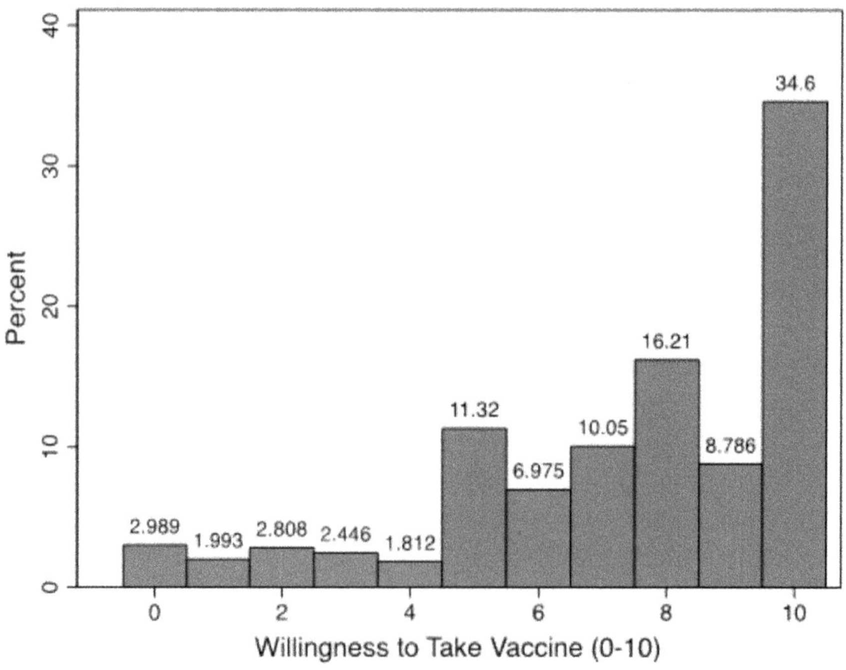

Figure 1.2. Willingness to Take Vaccine in May–June 2021

Source: Alumni Association of Election Study Center, National Chengchi University (2021).

vaccines could be the key reason to explain the significant drop of Tsai's approval around mid-2021.

As vaccination has become the most effective tool to fight against the spread of COVID-19, whether an individual can get vaccinated can be regarded as one of his/her major criteria to assess the government performance. In the following analysis, we use two waves of TEDS survey data to explore whether vaccination matters when people assess the performance of President Tsai Ing-wen administration.

DATA AND MODELS

The first dataset used in this study was obtained via a pseudo-probability sample web survey administrated by TEDS (that is, TEDS2021_SE07). Specifically, the panelists of the TEDS web survey are invited via previous telephone interviews. That is, in order to join in the web survey panel, one needs to be randomly selected via a telephone survey first. As not everyone can become a panelist with no restriction, the TEDS web survey should not be regarded as an opt-in survey. Yet joining in the panel certainly depends on one's agreement. Thus, some kind of self-selection mechanism still exists in terms of sample representation. In other words, while the TEDS web survey panel comprises randomly selected samples, it cannot fully represent the general population.

Due to the outbreak of COVID-19, TEDS was not able to conduct its quarterly survey via regular telephone interview. Instead the TEDS web survey was conducted in July 2021 as a replacement. About 12,000 email invitations were sent out through the TEDS web survey panel and 1,202 responses were collected.

This study focuses on three dimensions associated with the assessment of the government performance in the pandemic era—vaccination policy (that is, jab arrangement in particular), prevention of COVID-19, and President Tsai's approval rating. The actual wordings of the three questions are as follows: [Jab Arrangement] "How satisfied are you with the government's immunization schedule?" [COVID-19] "How satisfied are you with the government's performance in handling the COVID-19 pandemic?" [Approval] "How satisfied are you with Tsai Ing-wen's overall performance as president since her inauguration?"

Figure 1.3 demonstrates that only about 35 percent and 38 percent of the respondents were satisfied with the government's jab arrangement and overall performance on COVID-19 prevention, respectively. As the survey was conducted at the time right after the acceleration of the number of confirmed diagnoses, such a low level of satisfaction with the government's handling of the COVID-19 pandemic was not surprising. Under such circumstances, a low level of Tsai's approval rating appeared to be inevitable—only 35 percent of the respondents were satisfied with her overall performance while more than 54 percent were not satisfied.

As we focus on whether people who got vaccinated are more likely to favor the government performance, our key independent variable is whether or not the respondent has already got the first jab of any vaccine.[6] Figure 1.4 shows the differences on the assessment of government performance between the respondents who did not have any jab and those who got at least the first jab. Clearly, the respondents who did not have any jab of vaccine were less likely to be satisfied with the government performance with respect to all the three measures than their counterparts. For example, 31 percent of the respondents who did not have any jab were satisfied with the government's jab arrangement while 43 percent of those who had at least one jab were satisfied. A similar difference can also be observed regarding President Tsai's approval rating. In other words, having the first jab of vaccine seemed to be relevant to one's assessment of government performance during the widespread outbreak of COVID-19 in 2021.

Next, we use multivariate analysis to see whether "having a jab" has any real impact on the three government performance measures by controlling other variables. Because all three satisfaction variables are dichotomous (that is, satisfied versus not satisfied), logit models are constructed (that is, jab equation, COVID-19 equation, and approval equation). Regarding control variables, we include three major political variables that determine the main political cleavage in Taiwan (that is, partisanship, Taiwanese identity, and attitudes toward future cross-Strait relations or the so-called unification-independence spectrum) as well as a number of demographic variables (that is, gender, age, education, and region of residential registration).[7,8] In table 1.1, the coefficients for the jab variable are significant with the expected positive sign in all the three equations. Additionally, the coefficients for all three political variables are also significant with the expected signs of directions.

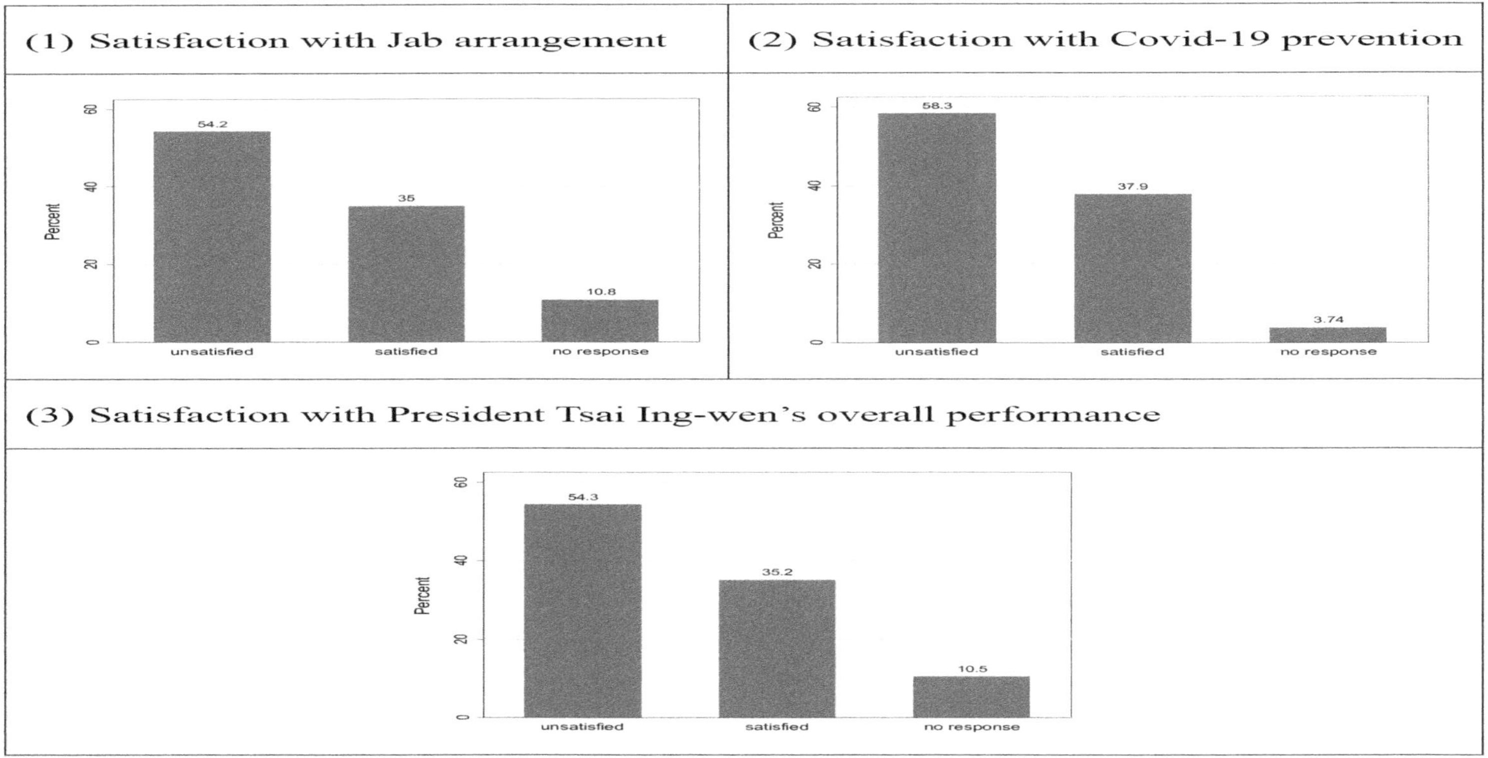

Figure 1.3. Assessment of Government Performance on Three Dimensions (July 2021)

Source: Taiwan's Election and Democratization Studies (TEDS2021_SE07).

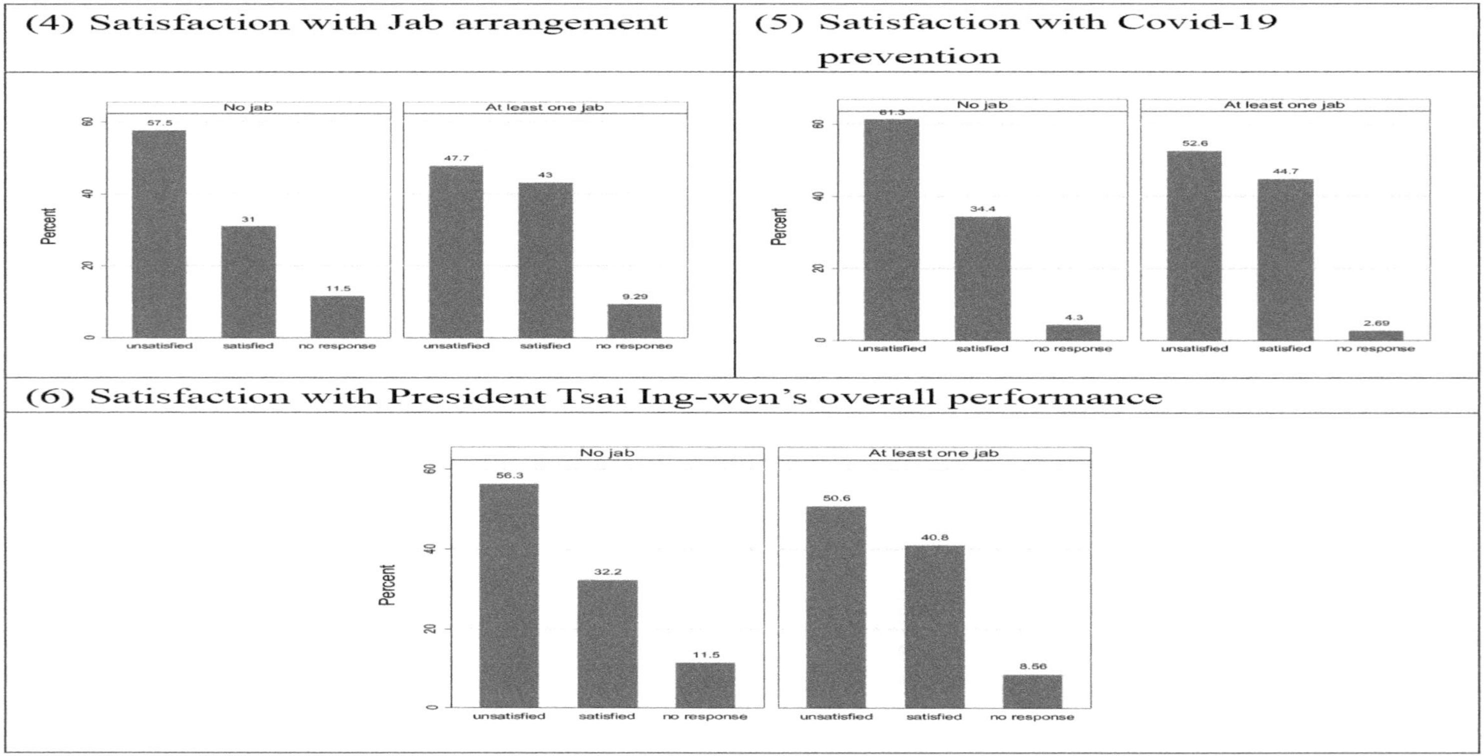

Figure 1.4. Assessment of Government Performance on Three Dimensions, by Jab (July 2021)

Source: Taiwan's Election and Democratization Studies (TEDS2021_SE07).

Table 1.1. Explaining the Level of Satisfaction with Government Performance (July 2021)

	Jab	*COVID-19*	*Approval*
Dep. Variable	*Coef. (Std. Err.)*	*Coef. (Std. Err.)*	*Coef. (Std. Err.)*
Jab	0.499**	0.466**	0.362*
	(0.177)	(0.183)	(0.215)
Female	–0.047	0.395**	0.343*
	(0.163)	(0.169)	0.198
Age (base: 20–29)			
30–39	–0.622**	–0.309	0.074
	(0.293)	(0.290)	(0.334)
40–49	–0.342	0.019	0.386
	(0.303)	(0.305)	(0.355)
50–59	0.047	0.053	0.659
	(0.342)	(0.351)	(0.416)
65+	0.235	0.604	1.358**
	(0.391)	(0.410)	(0.483)
College	–0.100	0.149	0.579**
	(0.216)	(0.230)	(0.275)
Region (base: Taipei Metropolitan)			
New Taipei Keelung	0.567*	0.351	0.610
	(0.314)	(0.320)	(0.375)
TaoChuMiao	0.014	0.020	0.508
	(0.257)	(0.265)	(0.311)
ChungChangTao	–0.096	0.015	0.013
	(0.238)	(0.244)	(0.296)
YunChiaNan	–0.201	0.039	–0.199
	(0.291)	(0.297)	(0.343)
KaoPingPeng	0.054	0.359	0.253
	(0.255)	(0.263)	(0.305)
YiHuaTung	0.582	1.212**	0.668
	(0.429)	(0.465)	(0.523)
Camp			
Blue	–0.995**	–1.422**	–2.146**
	(0.295)	(0.343)	(0.477)
Green	1.177**	1.197**	1.718**
	(0.191)	(0.190)	(0.219)
TPP	–0.826**	–1.178**	–1.535**
	(0.252)	(0.259)	(0.309)
Taiwanese	0.869**	1.214**	1.955**
	(0.240)	(0.247)	(0.323)

(continued)

Table 1.1. *Continued*

	Jab	*COVID-19*	*Approval*
Dep. Variable	*Coef.* *(Std. Err.)*	*Coef.* *(Std. Err.)*	*Coef.* *(Std. Err.)*
Uni-Ind			
SQ	0.448	0.715	–0.139
	(0.372)	(0.475)	(0.542)
Independence	1.477**	1.956**	1.248**
	(0.402)	(0.494)	(0.560)
Constant	–2.001**	–3.259**	–4.001**
	(0.535)	(0.619)	(0.712)
N	1034	1112	1039
Log likelihood	–492.770	–469.764	–351.246
Pseudo R2	0.290	0.372	0.497

Note: * $p<0.1$; ** $p<0.05$

Source: Taiwan's Election and Democratization Studies (TEDS2021_SE07).

Given the coefficients for the logit models shown in table 1.1, we calculate the probability changes of the three government performance measures by switching the jab variable from "no jab" to "at least one jab" (that is, from 0 to 1), holding other variables constant. Table 1.2 shows that the respondent who took at least one jab increases his/her level of satisfaction with jab arrangement, COVID-19 prevention, and Tsai's overall performance by about 11.5, 10.2, and 7.1 percentage points, respectively, compared against his/her counterpart who has not taken any jab. It is clear that vaccination has substantial impacts on one's assessments of multiple related government performances.

As only a small proportion of the people have taken vaccines in July 2021, we also analyze whether one's expected time of taking vaccines may affect his/her assessment of government performance on jab arrangement, COVID-19 prevention, and Tsai's administration in general, respectively.[9] Table 1.3 indicates that the coefficients for the jab expectation variable are

Table 1.2. Probability Changes on Government Satisfaction from "No Jab" to "At Least One Jab" (July 2021)

Probability Change	*Satisfaction with Jab Arrangement*	*Satisfaction with COVID-19 Prevention*	*Satisfaction with Tsai's Performance*
From "no jab" to "at least one jab"	11.48	10.23	7.06

Source: Taiwan's Election and Democratization Studies (TEDS2021_SE07).

Table 1.3. Expectation of Jab and Level of Satisfaction with Government Performance (July 2021)

	Jab	*COVID-19*	*Approval*
Dep. Variable	*Coef.* *(Std. Err.)*	*Coef.* *(Std. Err.)*	*Coef.* *(Std. Err.)*
Expect	–0.146**	–0.263**	–0.211**
	(0.075)	(0.081)	(0.100)
Female	–0.370	0.209	0.252
	(0.265)	(0.273)	(0.340)
Age (base: 20–29)			
30–39	–0.738*	–0.589	–0.033**
	(0.446)	(0.458)	(0.555)
40–49	–0.777*	–0.618	–0.275
	(0.473)	(0.485)	(0.585)
50–59	–0.298	–0.915	0.283
	(0.565)	(0.592)	(0.732)
65+	0.470	–0.341	1.099
	(0.725)	(0.803)	(0.958)
College	0.350	0.363	0.949**
	(0.357)	(0.374)	(0.482)
Region (base: Taipei Metropolitan)			
New Taipei Keelung	0.376	0.350	0.336
	(0.527)	(0.515)	(0.642)
TaoChuMiao	0.117	0.284	0.298
	(0.425)	(0.437)	(0.544)
ChungChangTao	–0.123	0.791**	0.002
	(0.394)	(0.404)	(0.525)
YunChiaNan	–0.805*	0.122	–0.512
	(0.470)	(0.496)	(0.590)
KaoPingPeng	–0.401	0.504	–0.038
	(0.410)	(0.429)	(0.534)
YiHuaTung	0.751	1.130	0.302
	(0.772)	(0.823)	(0.916)
Camp (base: Independent voters)			
Blue	–1.320**	–1.959**	–1.660**
	(0.562)	(0.678)	(0.763)
Green	1.077**	1.236**	2.276**
	(0.310)	(0.309)	(0.391)
TPP	–0.783*	–1.224**	–1.231**
	(0.422)	(0.445)	(0.538)
Taiwanese	1.580**	1.230**	2.404**
	(0.429)	(0.420)	(0.647)

(continued)

Table 1.3. *Continued*

Dep. Variable	*Jab* Coef. (Std. Err.)	*COVID-19* Coef. (Std. Err.)	*Approval* Coef. (Std. Err.)
Uni-Ind (base: Unification)			
SQ	–0.048	0.190	–0.983
	(0.673)	(0.770)	(0.867)
Independence	0.718	0.951	0.281
	(0.709)	(0.783)	(0.874)
Constant	–1.110	–1.330	–2.779**
	(1.000)	(1.063)	(1.283)
N	411	433	397
Log likelihood	–188.784	–180.237	–122.710
Pseudo R2	0.324	0.389	0.549

Note: * $p<0.1$; ** $p<0.05$

Source: Taiwan's Election and Democratization Studies (TEDS2021_SE07).

significant with the expected negative signs in all the three equations. That is, the longer the time one expects to wait for vaccination, the less likely he/she would be satisfied with the related government performances.

Again, we use the coefficients for the logit models shown in table 1.3 to calculate the probability changes of the three government performance measures by switching the jab expectation variable from "within one month" to "six-plus months later" (that is, from 1 to 7), holding other variables constant. Table 1.4 shows that the respondent who expects to wait for six more months to take the first jab may decrease his/her level of satisfaction with jab arrangement, COVID-19 prevention, and Tsai's overall performance by about 18.7, 31, and 24 percentage points, respectively, compared against his/her counterpart who expects to take the first jab within a month. Additionally, waiting for one more month may, on

Table 1.4. Probability Change with the Change of the Expectation for the First Jab (July 2021)

Probability Change	*Satisfaction with Jab Arrangement*	*Satisfaction with COVID-19 Prevention*	*Satisfaction with Tsai's Performance*
Marginal effect	–3.28	–5.76	–4.36
Min →Max (1→7)	–18.71	–31.03	–23.96

Source: Taiwan's Election and Democratization Studies (TEDS2021_SE07).

average, decrease one's level of satisfaction with the three government performance measures by 3.3, 5.8, and 4.4 percentage points, respectively. In short, the expected waiting time for vaccination also has substantial impacts on one's assessments of multiple related government performances.

DURING THE DECLINE OF COVID-19 CASES

As shown in figure 1.1, President Tsai's approval rating rises in the third quarter of 2021. Indeed in September 2021, more than 40 percent of Taiwanese have already taken the first jab of vaccine. Older people even have started taking the second jab. In other words, the shortage of the vaccine is no longer a salient issue. And the number of diagnoses turned back to single digits a day. It seemed that Taiwan had got through the May outbreak and become safe again.

Thus, we expect that in the survey conducted in the third quarter of 2021 (that is, TEDS2021_PA09),[10] the extent to which "having a jab" affects the three government performance measures, if any, could be limited. By controlling demographic and political variables, table 1.5 indicates that the coefficients for the jab variable are still significant with the expected positive signs in the COVID-19 and approval equations, respectively. In the jab equation, the coefficient for the jab variable is not significant but positive as expected. In other words, even after the May outbreak, vaccination remains a salient issue when one assesses the government performance on COVID-19 prevention and Tsai's administration in general.

We then calculate the probability changes of the three government performance measures by switching the jab variable from "no jab" to "at least one jab," holding other variables constant. Table 1.6 shows that a respondent who took at least one jab increases his/her level of satisfaction with jab arrangement, COVID-19 prevention, and Tsai's overall performance by about 6, 12.4, and 10.4 percentage points, respectively, compared against his/her counterpart who has not taken any jab. Thus, even in September 2021, the impacts of "having a jab" on one's assessments of government performances remain substantive.

Again, by using the September data, we also analyze whether one's expected time of taking the vaccine may affect his/her assessment of govern-

Table 1.5. Explaining the Level of Satisfaction with Government Performance (September 2021)

	Jab	*COVID-19*	*Approval*
Dep. Variable	*Coef.* *(Std. Err.)*	*Coef.* *(Std. Err.)*	*Coef.* *(Std. Err.)*
Jab	0.241	0.500**	0.448**
	(0.160)	(0.173)	(0.198)
Female	–0.065	0.251	–0.049
	(0.149)	(0.161)	(0.193)
Age (base: 20–29)			
30–39	–0.013	–0.020	–0.303
	(0.251)	(0.271)	(0.324)
40–49	0.013	0.372	–0.113
	(0.238)	(0.255)	(0.298)
50–59	0.117	0.221	–0.105
	(0.261)	(0.273)	(0.316)
65+	–0.124	0.243	–0.351
	(0.282)	(0.297)	(0.354)
Education (base: Elementary and below)			
Junior high	–0.046	–0.106	–0.363
	(0.368)	(0.442)	(0.504)
Senior high	–0.261	–0.421	–0.468
	(0.317)	(0.390)	(0.408)
Junior college	–0.219	–0.699*	–0.926**
	(0.343)	(0.417)	(0.457)
University	–0.225	–0.208	–0.278
	(0.327)	(0.398)	(0.419)
Region (base: Taipei Metropolitan)			
New Taipei Keelung	0.590**	0.135	0.391
	(0.291)	(0.317)	(0.382)
TaoChuMiao	0.203	–0.099	–0.589
	(0.242)	(0.269)	(0.324)
ChungChangTao	0.053	0.090	–0.086
	(0.240)	(0.252)	(0.299)
YunChiaNan	0.428*	0.804**	0.232
	(0.244)	(0.280)	(0.303)
KaoPingPeng	0.480**	–0.008	–0.415
	(0.241)	(0.260)	(0.305)
YiHuaTung	–0.184	0.096	–0.579
	(0.373)	(0.372)	(0.449)
Camp (base: Independent voter)			
Blue	–0.525**	–0.686**	–1.390**
	(0.221)	(0.230)	(0.272)
Green	1.306**	1.482**	2.553**
	(0.176)	(0.193)	(0.272)

	Jab	*COVID-19*	*Approval*
Dep. Variable	*Coef.* *(Std. Err.)*	*Coef.* *(Std. Err.)*	*Coef.* *(Std. Err.)*
TPP	–0.262	–1.017**	–1.118**
	(0.276)	(0.297)	(0.333)
Taiwanese	0.644**	0.907**	1.022**
	(0.177)	(0.184)	(0.207)
Uni-Ind (base: Unification)			
SQ	0.221	–0.020	–0.200
	(0.333)	(0.328)	(0.375)
Independence	0.377	0.609*	0.297
	(0.351)	(0.347)	(0.401)
Constant	–1.325	–1.345**	–0.144
	(0.521)	(0.560)	(0.602)
N	1066	1081	999
Log likelihood	–612.493	–549.243	–407.766
Pseudo R2	0.157	0.258	0.392

Note: * *p*<0.1; ** *p*<0.05

Source: Taiwan's Election and Democratization Studies (TEDS2021_PA09).

ment performance on jab arrangement, COVID-19 prevention, and Tsai's administration in general, respectively. Contrary to the results shown in table 1.3, table 1.7 indicates that the coefficients for the jab expectation variable are no longer significant but with the expected negative signs in all the three equations. In other words, waiting time for vaccination does not affect one's satisfaction with the government performances as the shortage of vaccines has no longer been a problem in September 2021.

Regarding the substantive impacts of vaccine waiting time on the assessments of government performance, table 1.8 shows that the respondent who expects to wait for six more months to take the first jab may decrease his/her level of satisfaction with jab arrangement, COVID-19

Table 1.6. Probability Changes on Government Satisfaction from "No Jab" to "At Least One Jab" (September 2021)

Probability Change	*Satisfaction with Jab Arrangement*	*Satisfaction with COVID-19 Prevention*	*Satisfaction with Tsai's Performance*
From "no jab" to "at least one jab"	5.96	12.39	10.42

Source: Taiwan's Election and Democratization Studies (TEDS2021_PA09).

Table 1.7. Expectation of Jab and Level of Satisfaction with Government Performance (September 2021)

	Jab	*COVID-19*	*Approval*
Dep. Variable	*Coef.* *(Std. Err.)*	*Coef.* *(Std. Err.)*	*Coef.* *(Std. Err.)*
Expect	–0.005	–0.054	–0.203
	(0.121)	(0.129)	(0.180)
Female	–0.494	0.391	0.110
	(0.342)	(0.348)	(0.489)
Age (base: 20–29)			
30–39	–0.486	–0.196	–1.009
	(0.469)	(0.499)	(0.694)
40–49	–1.139**	–0.134	–0.978
	(0.570)	(0.520)	(0.719)
50–59	–1.325**	–0.710	–1.181
	(0.591)	(0.575)	(0.839)
65+	–0.476	0.733	–1.329
	(0.771)	(0.751)	(1.000)
Education (base: Elementary and below)			
Junior high	0.299	1.486	0.419
	(0.933)	(0.981)	(1.215)
Senior high	–0.158	1.026	1.084
	(0.826)	(0.894)	(1.045)
Junior college	–0.462	0.885	1.041
	(0.932)	(0.980)	(1.266)
University	–0.804	0.626	0.944
	(0.836)	(0.902)	(1.019)
Region (base: Taipei Metropolitan)			
New Taipei Keelung	–0.008	–0.724	0.454
	(0.948)	(0.917)	(1.347)
TaoChuMiao	–0.754	–0.587	–1.225
	(0.551)	(0.553)	(0.748)
ChungChangTao	–0.121	–0.488	–0.555
	(0.569)	(0.538)	(0.672)
YunChiaNan	0.040	–0.168	–1.225*
	(0.592)	(0.609)	(0.687)
KaoPingPeng	0.065	–0.448	–2.731**
	(0.608)	(0.607)	(0.923)
YiHuaTung	–0.928	–0.291	–0.852
	(0.780)	(0.923)	(1.242)
Camp (base: Independent voter)			
Blue	–0.112	–0.824*	–2.369**
	(0.510)	(0.489)	(0.737)
Green	1.279**	1.381**	3.882**
	(0.439)	(0.433)	(0.833)

	Jab	*COVID-19*	*Approval*
Dep. Variable	*Coef.* *(Std. Err.)*	*Coef.* *(Std. Err.)*	*Coef.* *(Std. Err.)*
TPP	0.241	–0.701	–1.230**
	(0.476)	(0.510)	(0.628)
Taiwanese	0.079	0.033	0.451
	(0.403)	(0.411)	(0.487)
Uni-Ind (base: Unification)			
SQ	–0.103	–0.671	0.014
	(0.668)	(0.541)	(0.748)
Independence	–0.393	–0.058	0.197
	(0.740)	(0.621)	(0.819)
Constant	0.973	–0.364	0.778
	(1.237)	(1.240)	(1.493)
N	212	211	195
Log likelihood	–124.305	–120.426	–70.149
Pseudo R2	0.139	0.168	0.471

Note: * $p<0.1$; ** $p<0.05$

Source: Taiwan's Election and Democratization Studies (TEDS2021_PA09).

prevention, and Tsai's overall performance by about 0.46, 5.2, and 20.2 percentage points, respectively, compared to his/her counterpart who expects to take the first jab within a month. Additionally, waiting for one more month, on average, may decrease one's level of satisfaction with the three government performance measures by 0.12, 1.31, and 5.06 percentage points. In short, the expected waiting time for vaccination has relatively limited impacts on one's assessments of government performance on jab arrangement and COVID-19 prevention in September 2021. Yet it still appears to affect one's satisfaction with Tsai's overall performance in a substantive way.

Table 1.8. Probability Change with the Change of the Expectation for the First Jab (September 2021)

Probability Change	*Satisfaction with Jab Arrangement*	*Satisfaction with COVID-19 Prevention*	*Satisfaction with Tsai's Performance*
Marginal effect	–0.12	–1.31	–5.06
Min →Max (1→7)	–0.46	–5.20	–20.02

Source: Taiwan's Election and Democratization Studies (TEDS2021_PA09).

CONCLUDING REMARKS

This paper analyzes the extent to which the demand of vaccine affects one's satisfaction with the government performance by comparing two waves of surveys conducted during and after the May outbreak of COVID-19 in 2021. Our findings are mainly twofold:

First, when the vaccine shortage became a salient issue during the COVID-19 outbreak in May 2021, those who had the first jab were more likely to be satisfied with the government performance. Even when the number of COVID-19 cases significantly dropped in September, "having a jab" still substantively affected one's satisfaction with the assessments of government performance though such impact somehow decreases in magnitude.

Second, when the demand for vaccines was high, the expected waiting time for vaccines also affected one's assessment of government performance. That is, the longer the time one expected to take the first jab, the less likely he/she would be satisfied with the government performance. Yet when the demand has been fulfilled, waiting time for vaccines has no longer been an important issue and its impacts on one's assessments of government performance became limited.

Overall, this analysis demonstrates that when a salient issue or a certain policy demand emerges, it is crucial for the government to solve the issue or fulfill the demand in time. Indeed, some argue that most of the time, the president's approval rating is mainly determined by partisanship or ideology rather than by performance (Mueller 1973; Sigelman and Conover 1981; Schmitt 1983; Callaghan and Virtanen 1993; Dalton 2019). Yet our finding shows that citizens are still rational. It is important for a government to fulfill citizens' needs and distribute specific benefits in particular during crises.

NOTES

1. Most of the data analyzed in this article were from surveys conducted by Taiwan's Election and Democratization Study (TEDS) between 2016 and 2021, including telephone and web surveys. The coordinator of the multiyear project of TEDS is Professor Chi Huang (2016–2020, National Chengchi University)

and Professor Lu-huei Chen (2020–, National Chengchi University). For more information, please refer to the TEDS website (http://www.tedsnet.org). The authors appreciate the assistance in providing data by the institute and individuals aforementioned. The authors are alone responsible for views expressed herein.

2. For more information about Taiwan's COVID-19 cases report, please refer to https://covid-19.nchc.org.tw/dt_005-covidTable_taiwan.php?language=en (accessed July 25, 2022).

3. The survey was actually conducted in mid-July, at the time that the accumulated confirmed diagnoses was about fifteen thousand.

4. The survey was sponsored by the Alumni Association of Election Study Center at National Chengchi University and conducted by using the same method as that of the TEDS web survey.

5. The question wording is: "If 0 means 'you have completely no intention to take the vaccine of COVID-19' and 10 means 'you have full intention to take the vaccine of COVID-19,' on a 0–10 scale, where are you located?"

6. The wording of the question is: "Have you gotten any COVID-19 vaccine in Taiwan?"

7. The respondents' partisanships include four categories: Blue camp (for example, Kuomintang, People First Party, and New Party), Green camp (for example, Democratic Progressive Party, New Power Party, and Taiwan Radical Wing), Taiwan People's Party, and Independent voters. Identity is coded as a dichotomous variable: Taiwanese identity and others. And attitudes toward future cross-Strait relations are classified into three categories as follows: unification, independence, and maintaining the status quo.

8. In the web survey, a great proportion of the respondents have obtained college-level education (about 79 percent). Thus, the respondents' education levels are classified into only two categories (that is, college or not). But in the following analysis of the TEDS telephone survey data, the respondents' education level is classified into the normal five categories (for example, 20–29; 30–39; 40–49; 50–59; and 60 and above). Regarding the variable of regions of residential registration, respondents are classified into seven regions include Taipei Metropolitan, New Taipei and Keelung, TaoChuMiao, ChungChangTao, YunChiaNan, KaoPingPeng, and YiHuaTung.

9. For the jab expectation variable, we used the following question: "When do you expect to be vaccinated?" We then coded the responses from 1 to 7 indicating "within one month" to "six-plus months later."

10. The dataset used here is TEDS telephone survey of presidential approval rating conducted in September 2021.

REFERENCES

Baker, William D., and John R. Oneal. 2001. “Patriotism or Opinion Leadership? The Nature and Origins of the ‘Rally ’Round the Flag’ Effect.” *The Journal of Conflict Resolution* 45 (5): 661–87.

Boin, Arjen, Paul t’ Hart, Eric Stern, and Bengt Sundelius. 2017. *The Politics of Crisis Management: Public Leadership Under Pressure.* Cambridge: Cambridge University Press.

Callaghan, Karen J., and Simo Virtanen. 1993. “Revised Models of the ‘Rally Phenomenon’: The Case of the Carter Presidency.” *Journal of Politics* 55 (3): 756–64.

Dalton, Russell. 2019. *Citizen Politics: Public Opinion and Political Parties in Advanced Industrial Democracies*. Washington, DC: Congressional Quarterly Press.

Dennison, James. 2019. “A Review of Public Issue Salience: Concepts, Determinants and Effects on Voting.” *Political Studies Review* 17 (4): 436–46.

Doty, Richard M., Bill E. Peterson, and David G. Winter. 1991. “Threat and Authoritarianism in the United States, 1978–1987.” *Journal of Personality and Social Psychology* 61 (4): 629–40.

Edwards, George C. III, William Mitchell, and Reed Welch. 1995. “Explaining Presidential Approval: The Significance of Issue Salience.” *American Journal of Political Science* 39 (1): 108–34.

Edwards, George C. III, and Tami Swenson. 1997. “Who Rallies? The Anatomy of a Rally Event.” *Journal of Politics* 59 (1): 200–212.

Esaisson, Peter, Jacob Sohlberg, Marina Ghersetti, and Bengt Johansson. 2021. “How the Coronavirus Crisis Affects Citizen Trust in Institutions and in Unknown Others: Evidence from ‘the Swedish Experiment.’” *European Journal of Political Science* 60: 748–60.

Gronke, Paul, and Brian Newman. 2003. “FDR to Clinton, Mueller to ?: A Field Essay on Presidential Approval.” *Political Research Quarterly* 56 (4): 501–12.

Hetherington, Marc, and Michael Nelson. 2003. “Anatomy of a Rally Effect: George W. Bush and the War on Terrorism.” *PS: Political Science & Politics* 36 (1): 37–42.

Johansson, Bengt, David Nicolas Hopmann, and Adam Shehata. 2021. “When the Rally-Around-The-Flag Effect Disappears, or: When the Covid-19 Pandemic Becomes ‘Normalized.’” *Journal of Elections, Public Opinion, and Parties* 31 (S1): 321–34.

Krosnick, Jon A. 1990. “Government Policy and Citizen Passion: A Study of Issue Publics in Contemporary America.” *Political Behavior* 12 (1): 59–92.

Lambert, Alan J., J. P. Schott, and Laura Scherer. 2011. "Threat, Politics, and Attitudes: Toward a Greater Understanding of Rally-Around-the-Flag Effects." *Current Directions in Psychological Science* 20 (6): 343–48.

Mueller, John E. 1973. *War, Presidents, and Public Opinion.* New York: Wiley.

Schmitt, Hermann. 1983. "Party Government in Public Opinion: A European Cross-National Comparison." *European Journal of Political Research* 11 (4): 353–76.

Sigelman, Lee, and Pamela Johnston Conover. 1981. "The Dynamics of Presidential Support during International Conflict Situations: The Iranian Hostage Crisis." *Political Behavior* 3 (4): 303–18.

Tajfel, Henri. 1982. "Social Psychology of Intergroup Relations." *Annual Review of Psychology* 33: 1–39.

Wang, T. Y., and Su-feng Cheng. 2021. "Covid-19 and the Anatomy of the Rally Effect in Taiwan." *Asian Survey* 61 (3): 388–410.

Yam, Kai Chi, Joshua Conrad Jackson, Christopher M. Barnes, Jason Lau, Xin Qin, and Hin Yeung Lee. 2020. "The Rise of Covid-19 Cases Is Associated with Support for World Leaders." *Proceedings of the National Academy of Sciences* 117: 25429–33.

2

Government Performance and Political Trust

Chiung-Chu Lin

INTRODUCTION AND RESEARCH BACKGROUND

To combat the COVID-19 pandemic that began in early 2020, different countries adopted various policies to prevent and solve this global crisis. Some governments controlled the crisis well while some other countries were less able to do so.[1] Since the COVID-19 outbreak in early 2020 around the world, the Taiwanese government and public health authorities have adopted significant policies to guide society safely through the pandemic. According to the statistics from the Taiwan Centers for Disease Control, Taiwan had 1,023 COVID-19 confirmed cases by the end of March 2020 while many countries have had more than 120,000 confirmed cases.[2] It was only in mid-May 2021 with a wider community outbreak in Taipei City and New Taipei City that Taiwanese society faced a greater threat from this pandemic.

How the public evaluates the performance of the government in dealing with the pandemic is related to people's willingness to follow instructions. It is also worth highlighting that political trust is associated with people's willingness to be vaccinated and to wear face masks (Chuang et al. 2015). Therefore, the concept of political trust becomes a core concept in understanding government's ability to control the spread of COVID-19 in different countries. For example, some studies on the COVID-19 outbreak focused on the perspective of the association between political trust and confirmed cases. Other studies examined the relationship between social capital and the spread of the cases (Kye and Hwang 2020). Some research has also asked whether authoritarian regimes are more capable of confronting pandemics than democratic regimes (Brzechczyn 2020). Research evidence also suggests that trust in government is expected to increase regardless of policies enacted during crises (Muller 1970, 1973). Furthermore, the existing research pointed out that trust in the government plays an important role during emergencies (Siegrist and Zingg 2014).

This paper aims to study how Taiwanese people respond to the government's performance in tackling the COVID-19 pandemic. It focuses on the public's attitudes toward the government's actions on COVID-19 and how those attitudes were associated with political trust in government. It will first present how trust in government changed as the pandemic unfolded since 2020 and how the evaluation of the government's actions in response to the pandemic shaped the public's political support. By doing so, this paper aims to contribute to a better understanding of performance evaluation and the role of political trust during the COVID-19 crisis in Taiwan.

This paper proceeds as follows. It first reviews relevant literature on political trust and its association with the approval of government actions or performance. It then introduces the survey data that was used in this paper. The following sections present the public's evaluations of government performance in dealing with the pandemic. It further examines the relationship between performance evaluations and trust in government by building a regression model. The last section presents the conclusion and discussion.

POLITICAL TRUST DURING THE PANDEMIC

Rudolph (2017, 197) has noted that "political trust functions as a heuristic or decision rule that helps people decide whether to support or oppose government action." This shows that political trust is an important factor in terms of understanding political legitimacy. The concept of political trust refers to the definition by David Easton (1975) who posited two different kinds of support for the political system. On one hand, specific support is toward the government or political leaders, while on the other diffuse support refers to support for the political regime. In this paper, political trust refers to specific support.

There are several approaches to discussing trust (Uslaner 2018, 5–6). Taken from a sociopsychological approach, it emphasizes individual characteristics and personal experience to shape the degree of trust an individual holds (Newton 2007, 350). An individual's trust in political institutions is shaped by his/her evaluations of what and how the political institutions or political leaders go about their actions. Thus, political trust is also influenced by the operation of political institutions (Newton 2007, 357).

Why does political trust matter during the COVID-19 crisis? Research has shown that political trust plays a role in an individual's political behavior. It has a positive impact on encouraging individuals to have more electoral participation and willingness to obey laws. Individuals with high levels of political trust tend to vote for the ruling party and follow the rules and regulations imposed by the governments (Bol et al. 2021; Marien and Hooghe 2011). Political trust, therefore, reflects a relationship between the citizens and political institutions.

Therefore, understanding the role of political trust during the extraordinary and sudden nature of the pandemic is especially important. Several studies have examined the role of political trust during the COVID-19 pandemic (Davies et al. 2021; Belchior and Teixeira 2021; Bol et al. 2021; Yang and Tsai 2020; Kye and Hwang 2020; Wu 2021). On one hand, trust is an individual's confidence in institutions. Marien and Hooghe (2011) indicated that "the level of political trust is associated with the level of obedience to the law. Those with a low level of political trust tend to break the law." Thus, trust encourages an individual's willingness to get vaccinated, follow regulations, and comply with strict control measures in combating the COVID-19 pandemic (Siegrist and Zingg 2014; Wu 2021, 46; Marien and Hooghe 2011). In Wu's study (2021, 30) on the role of social capital during the pandemic in China, she found that "political trust plays a greater role than social trust in slowing the community spread of COVID-19." By analyzing the latest wave of the WVS (2016–2020) data, Wu (2021, 29) also found that political trust had a significant impact on reducing the COVID-19 spread. Therefore, a higher level of trust yields better results in curbing the spread of the disease.

On the other hand, strict measures such as "home quarantine," "stay home," or "lockdown" policies have increased trust in the government

(Bol et al. 2021). Nielsen and Lindvall (2021, 1191) compared the political trust in Sweden and Denmark during the pandemic and argued that trust in government was influenced by the respondent's evaluation of the government's capability in handling the pandemic. People's satisfaction with government performance in handling the pandemic has a positive impact on political trust. It seems that one's satisfaction with government performance is associated with trust in government. Holding trust in government and health authorities, an individual is more likely to obey the regulations or laws during the COVID-19 pandemic. Furthermore, this reduces the spread of the disease.

In terms of studying pandemic politics, a considerable body of literature on the COVID-19 crisis has studied whether rally-around-the-flag or lockdown effects generated political trust (Kritzinger et al. 2021; Schraff 2020; Sibley et al. 2020). Extending from previous research, some scholars further examined whether emotional factors or cognitive factors determined changes in political trust (Schraff 2020; Belchior and Teixeira 2021). Schraff (2020) argued that an anxiety effect rather than a lockdown effect drives the rise in diffuse political support during the COVID-19 pandemic. With daily headlines on infection cases and numbers of deaths, the public was being constantly reminded of living in strange times. In the early phase of the pandemic, a majority of people in society found life to be fearful and filled with uncertainty. It is under such shocking and unexpected circumstances that individuals tend to have more psychological reactions than cognitive evaluations when they are invited to respond to their trust in political institutions (Schraff 2020, 2).

By contrast, having examined the relationship between individuals' assessments of the economic performance and the policy response to the crisis and trust in political leaders in Spain, Belchior and Teixeira (2021) argued that cognitive factors, that is, performance evaluations, rather than emotional reasons drive the increase of trust in the prime minister. It should be further noted that Belchior and Teixeira (2021) did not deny the emotional effects in explaining the rise of political trust. In short, both emotional and cognitive factors account for the increase of political trust during the early months of the COVID-19 pandemic.

Most studies have pointed out that trust in government is a key factor in combating the spread of viruses. Some literature has shown that measures adopted in response to the COVID-19 pandemic increased vote intention for the ruling party candidates, trust in government, and satisfaction with democracy (Bol et al. 2021; Belchior and Teixeira 2021). In short, satisfaction with government actions in combating the COVID-19 pandemic increases trust in the government.

When confronted with major serious health threats such as the COVID-19 pandemic crisis, the public was worried about being infected or unable to get enough protection. Fear and anxiety became a part of daily life. Under such critical and unusual periods, how the government responds to the COVID-19 pandemic will shape the public's trust in government. The concept of political trust has been measured in different ways. Some surveys measure the concept by asking respondents to express how much confidence or trust they have in different political institutions. By contrast, some surveys measure the concept by asking if they approve or disapprove of the job performance of government or political leaders.[3] It appears that both evaluations on government performance and trust in government were used interchangeably to unpack the concept of political trust in different survey projects. In this paper, we treat trust in government as a dependent variable and government policies/measures in response to the epidemic as independent variables. This paper expects policy evaluations to have a positive relationship with political trust.

In addition to factors determining the level of political trust, a variety of studies noted that partisanship and ideology shaped individuals' trust in government or leaders (Sheng 2003; cited from Bol et al. 2021, 498). Those who are supporters of the ruling party tend to have a higher level of political trust, and vice versa. Furthermore, researchers have argued that successful crisis communication is also related to people's trust in government. Any uncertain or unknown risk information will trigger unnecessary fears and anxiety and thus will decrease trust in government (Siegrist and Zingg 2014, 29). Therefore, we could expect that people who pay more attention to the COVID-19 pandemic news or agree that the government provides the citizens with enough risk information are more likely to have a higher trust in the government.

In a nutshell, political trust is especially important for a country when facing a serious threat. This literature review gives us theoretical and empirical grounds to assume that trust in government during the pandemic is largely determined by government policies/measures evaluations, partisanship, and political communication.

DATA AND RESEARCH METHOD

To combat this global pandemic, many governments announced a set of measures to restrict the public's movements and economic activities. Doing so may further deteriorate the economic situation domestically. It is possible that the government would be blamed for bad economic performance and the high unemployment rate. In the meantime, the public expects the government to handle the crisis quickly to return life to normal. Without trust, people may not follow any measures or even break laws. Therefore, trust in government may vary according to the situation.

To understand what factors influence people's trust in government during the pandemic crisis, this paper first presents descriptive statistics that were conducted by the TVBS Polls Center during the period between February 2020 and September 2021. All results from those surveys were taken from the TVBS Poll Center website (https://www.tvbs.com.tw/poll-center). This paper also analyzes web survey data to answer questions posited in this paper. Since the epidemic alert increased to level 3 nationwide on May 15, it was impossible to conduct a telephone interview during the early stages of the community epidemic outbreak since mid-May 2021. Internet surveys became a more appropriate method for collecting public opinion. The internet survey was conducted during the period between June 3 and June 9, 2021, by the Election Study Center, National Chengchi University, with 1,100 successful cases. Given that there was a nationwide epidemic alert in response to the continued threat of COVID-19, the internet survey provides us with timely results in understanding public opinion during a sudden and shocking period of the pandemic crisis.

Last, this paper presents the results of the association between trust and behavior by using data from a telephone interview that was conducted in November 2021. The data provide further evidence that trust is related to an individual's willingness to follow government's regulations.

Based on the theoretical grounds discussed in the literature review, we expect the public's evaluations of the government's policies/measures in response to the COVID-19 pandemic will have an influence on their trust in the government during the crisis. Hence, the main hypothesis is as follows:

H1: People who agreed that the government provided enough information in preventing the COVID-19 pandemic tend to have higher political trust.

H2: People who agreed that the government adopted appropriate measures to prevent the spread of the epidemic tend to have higher political trust.

The response variable is the political trust, which reads, "If 0 represents very unsatisfied and 10 represents very satisfied, from 0 to 10 how much will you give regarding the government's performance in controlling the COVID-19 pandemic now?" A larger value represents a higher level of trust in government. There are two questions to measure the concept of evaluations of government policies/measures: "Does the government provide enough epidemic information or not?" and "Does government control too much or too little?" Given the numerical nature of the dependent variable, this paper uses a regression model to test the hypothesis. The regression model also includes variables of partisanship, political interest, and news attention as control variables.[4]

ATTITUDE TOWARD GOVERNMENT'S PERFORMANCE AND TRUST IN GOVERNMENT

The outbreak of COVID-19 around the world since early 2020 has created challenges to the government and political system. At the beginning of the outbreak of the pandemic, the government in Taiwan immediately adopted measures such as border control and quarantine, nationalized production and distribution of masks, daily press briefings, and postponing the first day of the new semester until February 25, 2020. In addition, the government also constantly encouraged people to wash their hands frequently and wear masks in closed areas. Taiwan has controlled the pandemic better than Western democracies in terms of the deaths during the year 2020. It was not until early May 2021 that a community outbreak in northern Taiwan led the government and health authorities to adopt stricter measures. The Central Epidemic Command Center (CECC) raised the epidemic warming to level 3 both in Taipei City and New Taipei City on May 15, 2021.[5] It was on May 19 that the CECC announced a nationwide epidemic alert in response to the continued threat of COVID-19.

In the meantime, the public has been urged to continue to abide by and cooperate with level 3 epidemic prevention and control measures such as mandatory mask wearing outdoors, providing real-name identification when entering public spaces, a ban on gatherings of more than five people indoors and ten people outdoors, suspension of some business operations, moving to online teaching, no dine-ins, etc.

As mentioned before, threat perceptions during crises will increase people's trust in government. Polls have shown that the COVID-19 pandemic has given political leaders a rise in popularity, especially in Australia, Canada, and Germany.[6] This is also the case in Taiwan. With concerns over the coronavirus epidemic in early February 2020, people were panic lining up to purchase face masks everywhere. In order to have enough face masks to distribute to every citizen, the government helped manufacturers to increase mask production capacity and later nationalized mask distribution and banned mask exports.

According to surveys conducted by the TVBS Poll Center between the period of February 2020 and May 2021,[7] 56 percent of Taiwanese people were satisfied with the government's response to the COVID-19 crisis (see figure 2.1). The survey was conducted during the time that the government announced the policy of name registration in purchasing face masks. Later on, the government launched a name-based mask distribution system on March 12, making it much easier for citizens to purchase masks online. The government also announced an entry ban on foreign nationals and a fourteen-day quarantine for all inbound Taiwanese

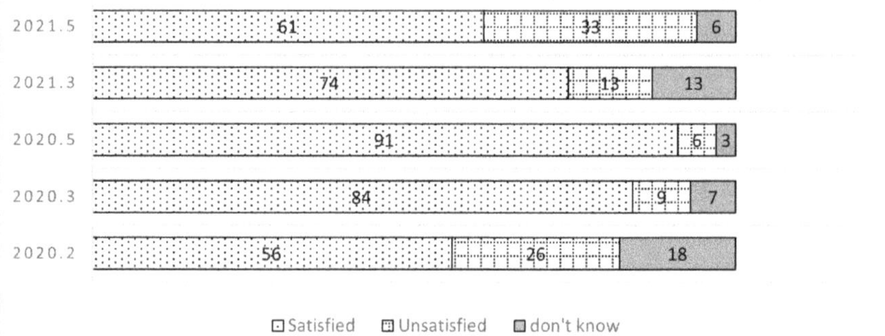

Figure 2.1. Overall, are you satisfied or unsatisfied with government performance in dealing with the COVID-19 pandemic?
Source: TVBS Poll Center.

travelers. By the end of March 2020, Taiwan only had 1,030 confirmed cases with 914 imported cases and 77 domestic cases, in contrast to other countries. Overall, the government has controlled epidemics better than most countries in the world.

The Taiwanese people gave a high approval rate to the government's good performance in combating the epidemic. Eighty-four percent of the respondents were satisfied with government performance in dealing with the COVID-19 pandemic in March 2020. The results from TVBS Polls display that the government has enjoyed a high level of approval before the sudden community outbreak in May 2021. In this circumstance, there is no doubt that we can expect a higher level of trust in government during the period between March 2020 and April 2021.

Since the outbreak of the epidemic, the CECC and the Minister for Health and Welfare Shih-Chung Chen held daily 2:00 p.m. news conferences. Watching the daily report from the CECC press conference either online or on TV channels also became a habit for many Taiwanese. The daily press conference provides clear statistics of confirmed cases, epidemic analysis, and new government pronouncements in combating the COVID-19 pandemic. By doing so, the daily press conference brings transparent and updated epidemic news and information. The openness enables the public to ease a certain level of anxiety over their risk perception. Public trust in government will increase under conditions of good perception on the government's competence. Thus, we should identify a high approval rate of the authorized institution in early 2020. Figure 2.2 confirms this trend. Taiwanese people gave Minister Shih-Chung Chen a high approval rate in early 2020 at the outbreak of the coronavirus epidemic in the world. More than 90 percent of the respondents were satisfied with his performance in response to the COVID-19 pandemic. Compared with figure 2.1 and figure 2.2, it is interesting to find that Taiwanese people have rated the minister performing better than the government. However, when the nation experienced a sudden community transmission in May 2021, the percentage of dissatisfaction with his performance went up from 14 percent in March 2021 to 43 percent in June 2021 (see figure 2.2).

Taiwan society faced a severe epidemic situation after May 2021 with the total confirmed cases reaching their peak during late May and June (see figure 2.3). The most serious period happened in late May with

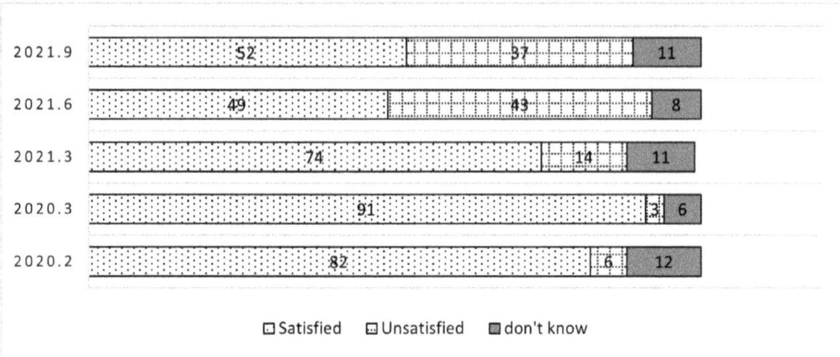

Figure 2.2. Overall, are you satisfied or unsatisfied with the Minister of the Ministry of Health and Welfare Shih-Chung Chen's performance in dealing with the COVID-19 pandemic?

Source: TVBS Poll Center.

more than seven hundred total confirmed cases, which were five hundred domestic confirmed cases per day. With the less than 1 percent vaccination rate and shortage of available vaccines at that moment, the public was worried about being infected and their chances of being vaccinated. Therefore, the percentage of satisfaction with the government and minster's performance went down significantly.

In the meantime, the public's confidence in the government's ability in combating the outbreak pandemic was being seriously questioned. Although more than half of the respondents expressed their confidence in the government on preventing the spread of the COVID-19 pandemic in June 2021, the confidence rate in fact decreased significantly since March

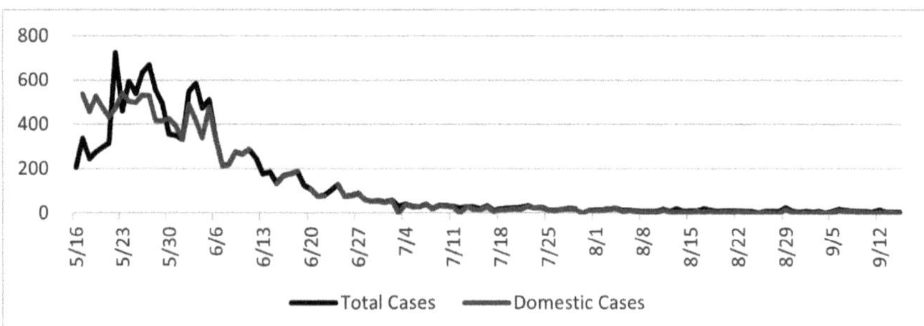

Figure 2.3. Statistics of Confirmed Cases in Taiwan (May 16, 2021 to September 15, 2021)

Sources: Daily press releases from the CESS and UDN News.

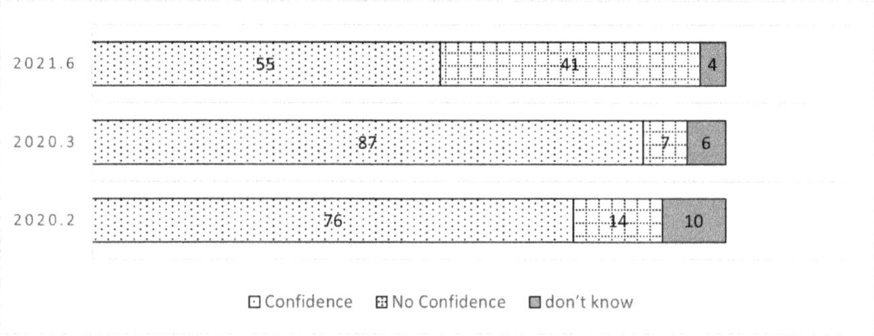

Figure 2.4. Do you have confidence or not in the government in preventing the spread of the pandemic?
Source: TVBS Poll Center.

2020, with a difference of 32 percent (see figure 2.4). The percentage of people who were worried about being infected reached a peak in June 2021 as well (see figure 2.5). Although the total confirmed cases went down to less than twenty cases with domestic confirmed cases below ten cases in early September 2021 (see figure 2.3), there was still more than 60 percent of the respondents who were worried about being infected. To address this issue, it could be that roughly 43 percent of the population received the first dose of a vaccine and only 4 percent of the population were fully vaccinated by the end of August 2021.

All results taken together, it showed that the government and minister have enjoyed a high approval rate during 2020. However, the public felt a critical threat arising from the community outbreak and was not satisfied

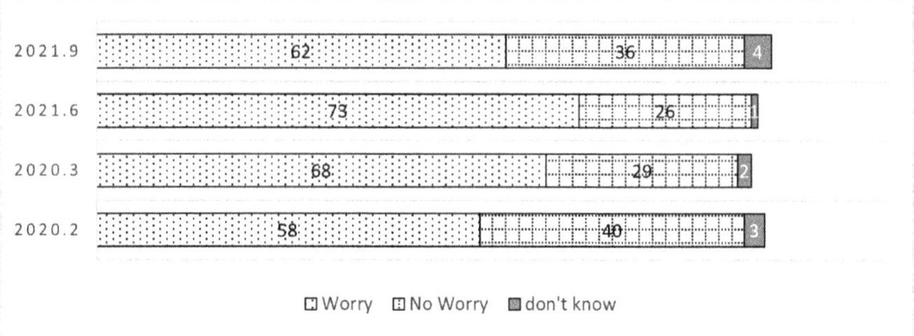

Figure 2.5. Do you worry or don't worry that you will be infected with the COVID-19 virus?
Source: TVBS Poll Center.

Table 2.1. Political Trust by Measuring Approval of the Government's Performance

Date	*Mean*	*Std.*	*N*
May 2020	8.4	1.6	1,209
June 2021	4.1	3.1	1,100

Source: Tsai 2020, 2021.

with what the government did. Despite the fact that TVBS Polls featured the public's evaluations of the Taiwanese government's performance in confronting the COVID-19 pandemic since February 2020, the surveys provided no further details beyond that.

In the following section, we first compare two waves of surveys conducted by the ESC and present the results in table 2.1. One thing that needs to be highlighted is that the first survey was conducted by telephone interview while the second one collected opinions via the internet. It displays similar findings to the TVBS Poll results, which mentioned earlier that the Taiwanese gave a high approval rate to the government. Table 2.1 shows that the average score was 8.4 in May 2020, which is the period that the total cumulative cases were less than 450 cases[8] and no more new domestic cases were confirmed during that period. As mentioned earlier, with a correlating community epidemic outbreak in early May 2021, the results from the internet survey show that the Taiwanese were unsatisfied with the government. The average score was 4.1.

The internet survey that was conducted in June 2021 also asked respondents to evaluate the measures that the government adopted in response to the epidemic situation. For example, having correct and enough information is important for the public to know about the pandemic crisis. Knowing the risk is likely to encourage the public to follow the regulations and get vaccinated (Siegrist and Zingg 2014). According to table 2.2, it is clear that a majority of the respondents agreed that the government provided enough information. The perception may partly come from the CECC daily press conference and reports that facilitate transparent practices on disease control. As noted earlier a nationwide epidemic alert raised to level 3 continued through June 2021. The daily confirmed cases gradually decreased from more than five hundred to less than three hundred during the period of the internet survey (see figure 2.3).[9] It seems that the local

Table 2.2. Attitudes Toward Government Measures in Response to the Epidemic

Do you agree or disagree that the government did provide the citizens with enough epidemic prevention information in the recent COVID-19 epidemic crisis?

	n	%
Disagree	443	40.3
Agree	657	59.7

If the COVID-19 pandemic is getting worse, do you support or do not support the government adopting a home quarantine policy?

	n	%
Don't support	178	16.2
Support	922	83.8

Do you think it is too much, too little, or appropriate for the government's measures in limiting individual liberty to stop the spread of the pandemic?

	n	%
Too much	24	2.2
Too little	487	44.3
Appropriate	589	53.5

Some people say, "The government should communicate with people first instead of requiring directly the public to obey regulations in terms of closing down schools during the period of COVID-19 pandemic." Do you agree or disagree with the statement?

	n	%
Disagree	810	73.6
Agree	290	26.4

Source: Tsai 2021.

transmission of the coronavirus was under control. Even so, more than 80 percent of the respondents supported the government adopting a home quarantine policy to control the situation.

In the meantime, 53.5 percent of the respondents agreed that the prevention measures that the government adopted are appropriate, while 44.3 percent reported that the government did too little. This figure displays a consistent public opinion toward accepting a home quarantine policy. Last, more than 70 percent of the respondents agreed the government has the authority to take stricter policies based on the condition of the epidemic. The results, to some extent, reflect a certain level of public trust in government as well.

POLICIES/MEASURES EVALUATIONS AND POLITICAL TRUST

During a health crisis, the unknown and new virus causes fear and uncertainty. People will want to know the real situation and what has happened. In the meantime, the government also needs to make sure any necessary precautions or measures are known by its citizens. As noted earlier, the CECC held a daily press conference in the afternoon that reported statistics of confirmed cases and announced new practices on disease control. The daily press conference brought transparency to the public with updated news and information. Therefore, those who have a feeling of receiving enough information should hold a higher trust in the government. Table 2.3 confirmed that those who agree to receive enough information tend to have a higher trust in the government. Table 2.3 shows that the average score of political trust for those who agree the government had provided enough prevention information is 5.53, which is higher than those who disagree significantly.

When confronted with a serious health crisis, the government had to take fast measures to respond. Those who appraise the government had taken appropriate measures to stop the spread of the pandemic should have a higher trust in the government than others. Table 2.4 shows that people who believe the government took appropriate action in preventing the spread of the epidemic have the highest point in political trust. The mean is 4.79, followed by those who think the government took too little action (the mean is 3.37). Those who have the lowest trust in the government are the respondents who identified the government took too many measures that infringed on individuals' liberty. In other words, the higher political trust people have, the more willingness to trade off civil liberties for greater personal safety (Davis and Silver 2004).

In the context of a country experiencing a serious epidemic, the society may have different thoughts on how the government should communicate with the public in advance or if the government made the decision on its own. Under the critical situation in combating the COVID-19 pandemic, people with a high level of trust in the government will tend to support the government taking an action on its own first. The results displayed in table 2.5 confirm that those who don't think the government has to communicate with the public in advance to respond to the health crisis have a higher level of trust in the government with an average score of 4.4.

Moreover, when the epidemic situation got worse, the authorities might have to adopt a home quarantine policy. Doing so means that the government did not do well in preventing the spread of the COVID-19 epidemic. Therefore, those who support a home quarantine policy may have lower trust in the government. Table 2.6 confirmed this. Those who support the government to adopt a home quarantine policy have an average score of 3.9 in trust of the government, in contrast to those who did not support the policy with an average score of 5.15.

Table 2.3. The Government Provided Enough Epidemic Information

	N	*Mean*	*Std. deviation*	*t Test*
Disagree	443	1.98	2.19	*P*<0.001
Agree	657	5.53	2.79	

Note: The question read, "Do you agree or disagree that the government did provide the citizens with enough epidemic prevention information in the recent COVID-19 epidemic crisis?"

Source: Tsai 2021.

Table 2.4. The Government's Actions to Stop the Spread of the Pandemic

	N	*Mean*	*Std. deviation*	*ANOVA*
Too much	24	1.96	2.61	*P*<0.001
Too little	487	3.37	2.89	
Appropriate	589	4.79	3.11	

Note: The question read, "Do you think it is too much, too little, or appropriate for the government's measures in limiting individual liberty to stop the spread of the pandemic?"

Source: Tsai 2021.

Table 2.5. The Government Should Consult with People Before Announcing Regulations

	N	*Mean*	*Std. deviation*	*t Test*
Disagree	810	4.40	3.09	*P*<0.001
Agree	290	3.27	2.99	

Note: The question read, "Some people say, 'The government should communicate with people first instead of requiring directly the public to obey regulations in terms of closing down schools during the period of COVID-19 pandemic.' Do you agree or disagree with the statement?"

Source: Tsai 2021.

Table 2.6. The Government Should Adopt a Home Quarantine Policy

	N	*Mean*	*Std. deviation*	*t Test*
Don't support	178	5.15	3.31	*P*<0.001
Support	922	3.90	3.02	

Note: The question read, "If the COVID-19 pandemic is getting worse, do you support or do not support the government to adopt a home quarantine policy?"

Source: Tsai 2021.

So far, this paper identified the public' attitudes toward the Taiwanese government in handling the health crisis. How did those attitudes influence individuals' trust in government? Do people's evaluations on the government's policies/measures play a role in their trust in the government? Table 2.7 presents the results from a multiple regression model. First, satisfaction with government policies/measures in controlling the pandemic has a significantly positive effect on the level of trust in government. Holding other variables as constant, people who agreed that the government provided enough epidemic information have higher political trust. The partial regression coefficient is 1.29, which means there is a 1.29 unit increase in the estimated mean of political trust for every one-unit increase in the government having provided enough epidemic information.

Table 2.7. Regression Analysis of Trust in Government

	Coeff.	*(se)*
Constant	2.90***	(0.69)
Political interest	0.23*	(0.10)
News attention	–0.48**	(0.16)
The government provides enough epidemic information	1.29***	(0.07)
Government should communicate with the society	0.32***	(0.08)
Government control (appropriate=0)		
Too much	–1.02*	(0.45)
Too little	–0.51***	(0.14)
Party identification (DPP=0)		
Pan-blue	–3.32***	(0.20)
TPP	–2.68***	(0.22)
NPP	–1.20**	(0.35)
Small party and independent	–1.65***	(0.18)
N		2000
Adj. R2		0.522

Source: Tsai 2021.

In addition, compared to people who agree the government had done an appropriate job, those who agree that the government controlled too much or too little have lower trust in the government. For instance, there is 1.02 unit decrease in the estimated mean of political trust for people who viewed that the government controlled too much as compared to those who regarded that the government performed appropriately. Like findings in other democracies, partisanship is found to significantly affect the trust in government. Compared to supporters of the DPP, supporters of the Pan-Blue (including the KMT, the NP, and the PFP) and supporters of the TPP tend to have less trust in government. In short, these findings from the survey shed light on the process of citizens' cognitive responses to the government's performance in explaining political trust during the community outbreak.

Furthermore, we analyzed another telephone survey data that asked people's opinions on following regulations imposed by the government. Ninety-two percent of the respondents indicated that they abided by the regulations almost all the time, with only less than 1 percent disregarding regulations (Cheng 2021). Research has shown that political trust plays a role in an individual's willingness and behavior in following the rules and regulations imposed by the government (Bol et al. 2021; Marien and Hooghe 2011). It suggests that individuals who have a higher level of trust in the government tend to abide by laws and regulations.

Table 2.8 presents the results of examining the relationship between political trust and abiding by laws. The two variables are dependent on each

Table 2.8. Crosstabs of Political Trust and Whether or Not Citizens Abide by the Rules and Regulations in the Prevention of the COVID-19 Pandemic

	Abide by the Rules and Regulations	*Disregard the Rules and Regulations*	*No Opinion*	*Total Cases*	
Trust in the government	92.8%+	6.8%	0.5%–	2,084	χ^2=14.436 df=2 *P*<0.01
Didn't trust the government	90.6%–	7.5%	1.9%+	840	
Total cases	2,694	204	26	2,924	

Note: "+" stands for the cell's adjusted residuals is significantly larger than would be expected if the null hypothesis were true, with a significance level of 0.05. "–" indicates that the number of cases in that cell is significantly smaller than would be expected if the null hypothesis were true.

Source: Cheng 2021.

other. There was 92.8 percent of the respondents trusted the government significantly to keep to regulations such as washing hands frequently, wearing masks, and keeping social distance, which is higher than the percentage of those who didn't trust the government. Compared to people who trust in government, those who don't trust the government significantly decline to offer clear answers on their behavior in abiding by the regulations. Altogether results from table 2.8 to further support the main findings that political trust plays an essential role in containing the spread of the COVID-19 pandemic.

CONCLUSION AND DISCUSSION

Taiwan learned lessons during the 2003 SARS crisis, therefore, the government responded to the COVID-19 pandemic quickly. Opinion polls showed the government's high approval rating in combating the COVID-19 crisis before the community outbreak in May 2021. In the early stages of the community outbreak in Taipei City and New Taipei City, the country recorded a high number of new daily cases, corresponding to the peak of the pandemic since 2020. The medical system in northern Taipei became overloaded to the point where hospitals were unable to admit COVID-19 patients. Having emphasized that it was proactive in preventing the virus, the sudden outbreak highlighted the government's unpreparedness and miscoordination in combating the pandemic. Will the public's evaluations of the government's reactions to the COVID-19 influence their trust in the government during the critical phase of the pandemic?

Previous studies have shown that people's trust in government was positively related to their intention to get vaccinated and to comply with regulations or laws. Thus, studying trust in government during the pandemic crisis is essential in understanding why some countries were able to control the crisis while some were not. Scholars indicated that both cognitive and emotional factors account for citizens' trust in government when the country is facing an extraordinary event such as the COVID-19 pandemic (Belchior and Teixeira 2021). While we do not have measurements on emotional factors, this paper investigates how cognitive factors such as policy evaluations play a role in shaping individuals' political trust after the community outbreak in May.

Our findings suggest that cognitive factors do play a role in shaping the public's trust in government. People who identified the government as having taken appropriate actions to stop the spread of the pandemic tend to have a higher level of trust in the government. Moreover, those who agree that the government provided the public with enough information in preventing the pandemic tend to have a higher level of trust in the government. In addition to the cognitive factors, partisanship also has a significant effect on the trust in government. The results show that supporters of the Pan-Blue and Taiwan People's Party tend to have less trust in the government. Individuals who have a higher level of trust in the government tend to abide by laws and regulations.

However, the data used in this paper have some limitations. The internet survey did not measure the emotional factors and economic evaluations. As such, this paper is unable to explore the roles played by emotional factors or economic evaluation during the periods of the pandemic. Overall, this paper found that performance evaluations play a significant role in the public's trust in government.

APPENDIX: FURTHER READING

Table 1. Questions wordings and the codebook

Variable	*Questions*	*Code*
Political Trust	**Q13:** If 0 represents very unsatisfied and 10 represents very satisfied. From 0 to 10 how much will you give regarding the government's performance in controlling the COVID-19 pandemic now?	
Political interest	**Q1:** In general, how interested would you say you are in politics?	Very interested=4 Somewhat interested=3 Not very interested=2 Not interested at all =1
News attention	**Q14:** How closely do you follow COVID-19 pandemic news?	Very closely=4 Fairly closely=3 Not very closely=2 Not closely at all=1

(continued)

Table 1. *Continued*

Variable	*Questions*	*Code*
The government provides enough epidemic information	**Q17:** Do you agree or disagree that the government did provide the citizens with enough epidemic prevention information in the recent COVID-19 pandemic crisis?	Strongly agree=4 Agree=3 Disagree=2 Strongly disagree=1
Government control	**Q18:** To prevent the spread of the pandemic this time, the government adopted many measures to restrict individual liberty such as home isolation and going abroad. Do you think the restrictions are too much, too little, and appropriate?	Too much=1 Too less=2 Appropriate=0
Home quarantine policy	**Q19:** If the spread of the COVID-19 pandemic keeps continuing, do you support or do not support the government adopting the lockdown policy?	Strongly support=4 Support=3 Don't support=2 Strongly don't support=1
Partisanship	**Q30:** Among all political parties in our country, which party do you think of yourself as close to any particular party? **Q30A:** (If Q30 answers yes) Do you feel very close to this party, somewhat close, or not very close? **Q30B:** (if Q30 answers no) Do you feel a little closer to one of the political parties than the others?	Pan-Blue=1 (includes the KMT, the NP, and the PFP) DPP=2 TPP=3 NPP=4 Small parties, Independents and don't know=9

NOTES

1. See https://www.bloomberg.com/news/features/2021-11-23/the-winners-and-losers-from-a-year-of-ranking-covid-resilience, accessed December 2, 2021.
2. For example, the United States has 30,398,049 confirmed cases, France has 4,585,385 confirmed cases, and Brazil has 12,658,109 confirmed cases. https://www.cdc.gov.tw/Bulletin/Detail/XRoVwbiFHMBGt2rY878zhg?typeid=9; https://www.cdc.gov.tw/Bulletin/Detail/6Gkh8vw-Urlyl0soflgBww?typeid=9, accessed March 4, 2022.

3. Afrobarometer survey or Asian Barometer, for example, measure the concept of political trust by asking respondents questions such as "I'm going to name a number of institutions. For each one, please tell me how much trust do you have in them? Is it a great deal of trust, quite a lot of trust, not very much trust, or none at all?" The institutions include the president or prime minister, courts, national government, political parties, police, local government, newspapers, television, and so on. The American National Election Studies in 2008 and 2012, for example, measure the concept of political trust by asking the questions, "Does the respondent approve or disapprove of the way the current U.S. president is handling the job?" or "Does the respondent approve or disapprove of the way the current U.S. Congress has been handling its job?" (Kumagai and Iorio, 2020, 31–38).

4. Please see the appendix for question wordings and variables codebook.

5. https://www.cdc.gov.tw/Category/ListContent/tov1jahKUv8RGSbvmzLwFg?uaid=R1K7gSjoYa7Wojk54nW7fg, accessed June 12, 2021.

6. https://www.economist.com/graphic-detail/2020/05/09/covid-19-has-given-most-world-leaders-a-temporary-rise-in-popularity, accessed April 3, 2022.

7. https://www.tvbs.com.tw/poll-center, accessed July 12, 2021.

8. https://www.cdc.gov.tw/Category/ListContent/tov1jahKUv8RGSbvmzLwFg?uaid=qaRsl59wDh-lB9D8iU8uoA, accessed June 12, 2021.

9. https://covid-19.nchc.org.tw/dt_005-covidTable_taiwan.php, accessed June 12, 2021.

REFERENCES

Altiparmakis, Argyros, et al. 2021. "Pandemic Politics: Policy Evaluations of Government Responses to COVID-19." *West European Politics* 44 (5–6): 1159–79.

Belchior, Maria, and Conceicao Pequito Teixeira. 2021. "Determinants of Political Trust during the Early Months of the COVID-19 Pandemic: Putting Policy Performance into Evidence." *Political Studies Review*. https://doi.org/10.1177/14789299211056193.

Bol, Damien, et al. 2021. "The Effect of Covid-19 Lockdowns on Political Support: Some Good News for Democracy." *European Journal of Political Research* 60 (May): 497–505.

Brzechczyn, Krzysztof. 2020. "The Coronavirus in Liberal and Illiberal Democracies and the Future of Globalized World." *Society Register* 4 (2): 83–94. https://doi.org/10.14746/sr.2020.4.2.06.

Cheng, Su-Feng. 2021. "The Taiwan Identity Under Threat: Its Development and Implications." Ministry of Science and Technology Research Project. MOST 110-2410-H-004-059-SS3.

Christensen, Tom, and Per Lægreid. 2005. "Trust in Government: The Relative Importance of Service Satisfaction, Political Factors, and Demography." *Public Performance & Management Review* 28 (4): 487–511.

Chuang, Ying-Chih, et al. 2015. "Social Capital and Health-Protective Behavior Intentions in an Influenza Pandemic." *PLoS One* 10 (4): e0122970. doi: 10.1371/journal.pone.0122970.

Davies, Ben, et al. 2021. "Changes in Political Trust in Britain during the COVID-19 Pandemic in 2020: Integrated Public Opinion Evidence and Implications." *Humanities & Social Sciences Communications* 8 (166). DOI https://doi.org/10.1057/s41599-021-00850-6.

Davis, Darren W., and Brian D. Silver. 2004. "Civil Liberties vs. Security: Public Opinion in the Context of the Terrorist Attacks on America." *American Journal of Political Science* 48 (1): 28–46.

Easton, David. 1975. "A Re-Assessment of the Concept of Political Support." *British Journal of Political Science* 5 (4): 435–57.

Hetherington, Marc J. 1998. "The Political Relevance of Political Trust." *American Political Science Review* 92 (4): 791–808.

Kritzinger, Sylvia, et al. 2021. "'Rally Round the Flag': The COVID-19 Crisis and Trust in the National Government." *West European Politics* 44 (5–6): 1205–31.

Kumagai, Saki, and Federica Iorio. 2020. *Building Trust in Government through Citizen Engagement*. World Back Group.

Kye, Bongoh, and Sun-Jae Hwang. 2020. "Social Trust in the Midst of Pandemic Crisis: Implications from COVID-19 of South Korea." *Research in Social Stratification and Mobility* 68. https://doi.org/10.1016/j.rssm.2020.100523.

Marien, Sofie, and Marc Hooghe. 2011. "Does Political Trust Matter? An Empirical Investigation into the Relation between Political Trust and Support for Law Compliance." *European Journal of Political Research* 50 (2): 267–91.

Muller, John E. 1970. "Presidential Popularity form Truman to Johnson." *American Political Science Review* 64 (1): 18–34.

Muller, John E. 1973. *War, Presidents, and Public Opinion*. New York: John Wiley & Sons.

Newton, K. 2007. "Social and Political Trust." In *The Oxford Handbook of Political Behavior*, edited by R. J. Dalton and H.-D. Klingemann, 342–61. Oxford: Oxford University Press.

Nielsen, Julie Hassing, and Johannes Lindvall. 2021. "Trust in Government in Sweden and Denmark during the COVID-19 Epidemic." *West European Politics* 44 (5–6): 1180–204.

Rudolph, Thomas J. 2017. "Political Trust as a Heuristic." In *Handbook on Political Trust*, edited by Sonja Zmerli, 197–211. Cheltenham: Edward Elgar.

Schraff, Dominik. 2020. "Political Trust during the COVID-19 Pandemic: Rally Around the Flag or Lockdown Effects." *European Journal of Political Research*. https://doi.org/10.1111/1475-6765.12425.

Sheng, Emile C. J. 2003. "A Study of Taiwanese Democratic Value and Political Trust: A Comparison Before and After the Alternation of Power." *Journal of Electoral Studies* 10 (1): 115–69.

Sibley, C. G., Greaves, L. M., Satherley, N., Wilson, M. S., Overall, N. C., Lee, C. H. J., Milojev, P., Bulbulia, J., Osborne, D., Milfont, T. L., Houkamau, C. A., Duck., I. M., VickersJones, R., & Barlow, F. K. 2020. "Effects of the COVID-19 Pandemic and Nationwide Lockdown on Trust, Attitudes toward Government, and Well-being." *American Psychologist* 75(5), 618–630.

Sigrist, Michael, and Alexandra Zingg. 2014. "The Role of Public Trust During Pandemics: Implications for Crisis Communication." *European Psychologist* 19 (1): 23–32.

Tsai, Chia-Hung. 2020. 2020 Taiwan Democratic Values and Governance Survey.

Tsai, Chia-Hung. 2021. Civic Consciousness, Polarized Politics, and Communicative Democracy. Ministry of Science and Technology Research Project. MOST109-2410-H004-048-SS2.

Uslaner, Eric M. 2018. "The Study of Trust." In *The Oxford Handbook of Social and Political Trust*, edited by Eric M. Uslaner. Oxford: Oxford University Press.

Wu, Cary. 2021. "Social Capital and COVID-19: A Multidimensional and Multilevel Approach." *Chinese Sociological Review* 53 (1): 27–54.

Yang, Wan-Ying, and Chia-hung Tsai. 2020. "Democratic Values, Collective Security, and Privacy: Taiwan People's Response to COVID-19." *Asian Journal for Public Opinion Research* 8 (3): 222–45.

3

The Role of Partisan Opposition

Nathan F. Batto

INTRODUCTION

It is common to think of the COVID-19 pandemic as a crisis, and this framing affects how we evaluate different countries' responses. Crises are immediate and demand fast responses, so one way to think about responses is to ask whether governments were able to implement coercive emergency measures and obtain widespread compliance. A different crisis-oriented approach is to examine short-term public opinion such as a rally-around-the-flag effect, in which ordinary partisan strife is momentarily set aside to form a surge in support for the government.

However, COVID has not been a short-term emergency that could be resolved with an effective rapid response. More than two years into the pandemic, the world is still grappling with it. The challenge of stopping the initial wave has long since faded into memory. Several subsequent waves have battered the planet, and more are likely to appear. Any hopes that this would all be over by the summer, the end of the year, when vaccines arrive, or any other concrete deadline have been proven wishful thinking.

As the pandemic timeline has stretched out, any rally-around-the-flag effect has long since faded, and politics have shifted back to more normal patterns. For democracies, this has meant a reemergence of normal, partisan politics. Democratic governments must figure out how to respond to the continuing challenges of the pandemic while also navigating contentious domestic politics. More generally, good democratic governance must be grounded in partisan struggles. Many countries have found partisan divides to be a serious obstacle. For example, Americans have been quick to blame low vaccination rates on the partisan divide.[1]

Taiwan's effort to vaccinate its population demonstrates that intense partisanship does not necessarily undermine good public policy. Partisan conflict was not suspended in some grand, unified effort to achieve the national goal of universal vaccination. Quite the contrary. The main opposition KMT repeatedly questioned and criticized the governing DPP. Some of these attacks were opportunistic—the KMT leapt at every available failure. However, they were also grounded in the deeper partisan structure—an undercurrent of national identity ran through these attacks.

Taiwan has achieved vaccination rates comparable or even superior to most established democracies, and democratic conflict played a central role in this. The two main parties disagreed bitterly on many things. However, the process of partisan conflict taught everyone that they wanted a vaccine, even if they didn't want the same ones. Taiwan's successful governance, which was based entirely on voluntary compliance, was built on this very narrow consensus forged in the fires of ordinary democratic conflict.

POLITICS IN THE COVID ERA

In the aftermath of the global spread of COVID, many scholars rushed to ask how various countries had met the challenge. This was often framed in terms of whether democratic or authoritarian countries had performed better and what the implications of those answers might be.[2] Given the short time between the events and the publication of this first wave of research, it was natural that they often focused on the initial responses to the pandemic.

Sheng, for example, evaluates responses in terms of crisis management. Authoritarian regimes are said to have two key advantages in responding to crises. First, they are able to make decisions quickly, without the need to slowly build consensus. Second, they have far superior coercive capacity, so they can force the population to comply with emergency policies. China is used to illustrate of swift, successful crisis response. It was able to ruthlessly lock down Wuhan and surrounding

Hubei Province while dramatically building and opening a massive field hospital in just a few days.[3] However, democracies are founded on the principle that the legitimacy of the government rests on the active consent of the governed. Imperiously implementing heavy-handed coercive tactics is not an option.

A different short-term approach more consistent with democratic principles is to look at public opinion. It was widely noted that in many countries around the world, support for the government and people in power went up in the early days of the pandemic.[4] This was widely understood as a rally-around-the-flag effect, a well-known phenomenon in the context of foreign policy emergencies such as a military conflict. In such cases, the government's surge in short-term popularity is driven by cues from the opposition. If the opposition supports, or at least does not attack, the government, citizens who would normally oppose the government pick up on these cues and put aside their normal partisan grievances.[5]

However, the COVID pandemic has not turned out to be a short-term crisis that could be resolved with short-term emergency measures, regardless of whether those measures were highly coercive or buoyed by strong public support. After the immediate jolt faded, the willingness of populations to uncritically endure extraordinary measures has also waned. Any opposition ceasefire was temporary. After the adrenaline rush wears off, then what?

In Taiwan, surveys show a surge in support for the government in the first few months of the pandemic. In April 2020, a Formosa poll found 70.3 percent of respondents were satisfied with President Tsai's performance in office, and only 24.1 percent were dissatisfied. However, these astronomical approval ratings gradually faded to more normal levels. By the time debates over vaccine policy took center stage nearly a year later, the rally-around-the-flag effect had vanished.[6]

As the sense of emergency fades, the normal partisan divisions reassert themselves, and opposition parties go back to active opposition. Instead of overlooking government shortcomings in a unified effort to meet the emergency, opposition parties are more likely to highlight those shortcomings in an effort to convince voters that the government is incompetent and should be replaced at the next election.

Part of normal democratic politics is that the successes and failures of different government initiatives are often defined differently by different parties. The ideological lens of each party shapes their interpretations and helps to determine where opposition parties will attack. In the United States, for example, conservative Republicans and progressive Democrats have expressed very different understandings of the pandemic. Conservatives, who traditionally value individual freedom over collective benefits, have been much less willing to tolerate limits to those individual freedoms, such as lockdowns, social distancing, and mask and vaccine mandates. The anti-elitist strain in the modern Republican Party has also led to a heightened skepticism of science and science elites. These different impulses have been further exacerbated by consumption of different media.[7] In short, the preexisting political fault lines shape how the battles over COVID are fought.

In Taiwan, the COVID battles should reflect Taiwan's distinct partisan fault lines. The left and right divisions common in many democracies do not feature prominently in Taiwan.[8] Instead, politics are organized around questions of national identity.[9] To greatly simplify, whereas DPP supporters tend to reject the notion that they are Chinese, KMT supporters are more likely to think that their Taiwanese identity is compatible with also being Chinese. This basic difference in how most supporters of the two main parties think about themselves has concrete policy implications that pervade the entire system. The KMT tends to be more enthusiastic about interaction and cooperation with China, while the DPP generally wants to hold China at arm's length. Even though the COVID virus is itself blind to questions of national identity, these questions have played a major role in shaping how people in Taiwan dealt with the virus.

KMT ATTACKS

In this section, I examine KMT rhetoric on vaccines in 2021 in order to demonstrate that Taiwan's vaccination campaign was conducted amid intense partisan bickering. I pay special attention to the May to July period because this was the height of the outbreak and mass vaccination efforts were just beginning.

I focus on KMT attacks because the rally-around-the-flag literature identifies the absence of such attacks from the opposition as the key mechanism. I do not limit the focus to official KMT spokespeople.

Rather, I assume that citizens will consider statements from any prominent KMT figure as representing the party's positions unless those statements are subsequently repudiated or corrected by an even more authoritative party source. If a high-profile KMT figure says something and no one else in the KMT objects, it is fair for citizens to think that represents KMT mainstream thought.

The point here is not that the KMT was unreasonable, intransigent, or obstructionist. The point is that they were behaving like a normal opposition party in any democracy. Opposition parties do not generally prosper when the governing party is seen as performing well, so opposition parties do not have strong incentives to help them out. Opposition parties are supposed to take every opportunity to make life difficult for governing parties. In fact, this review of several prominent lines of attack shows energetic opposition by the KMT that was often, though not always, embedded in the national identity cleavage. This was democratic politics as usual.

Why Not Use Chinese Vaccines?

Throughout the first half of 2021, Taiwan faced a vaccine supply shortage, and various KMT figures suggested turning to China. This idea was anathema to the DPP government because it would have required official contacts with the PRC that, in turn, would almost certainly have required accepting a One China policy, a repudiation of the DPP's longstanding insistence on Taiwan sovereignty. In contrast, One China is one of the KMT's (literally: Chinese Nationalist Party) founding principles and was the cornerstone of Ma Ying-jeou's 馬英九 presidency. Unlike the DPP, the KMT did not see Chinese vaccines as a threat to sovereignty or their national identity. Calls for Chinese vaccines were never the KMT's main message, perhaps because there was never much evidence that the population was eager for Chinese vaccines. Nevertheless, they popped up several times.

Former president Ma was the first major figure to advocate using Chinese vaccines. At a temple visit during Lunar New Year, Ma said that if China offered vaccines, the government should not reflexively refuse them.[10] Ma returned to this theme a few days later at KMT headquarters, saying that the world had high hopes for Mainland, Russian, and Indian vaccines, and, given its difficulties and delays in procuring vaccines, Taiwan should not rule out this option. Ma's office also issued a press release complaining that the DPP was unable to face cross-Straits issues rationally due to its ideological biases.[11] Legislator Lai Shih-pao 賴士葆 concurred with Ma, accusing the government of making choices by political correctness and leaving no room for a rational discussion of scientific merits.[12]

In May as the outbreak started, former legislator Ting Shou-chung 丁守中 made an explicit call for Chinese vaccines. Because the international vaccines had not yet arrived and the domestic vaccines were not yet ready, Taiwan needed a supply from China. Ting further proclaimed that he would be first in line to get a Chinese vaccine.[13] A few people went beyond just calling for the government to obtain Chinese vaccines. Chang Ya-chung 張亞中, who was running for KMT party chair, claimed he had secured five million doses of Chinese vaccines, and former legislator Alex Tsai 蔡正元 added that even if Chinese vaccines were not as good as Moderna and Pfizer they were definitely better than AstraZeneca.[14] Former KMT party chair Hung Hsiu-chu 洪秀柱 offered herself as a bridge to go to China and get Chinese vaccines. The vaccines had been approved by the WHO, Hung noted, so there should not be any biases against them.[15] A month later, Hung posted on her Facebook page that she was in China and planned to get a Chinese vaccine in the next few days.[16]

In late June, the KMT legislative caucus introduced a bill requiring the government to purchase thirty million doses of WHO-approved vaccines. The bill did not explicitly mention Chinese vaccines, but the DPP charged that the bill was a sneaky effort to force purchases of Chinese vaccines because those were the only WHO-approved vaccines available on such a short timeline.[17] The bill had no hope of passing, so it is fair to consider it as a device for political communication.

Given the lack of public enthusiasm for Chinese vaccines, this repeated appeal seems unexpected. It only makes sense in light of the larger partisan framework in which KMT politicians assume that increased cooperation with China is natural and desirable.

Concerns about AstraZeneca

Prior to the outbreak, AstraZeneca (AZ) was the only vaccine available in Taiwan. Rather than presenting a unified front and encouraging everyone to get a shot, as might be expected in a rally-around-the-flag environment, the KMT repeatedly and consistently expressed doubts about AZ.

In late February as the government was preparing to start the first wave of vaccinations, KMT legislators questioned whether AZ was effective. Alex Fai 費鴻泰 pointed to doubts about AZ in many countries, saying, "if it isn't good, don't import it, we'll wait."[18] Lin Wei-chou 林為洲 wondered why President Tsai, Premier Su, and Minister Chen hadn't publicly gotten shots, adding that everyone was confident in Pfizer and Moderna but less so in AZ.[19]

Over the spring, the KMT questioned whether the government had purchased *too much* AZ. When only 30 to 40 percent of frontline medical workers immediately signed up for an AZ shot, former legislator Sun Ta-chien 孫大千 wondered if the current stock would expire and become garbage.[20] A few weeks later, Sun went further. Given concerns about AZ from Denmark and other countries, Sun called for an immediate halt to all further purchase of AZ, saying that the government should not gamble with people's health and safety. Besides, because the people were hesitant to take AZ, amassing stockpiles that would expire before use would be a big waste of resources and might also cause the country to miss out on purchasing other vaccines.[21] Legislator Wu Sz-huai 吳斯懷 worried that the government would deal with the excess of AZ vaccines by forcing the military to take it.[22]

Even as concerns about the outbreak started growing in early May, the KMT continued to cast doubts on AZ. KMT Culture and Communications Director Wang Yu-min 王育民 held a press conference to state that people were still skeptical about AZ and reluctant to take it.[23] As late as May 12, KMT legislator Cheng Li-wen 鄭麗文 stated that AZ was completely ineffective against the UK variant and wondered where the BNT and Moderna shots were.[24]

During the spring, it was hard to find any KMT figure saying anything positive about AZ. They might not work, no one wanted them, and they were destined to end up in the garbage pile. The government had clearly bought the wrong vaccines; anything else would have been better.

The Pandemic Is Here! We Need Vaccines Right Now!

When realization of the scope of the outbreak crashed into public consciousness in May, the way the KMT talked about vaccines changed almost overnight. Suddenly, the KMT stopped complaining about rotting stockpiles and started screaming about shortages. It still did not have many nice things to say about AZ, but it said the negative things far less often. With the population now scared of the virus and clamoring for vaccines, the KMT focused squarely on the issue of supply.

Just two days after his colleague painted AZ ineffective, legislator Cheng Cheng-chien 鄭正鈐 openly worried that the next shipment of AZ might be delayed. While he still wasn't completely sure about AZ, he nonetheless now wanted prompt delivery of it.[25] Similarly, Wang Yu-min 王育民, who had previously been a skeptic, now excoriated the government for failing at its legal responsibility to acquire vaccines. Where other countries took the challenge seriously, Wang charged, Taiwan's government didn't do enough and could now only feebly tell people that "there are no new developments."[26]

In early June, the KMT organized a virtual protest with the theme, "support medical workers, we want vaccines," featuring twenty empty buses and several banners outside the presidential building.[27] Three days later, the KMT held a press conference to voice concerns for the "forgotten 10m Taiwanese youths." Wang Yu-min 王育民 noted that the government had set up eleven priority categories covering thirteen million people. She then wondered why the other ten million people hadn't been included in the priority rankings and worried there would only be domestic vaccines left for them.[28] Of all the various KMT attacks, this was perhaps the most transparently cynical. Young people were at the bottom of every country's priority list, and Wang certainly didn't argue that another group should be bumped down. Young voters had overwhelmingly opposed the KMT in the 2020 election, so this was a clumsy attempt to pander to that demographic.

The KMT screamed about the lack of vaccines throughout May and early June, but the supply situation dramatically changed in June. On June 4, Japan sent 1.24 million doses of AZ to Taiwan. On June 6, the United States announced it would donate 750,000 doses, and on June 20, they actually sent 2.5 million doses of Moderna. The Japanese and American donations were absolutely critical to Taiwan's COVID response. With nearly four million doses on hand, the government was able to start a mass vaccination program for a population suddenly clamoring to get vaccines as soon as possible. These vaccines also provided an enormous psychological boost to a frightened population and gave Taiwan a little time to acquire vaccines from other sources. The gifts did not solve the supply crisis, but they did force the KMT modify its attacks.

KMT party chair Johnny Chiang 江啟臣 publicly thanked Japan for its gift, but other KMT figures were less gracious. KMT legislative caucus leader Alex Fai 費鴻泰 pointed out that vaccination rates in Japan were also low (6.9 percent at the time) and wondered why Japan was giving Taiwan the AZ that it didn't want.[29] Legislator Yeh Yu-lan 葉毓蘭 expressed disappointment at the quantity of vaccines from Japan, posting on her Facebook page that this was only 4 percent of the thirty million vaccines Japan was giving away to other countries, and she had expected Japan to give Taiwan at least 3.11 million doses.[30] The number 3.11 was a reference to the March 11, 2011, Fukushima earthquake and tsunami, after which Taiwanese enthusiastically donated to relief funds. The implication was that Japan owed Taiwan a debt of gratitude and the 1.24 million dose gift was miserly. This post was immediately criticized, and Yeh soon deleted it. As we have seen, the KMT had been talking down AZ for several months, so it is not surprising that Fai would complain that Japan was giving Taiwan the less desirable AZ vaccines while keeping the better Moderna and Pfizer for themselves. The long-term antipathy toward Japan among deep blue ideologues such as Fai and Yeh probably also played into this. This antipathy is rooted in KMT memories of the 1930s and 1940s in China, which are very different from the memories of people who spent that period in Taiwan.

The donation of Moderna from the United States elicited a different response from the KMT. Instead of focusing on the giver, they criticized the recipient. The KMT complained that the government hadn't bought enough vaccines and had to rely on gifts. KMT chair Johnny Chiang 江啟臣 pointed out that donations had far outnumbered purchases and asked if the government was just waiting for other countries to donate vaccines what it was good for.[31] Legislator Lai Shih-pao 賴士葆 wondered why the government had only bought 700,000 AZ and 300,000 Moderna doses so far because the legislature had approved NTD 34 billion for this purpose. He answered his own question, concluding that either the government was inept or it was engaged in a conspiracy to enrich domestic vaccine manufacturers at the expense of peoples' lives. Taipei city councilor Luo Chih-chiang 羅智強 lamented that Taiwan was becoming a "vaccine beggar."[32]

The Long Quest for BNT Vaccines

After spending May excoriating the central government for failing at its responsibility to purchase sufficient vaccine supplies, KMT chair Johnny Chiang 江啟臣 announced a shift in the party's position. Because the government was unable to purchase sufficient supplies, the KMT argued it should allow private groups and local governments to purchase vaccines, something the central government had steadfastly refused to consider.[33]

This theme was entwined with the government's failed attempts to buy BioNTech (BNT) vaccines and different partisan attitudes toward China. In February, a government deal to purchase five million doses of BNT fell apart at the last moment due to intervention by an "outside force."[34] For most of the spring and summer, the KMT complained that the "ideology" was preventing the government from completing a deal to purchase BNT. Legislator Lai Shih-pao 賴士葆 laid out the KMT argument concisely. The government had refused to deal with Shanghai Fosun, the company that held the rights to the Greater China market, because it insisted that BNT should deal directly with the Taiwan government rather than going through a Chinese agent. Because of the government's ideology, Taiwan had lost out on five million doses of BNT, which was the most effective of the vaccines.[35]

Several local governments led by KMT mayors or magistrates proposed buying vaccines for their local population. Nantou County magistrate Lin Ming-chen 林明溱 was the most aggressive. Lin claimed to have an agreement with China's Taiwan Affairs Office to purchase BNT/Pfizer vaccines through Shanghai Fosun on the condition that the central government authorized the Nantou County government to make the deal.[36] Former presidential candidate Han Kuo-yu 韓國瑜 then held a press conference with fourteen local heads of government who wanted to use their own channels to purchase vaccines.[37]

Several groups and individuals offered to purchase vaccines privately. I have already noted Chang Ya-chung's 張亞中 claim that he could obtain Chinese vaccines. Buddha's Light International Association 佛光山 expressed willingness to donate 500,000 doses of Johnson & Johnson.[38] Tzu Chi 慈濟 also expressed interest in purchasing vaccines.[39] However, the most vocal and credible of all these was Hunghai (Foxconn) founder and 2020 presidential contender Terry Gou 郭台銘, who announced that his

Yungling Foundation 永齡基金會 would attempt to purchase five million doses of BNT directly from the German factory.[40]

KMT party chair Johnny Chiang 江啟臣 promoted these efforts energetically. Upon hearing news of the Japanese gift, he thanked Japan for its generosity and then called on the central government to apply the same standards it had used for Japan to allow local governments and private groups to try to acquire vaccines. "The Tsai government uses the false concerns over vaccine safety to block importation, and it is blind to the constant loss of lives," Chiang complained.[41] A month later at the KMT Central Standing Committee, Chiang reiterated that four counties still wanted to attempt to purchase BNT vaccines because, faced with the people's needs, the KMT should not wait for more donations but should take the initiative to take action.[42]

The central government took a skeptical view of these efforts. Officially, they were worried about quality control. Unofficially, they were probably also worried about the political implications of setting up multiple distribution systems in which people living in some places could get access to vaccines while those in other areas could not. But their most serious reservation was probably the concern that these actors would make statements supporting One China and undermining Taiwan's sovereignty in order to secure purchases.

However, there was significant popular pressure on the central government to procure vaccines as quickly as possible, and they hit on a deft compromise. On June 19, the government announced it was authorizing Gou to negotiate with BNT on its behalf. Notably, Gou promised not to use the name "Taiwan, China" or do anything else that might damage the country's sovereignty. Moreover, the government mitigated the potential of Gou—who might still have presidential aspirations—to claim heroic salvation of the country by jointly authorizing Taiwan Semiconductors (TSMC) and Tzu Chi as partners in this effort.[43]

The fifteen million BNT doses these negotiators would eventually secure proved to be a major element in Taiwan's vaccination efforts. They also deprived the KMT of a potent issue. When the TSMC/Yungling/Tzu Chi negotiators struck a deal with BNT, the KMT could only cry sour grapes, complaining that the government first blocked such deals and now wanted to take credit for them.[44]

Doubts About Medigen

While the KMT was extremely vocal about wanting more vaccines from abroad, this did not apply to domestic vaccines. They particularly focused their ire on Medigen 高端, which they suspected of receiving special treatment from the DPP government. Former legislator Chen Yi-min 陳宜民, reviewing the difficulties of the other competing domestic vaccine developers, speculated, "It seems like someone wants Medigen to be first [to the market]."[45] There was a steady flow of stories about Medigen's stock price with the unspoken insinuation that someone must be manipulating this price. As we have already seen, the KMT also accused the government of not aggressively purchasing other vaccines in order to protect the domestic manufacturers. When President Tsai and Vice President Lai pointedly insisted on waiting for the domestic vaccines before getting a shot, the KMT interpreted this as evidence of something nefarious.

When Medigen announced its successful phase 2 results, the KMT said that people still had many doubts and wondered when Medigen would do its phase 3 trial or get international approval. The people urgently needed safe, effective, and internationally recognized vaccines.[46] KMT legislative caucus leaders were blunter. Alex Fai 費鴻泰 argued it was improper to use phase 2 results as a substitute for phase 3. Cheng Li-wen 鄭麗文 said that the government's price for Medigen was too high, especially because they had already received a huge subsidy. Moreover, the government had not aggressively attempted to purchase vaccines and had even blocked AZ from manufacturing in Taiwan in an attempt to protect domestic vaccines. The puppet master, Cheng explained, was President Tsai herself.[47] When Medigen got its emergency use authorization, the KMT legislative caucus presented four major controversies surrounding Medigen: (1) the EUA process was a black box; (2) half the committee was suddenly replaced; (3) the standard for approval was extremely low; and 4) the government had only fined Medigen NTD30,000 for a fiasco in which a contract with a Malaysian company suddenly fell apart, causing the stock price to surge and then fall.[48]

The KMT message on Medigen was clear. It expensive, corrupt, scientifically unproven, might not even work, and it had prevented Taiwan from getting other vaccines. Medigen, the KMT argued, was a disaster.

DID THE KMT ATTACKS AFFECT TAIWAN'S VACCINATION PROGRAM?

We have seen the KMT make a variety of attacks against the DPP government's vaccination strategy, some of which were more reasonable than others. A few points are worth noting. First and most importantly, the KMT never made an antivaccination argument. It questioned individual vaccines, but it never questioned vaccination in general. One reason was that the vaccine shortage provided an easy and obvious appeal: we want vaccines and the government is failing to provide them. More importantly, unlike in many other countries, Taiwan has no party founded on libertarian principles or heavily invested in antiscience ideas. Either way, the important point is that there was no major party making or validating antivaccination appeals. Taiwanese of all partisan stripes learned that they wanted a vaccine.

Second, not all vaccines were equally desirable. The KMT consistently and forcefully talked down Medigen. Before the May outbreak, it also talked down AZ. This point may have lost some of its persuasiveness in June, when it emerged that many AZ critics had rushed to get AZ, and some had even pulled strings to jump ahead in line. One of these was Ting Shou-chung, who got an AZ vaccine at roughly the same time he was publicly promising to be first in line to get a Chinese vaccine.[49] However, the months of doubts about AZ probably had some effect. BNT and Moderna were almost universally treated as the two most effective and most desirable vaccines. However, even here, there was a difference. The KMT spent months talking about how the government refused to purchase BNT because of ideological difficulties. Essentially, they were implying that "BNT is the best, but you can't have it." In sum, the KMT rhetoric implied a clear rank ordering of the four vaccines that Taiwan eventually had access to: BNT, Moderna, AZ, Medigen, from best to worst.

We can see some of the effects of the KMT's attacks in polling data. A poll from Formosa in late June reveals some interesting patterns.[50] The most important number from this poll is that only 4.9 percent of respondents absolutely refused to be vaccinated. In comparison, this number ranged from 12 percent to 30 percent in eight other wealthy countries.[51] There was not much difference between blue party identifiers and green party identifiers on this point. Taiwan simply did not have much strong antivax sentiment.

Table 3.1. Preference for Vaccines in Late June 2021 by Party ID

	Green Camp	*Blue Camp*	*Others*	*All*
Already got first shot	7.2	8.1	5.7	6.7
Will not get vaccinated	4.0	4.7	5.6	4.9
First or second preference is Medigen	19.6	3.3	7.5	10.7
First or second preference is AZ	16.6	6.7	10.8	11.8
First preference is Moderna	32.2	43.1	32.4	34.7
First preference is BNT	17.6	32.5	27.4	25.2
N	364	233	478	1,075

Notes: Cells are column percentages. The green camp is led by the DPP, and the blue camp is led by the KMT. Both camps include several smaller, allied parties.

Source: Recalculated by author from Formosa June 2021 National Government Survey.

The poll asked respondents, if they could choose any one, which of five vaccines (Moderna, Pfizer/BNT, AZ, Medigen, or United Biomedical 聯亞) they would prefer. They were then asked for their second choice. Please remember that very few people had been vaccinated at this point, the contracts for BNT had not yet been signed, and Medigen had not yet been approved. The KMT repeatedly attacked Medigen while President Tsai insisted on waiting for Medigen to get her vaccine shot, so it should not be surprising that there are clear partisan preferences for Medigen: 10.7 percent of respondents expressed a preference for Medigen, but this was 19.6 percent among green camp identifiers and a mere 3.3 percent among blue camp identifiers. The KMT spent several months criticizing AZ, so it should not be surprising that there is a similar, though slightly smaller, partisan difference in preferences for AZ: 16.6 percent of green camp party identifiers named AZ either as their first or second preference, while only 6.7 percent of blue camp party identifiers did so. The partisan differences in preferences for BNT and Moderna are smaller but still visible. Because the KMT spent several months clamoring for BNT, we expect blue camp identifiers to be more likely to want BNT as their first preference. In fact, Moderna was the top choice among both blue and green identifiers, and BNT was the second favorite option in both groups. However, blue identifiers were more evenly split among these two options. The ratio of BNT to Moderna first preferences was 0.75 among blue identifiers but only 0.55 among green identifiers.

The June 2021 Formosa poll was carried out before most people had had an opportunity to be vaccinated, and it asks about preferences rather than behavior. By the time a September 2021 TEDS poll[52] was conducted, nearly everyone had been eligible for one vaccine or another, so we can look at actual behavior. Please note that the various vaccines were available to different groups at different times, so people could not simply choose their first preference. For many people, this was a choice between the immediately available choice (often AZ) and waiting an undetermined amount of time for a different vaccine to become available. Medigen became widely available in September, but some people who would have chosen it had already gotten a different vaccine. BNT shots would start being administered within days after this poll. Nonetheless, even if people could not simply choose their most preferred vaccine, their behavior shows clear partisan patterns.

Again, very few people (4 percent) refused to get vaccinated at all, and this was similar across partisan groups. However, the respondents who did get vaccinated opted for different vaccines: 9.3 percent of green identifiers reported getting a Medigen shot, while almost no (0.5 percent) blue identifiers did. AZ was the most widely available vaccine, and many blue identifiers took it. However, AZ was less popular among blue identifiers than green identifiers (35.5 percent to 44.8 percent). On the other hand, blue identifiers were more likely to get Moderna than green identifiers (24.3 percent to 17.3 percent) and they were less likely to have gotten a shot at all (60.8 percent to 72.3 percent). With months of KMT rhetoric criticizing Medigen and AZ, it is easy to imagine that many blue identifiers had insisted on Moderna or were still waiting on BNT.

Table 3.2. Vaccination Status in Late September 2021 by Party ID

	Green Camp	*Blue Camp*	*Others*	*All*
Already got first shot	72.3	60.8	56.9	62.6
Will not get vaccinated	2.0	5.1	5.0	4.0
First shot was AZ	44.8	35.5	37.3	39.4
First shot was Moderna	17.3	24.3	15.8	17.8
First shot was Medigen	9.3	0.5	3.3	4.8
N	400	214	603	1,217

Note: Cells are column percentages.

Source: September 2021 TEDS Presidential Satisfaction Survey.

All in all, these polls show patterns that are consistent with the messages the KMT had been sending its supporters for several months. Everyone wanted a vaccine, but they did not all want the same vaccines.

CONCLUSION

Taiwan's vaccination program has achieved considerable success. By February 2022, 82.8 percent of Taiwanese had received at least one shot, a vaccination rate comparable to or exceeding most industrialized democracies in Europe, North America, and East Asia and a feat that is more remarkable given Taiwan's later start.[53] The foundation for this program was laid earlier in the year when the parties argued about how to go about vaccinating the population. As we have seen, the two main parties reached a consensus that vaccinations were desirable—and not much more.

The opposition KMT attacked the DPP government at every opportunity. There weren't enough vaccines, they were the wrong vaccines, the vaccines were too expensive, people had to wait too long for their vaccine, the government constantly made bad decisions due to its misguided ideology, too many people were dying, and the government simply didn't care enough about the people. This was not an example of an opposition restraining itself in the face of a national crisis, as might be expected in a rally-around-the-flag environment. Instead, this was normal no-holds-barred democratic politics replete with intense partisan conflict.

Significantly, these opposition attacks did not include any general appeals against all vaccines. In this regard, Taiwan was fortunate that its politics are grounded in the national identity cleavage and not the left/right cleavage found in many other countries. There were no parties reflexively appealing to absolute individual liberties or validating the arguments made by antivax voices. Instead of abstract arguments about individual freedom, the KMT made arguments about ineffective governance and flawed policies guided by a misguided national identity. These were objections that could be answered by successful governance. Taiwan's ideological disputes did not create insurmountable barriers for mass vaccination.

The Tsai government responded to the different KMT attacks with varying degrees of pragmatism and flexibility. The government simply ignored the KMT's call for Chinese vaccines. There was almost no public support for Chinese vaccines, so the DPP was happy to let the KMT paint itself into an unpopular position. No serious response was necessary. The Tsai government also chose not to directly engage the KMT when it attacked the domestic Medigen vaccine. The Tsai government plowed ahead with its plans to utilize Medigen, insisting it was safe and effective. However, they did not launch a big public campaign to promote Medigen. Instead, they repeated that taking Medigen was entirely voluntary; no one was forced to take it. Rather than trying to persuade blue camp identifiers to change their minds about Medigen, the government focused on acquiring vaccines that were more acceptable to them and accepting that much of the population would never accept Medigen. The approach was similar with AZ, though the government was helped a great deal by the KMT's mixed messages on AZ. First the KMT didn't want AZ, then it wanted it immediately, and then it turned out that several KMT leaders had pulled strings to get AZ before it was their turn. For many people clamoring to get a vaccine during the outbreak, the choice was between AZ and waiting. With muddled messages from the main opposition party, many citizens decided that AZ was acceptable.

Acquiring BNT demanded flexibility from the government. The key to the soft-handed government approach was ensuring that everyone eventually had access to a vaccine they found acceptable. In short, the government needed to acquire large quantities of Moderna or BNT, and Moderna proved unable to provide adequate supply. Given the influence of Shanghai Fosun over BNT, insisting that all purchases be handled directly by the central government was unlikely to yield results. To secure BNT, the government had to compromise its position by authorizing a middleman who has good ties in China and who might run for the presidency against the DPP. Even with the additional agents and the guarantee that sovereignty would not be compromised, this was a difficult pill for the government to swallow. However, they swallowed it, and the BNT doses eventually proved a vital factor in Taiwan's vaccination drive, accounting for a third of all initial protocol shots.[54] These doses were almost all administered after September, so they presumably went disproportionally to Tsai's partisan opponents in the blue camp, who had lower vaccination rates in the September data.

Taiwan's vaccination experience holds a few lessons about good governance. First, the structure of ideological cleavages matters. In this case, Taiwan was fortunate that its primary division did not impede vaccination efforts. Second, this program relied on voluntary compliance, not obedience to coercive policies. Third, the voluntary compliance was possible because the government was able to solve supply problems and procure vaccines that people were willing to take. Fourth, procuring those vaccines required a degree of pragmatism. Fifth and finally, all this was carried out in a democratic environment grounded firmly in party politics and public opinion. Democracy, even in trying circumstances, is compatible with good governance.

NOTES

1. For example, see Philip Bump, "Vaccine Politics Only Worsened the Partisan Divide in Covid-19 Deaths," *Washington Post*, November 8, 2021, https://www.washingtonpost.com/politics/2021/11/08/vaccine-politics-only-worsened-partisan-divide-covid-19-deaths/; Chris Cillizza, "This Is How Badly Partisanship Has Poisoned the Conversation about the Covid-19 Vaccine," CNN, November 16, 2021, https://edition.cnn.com/2021/11/16/politics/covid-19-vaccine-partisanship/index.html; Dan Goldberg and Alice Miranda Ollstein, "The Partisan Divide in Vaccinations Is Starker than You Realize," Politico, June 5, 2021, https://www.politico.com/news/2021/06/05/partisan-divide-vaccinations-491947; Chris Stirewalt, "Partisan Gap on Vaccines Frees Dems to Push Shots, Not Restrictions," *AEI*, November 30, 2021, https://www.aei.org/op-eds/partisan-gap-on-vaccines-frees-dems-to-push-shots-not-restrictions/.

2. Kavanagh and Singh 2020; Mao 2021; Sheng 2022.

3. Sheng 2022.

4. Kritzinger et al. 2021; Yam et al. 2020.

5. Baker and Oneal 2001; Groeling and Baum 2008.

6. The monthly Formosa National Government Surveys can be found at the site's page of poll results. Formosa Online Newspaper 美麗島電子報, "美麗島民調" [Formosa surveys], http://www.my-formosa.com/Topical/formosapollster.

7. John Kerr, Panagopoulos, and van der Linden 2021, 110892.

8. Hsiao, Cheng, and Achen 2017.

9. Achen and Wang 2017a; Achen and Wang 2017b.

10. Hu Peng-sheng 胡蓬生, "Miaoli Majiazhuang Jizu Ma Yingjiu: Dui dalu yimiao ying baoliu tanxing" 苗栗馬家庄祭祖 馬英九：對大陸疫苗應保留彈性" [Worshiping at Miaoli Majia Village. Ma: Maintain flexibility toward

Mainland vaccines], *Lianhe Bao* 聯合報 [United Daily News], February 13, 2021, https://udn.com/news/story/120940/5249838.

11. Liu Kuan-ting 劉冠廷, "Ying wu ju Zhongguo yimiao reyi. Ma Yingjiu: bu yao paichu keneng xuanxian" 籲勿拒中國疫苗惹議 馬英九：不要排除可能選項 [Don't refuse Chinese vaccines. Ma Ying-jeou: Don't rule out possible options], Zhongyang She 中央社 [Central News Agency], February 17, 2021, https://www.cna.com.tw/news/aipl/202102170113.aspx.

12. Cheng Wei 鄭煒, "Dalu yimiao maibumai? Lai Shibao tan: zai Taiwan wu lixing tantao kongjian" 大陸疫苗買不買？賴士葆嘆：在台灣無理性探討空間 [Should we buy Mainland vaccines? Lai Shih-pao sighs: No room for rational discussion in Taiwan], *Lianhe Bao* 聯合報 [United Daily News], February 16, 2021, https://udn.com/news/story/120940/5253097.

13. "Tai xian? Ding Shouzhong zhuzhang jinkou Zhongguo yimiao hai yao daitou da. Bei wangyou kuang paohong" 太閒？丁守中主張進口中國疫苗還要帶頭打 被網友狂砲轟 [Too bored? Ting Shou-chung supports importing Chinese vaccines and will be the first to get one. Vigorously attacked by netizens], *Ziyou Shibao* 自由時報 [Liberty Times], May 12, 2021, https://news.ltn.com.tw/news/politics/breakingnews/3530029.

14. Chou Chih-hao 周志豪, "Sunwen xuexiao yu taishang chuansuo. Jiang Jingguo zhi waisun juan Tai 500 wan ji BNT yimiao" 孫文學校與台商穿梭 蔣經國侄外孫捐台500萬劑BNT疫苗 [Shuttling from Sun Yat-sen Academy and Taiwanese businessmen. Chiang Ching-kuo's relative will donate five million doses of BNT to Taiwan], *Lianhe Bao* 聯合報 [United Daily News], May 29, 2021, https://udn.com/news/story/122190/5494808.

15. Chou Chih-hao 周志豪, "Yimiao shi jiejue yiqing zuizhong shouduan. Hong Xiuzhu: Yuan zhengqu Dalu yimiao lai Tai" 疫苗是解決疫情最終手段 洪秀柱：願爭取大陸疫苗來台 [Vaccines are the ultimate solution to the pandemic. Hung Hsiu-chu: I'm willing to ask for Mainland vaccines for Taiwan], *Lianhe Bao* 聯合報 [United Daily News], May 21, 2021, https://udn.com/news/story/122173/5476216.

16. Lin Liang-sheng 林良昇, "Hong Xiuzhu fu Zhong canjia luntan, jiang da Zhongguo yimiao, cheng 'you xinxin'" 洪秀柱赴中參加論壇 將打中國疫苗稱「有信心」[Hung Hsiu-chu goes to China to participate in a forum. Will get a Chinese vaccine. Says, "I have confidence"], *Ziyou Shibao* 自由時報 [Liberty Times], June 28, 2021, https://news.ltn.com.tw/news/politics/breakingnews/3584448.

17. Lee Cheng-ying 李承穎, "Minjindang Liyuan dangtuan pi Guomindang ti an: bi Taiwan da Zhongguo yimiao" 民進黨立院黨團批國民黨提案：逼台灣打中國疫苗 [DPP legislative caucus criticizes KMT bill: It will force Taiwan to

use Chinese vaccines], *Lianhe Bao* 聯合報 [United Daily News], June 21, 2021, https://udn.com/news/story/122190/5546599.

18. Fan Cheng-hsiang 范正祥, "Lanwei zhi AZ yimiao you yilü. Chen Shizhong: ni keyi deng mei qiangpo da" 藍委指AZ疫苗有疑慮 陳時中：你可以等沒強迫打 [Blue legislators say there are doubts about the AZ vaccine. Chen Shih-chung: you can wait, no one is forced to get a shot], Zhongyang She中央社 [Central News Agency], February 26, 2021, https://www.cna.com.tw/news/aipl/202102260112.aspx.

19. Chu Chen-kai 朱真楷, Lin Chin-ming 林縉明, and Yang Meng-li 楊孟立, "Guomingdang qiang Cai Yingwen ganbugan daitou da yimiao! Bei suan bugan da AZ deng huirui. Su gaikou yuan xian jiezhong" 國民黨嗆蔡英文 敢不敢帶頭打疫苗！被酸不敢打AZ等輝瑞 蘇改口願先接種 [KMT challenges Tsai Ing-wen: Do you dare be first to get a vaccine? Suspected of not daring to take AZ and waiting for Pfizer, Su changes course and will get a shot], *Zhongguo Shibao* 中國時報 [China Times], February 27, 2021, https://www.chinatimes.com/newspapers/20210227000352-260102?chdtv.

20. Liu Yuan-lin 劉宛琳, "AZ yimiao yilü. Sun Daqian: qing Cai Yingwen, Su Zhenchang he Chen Shizhong xian da" AZ疫苗疑慮 孫大千：請蔡英文、蘇貞昌和陳時中先打 [Doubts over AZ. Sun Ta-chien asks Tsai Ying-wen, Su Tseng-chang, and Chen Shih-chung to get shots], *Lianhe Bao* 聯合報 [United Daily News], March 16, 2021, https://udn.com/news/story/120940/5320568.

21. Chou Chih-hao 周志豪, "Xiesuan fengxian nanjie. Sun Daqian: Weifubu ying liji tingzhi caigou AZ yimiao" 血栓風險難解 孫大千：衛福部應立即停止採購AZ疫苗 [Throbosis danger unresolved. Sun Ta-chien: Health Ministry should immediately stop purchases of AZ vaccine], *Lianhe Bao* 聯合報 [United Daily News], April 16, 2021, https://udn.com/news/story/120940/5392226.

22. Wang Tzu-hsuan 王子瑄, "Guojun jiang bei bi da AZ yimiao? Wu Sihuai xiangqi 2 jian shi qizha le" 國軍將被逼打AZ疫苗？吳斯懷想起2件事氣炸了 [Will the military be forced to take AZ? Wu Sz-huai explodes thinking about two cases], *Zhongguo Shibao* 中國時報 [China Times], April 21, 2021, https://www.chinatimes.com/realtimenews/20210421001448-260407?chdtv.

23. Liu Kuan-ting 劉冠廷, "Guomindang: guoren dui AZ you yilü zhengfu ying jinsu jinkou qitai yimiao" 國民黨：國人對AZ有疑慮 政府應儘速進口其他疫苗 [KMT: people have doubts about AZ; government should quickly import other vaccines], Zhongyang She中央社 [Central News Agency], May 4, 2021, https://www.cna.com.tw/news/aipl/202105040082.aspx.

24. Huang Chien-hao 黃建豪, "Jin kong sheng 3 ji jingjie. Zheng Liwen wen Chen Shizhong: Heshi quanmin kuaisai? BNT yimiao zai na?" 今恐升3級警戒 鄭麗文問陳時中：何時全民快篩？BNT疫苗在哪？[Fear today will raise to level 3 alert. Cheng Li-wen asks Chen Shih-chung: When will all people get rapid

testing? Where are the BNT vaccines?] *Xintouke* 新頭殼 [New Talk], May 12, 2021, https://newtalk.tw/news/view/2021-05-12/571925.

25. Wang Tzu-hsuan 王子瑄, "Chen Shizhong tuokou 'danxin yimiao bugou da' Lanwei bao houmian you geng da tiao de" 陳時中脫口「擔心疫苗不夠打」藍委爆後面還有更大條的 [Chen Shih-chung admits "I'm worried we won't have enough vaccines." Blue legislators expose the bigger person behind the scenes], *Zhongguo Shibao* 中國時報 [China Times], May 14, 2021, https://www.chinatimes.com/realtimenews/20210514001056-260407?chdtv.

26. Lin Liang-sheng 林良昇, "Guomindang: caigou yimiao shi zhongyang fading zeren. Qirong xieze" 國民黨：採購疫苗是中央法定責任 豈容卸責 [KMT: vaccine purchases are a legal responsibility of the central government. Shirking its responsibility is intolerable], *Ziyou Shibao* 自由時報 [Liberty Times], May 24, 2021, https://news.ltn.com.tw/news/politics/breakingnews/3544081.

27. Liu Yuan-lin 劉宛琳, "Guomindang ting yihu yao yimiao xingdong. Difang xiangying 20 liang youlanche rao zongtongfu" 國民黨挺醫護要疫苗行動 地方響應20輛遊覽車繞總統府 [KMT supports medical workers with "We want vaccines" demonstration. Local supporters send 20 tour buses to surround the presidential building], *Lianhe Bao* 聯合報 [United Daily News], June 6, 2021, https://udn.com/news/story/122190/5512858.

28. Liu Yuan-lin 劉宛琳, "Yimiao gu'er. Guomindang: 1000 wan nianqingren zhi sheng guochan yimiao keda ma?" 疫苗孤兒 國民黨：1000萬年輕人只剩國產疫苗可打嗎？[Vaccine Orphan. KMT: Are there only domestic vaccines left for ten million youths?], *Lianhe Bao* 聯合報 [United Daily News], June 9, 2021, https://udn.com/news/story/122190/5520370.

29. Chen Yun 陳昀, "Guomingdang ti san suqiu. Fei Hongtai qiang: feidiao zhihui zhongxin jizhe hui" 國民黨提三訴求 費鴻泰嗆：廢掉指揮中心記者會 [KMT raises three demands. Alex Fai: Abolish CECC press conference], *Ziyou Shibao* 自由時報 [Liberty Times], May 28, 2021, https://news.ltn.com.tw/news/politics/breakingnews/3549381.

30. Lin Pao-hung 林保宏, "Jiao Riben 'zhishao gei 311 wan ji yimiao.' Ye Yulan ji gaiwen daoqian" 叫日本「至少給311萬劑疫苗」葉毓蘭急改文道歉 [Calling on Japan to "give at least 3.11 million vaccine doses." Yeh Yu-lan hurriedly changes her post and apologizes], TVBS, June 4, 2021, https://news.tvbs.com.tw/politics/1522539.

31. Wu Si-shan 吳賜山, "Ganxie mei zeng Tai 250 wan ji yimiao. Jiang Qichen wen zhengfu cunzai gongneng shi shema? Ying guochan yimiao chen cishi sanqi shiyan!" 感謝美贈台250萬劑疫苗 江啟臣問政府存在功能是什麼？籲國產疫苗趁此時三期試驗！[Thanking USA for gift of 2.5 million vaccines, Johnny Chiang asks what function the government has? Calls for domestic vaccines to undergo

Phase 3 testing], *Xintouke* 新頭殼 [New Talk], June 20, 2021, https://newtalk.tw/news/view/2021-06-20/591787.

32. Huang Yi-tzu黃奕慈, "Meiguo juanzeng Taiwan 250 wan ji yimiao. Lanying paohong 'chaoqian bushu dang yimiao qigai'" 美國捐贈台灣250萬劑疫苗 藍營砲轟「超前部署當疫苗乞丐」[USA donates 2.5 million vaccines. Blue camp blasts "Advance preparation to become a vaccine beggar"], *Xintouke* 新頭殼 [New Talk], June 20, 2021, https://newtalk.tw/news/view/2021-06-20/591748.

33. Shih Hsiao-kuang 施曉光, "Guomindang zhongyang zhuangwan? Jiang Qichen: dajia yinggai fen'gong caigou yimiao" 國民黨中央轉彎？江啟臣：大家應該分工採購疫苗 [KMT changes direction? Johnny Chiang: Everyone should cooperate to purchase vaccines], *Ziyou Shibao* 自由時報 [Liberty Times], May 28, 2021, https://news.ltn.com.tw/news/politics/breakingnews/3549169.

34. Yang Ya-tang 楊雅棠, "Waili jieru! Chen Shizhong ren 5 baiwan ji BNT yimiao heyue han ka" 外力介入！ 陳時中認5百萬劑BNT疫苗合約受阻喊卡 [Outside force intervenes! Chen Shih-chung admits contract for 5 million doses of BNT is stalled], *Lianhe Bao* 聯合報 [United Daily News], February 17, 2021, https://udn.com/news/story/120940/5254626.

35. Chang Yu-han 張語涵, "Yimiao dabuwan. Lanwei hong Chen Shizhong: Buxie yu zhonghua daili shang da jiaodao, nongde quan pan jie shu" 疫苗打不完 藍委轟陳時中：不屑與大中華代理商打交道 弄得全盤皆輸 [Can't administer enough vaccines. Blue legislators blast Chen Shih-chung: Refusing to interact with agent for Greater China ends in a complete loss], *Xintouke* 新頭殼 [New Talk], April 15, 2021, https://newtalk.tw/news/view/2021-04-15/564096.

36. Lai Hsiang-shan 賴香珊 and Hei Chung-liang 黑中亮, "Guotaiban huiying le! Lin Mingzhen jieqia dalu ni mai huirui yimiao 'jiu Nantou Xianmin'" 國台辦回應了！林明溱接洽大陸擬買輝瑞疫苗「救南投縣民」[Taiwan Affairs Office responds! Lin Ming-chen contacts Mainland about buying Pfizer vaccines to "rescue the people of Nantou County"], *Lianhe Bao* 聯合報 [United Daily News], February 17, 2021, https://udn.com/news/story/122173/5484569.

37. Su Yen-nan 蘇晏男, "Han Guoyu haozhao 14 wei guomingdang xianshizhang 'zixing goumai yimiao': Tairen congmei ruci haipa" [Han Kuo-yu calls for 14 KMT mayors to "buy vaccines on their own": Taiwanese people have never been this scared], *ETtoday*, May 26, 2021, https://www.ettoday.net/news/20210526/1991958.htm.

38. Yeh Wei-chen 葉韋辰, "Juan 50 wan ji qiaoshen yimiao! Foguangshan: yi mu de hanqing weifubu hezhun" 捐50萬劑嬌生疫苗！佛光山：已募得函請衛福部核准 [Donating 500,000 doses of Johnson & Johnson vaccine! BLIA: Already submitted request for approval to Ministry of Health], TVBS, May 28, 2021, https://news.tvbs.com.tw/life/1518227.

39. Chen Yu 陳煜, "Ciji genjin juanzeng yimiao? Shoudu shengming biaotai '2 fang'an' yu shijian saipao" 慈濟跟進捐贈疫苗？首度聲明表態「2方案」與時間賽跑 [Tzu-chi joins in donating vaccines? First statement says they have two proposals and are in a race with time], *Fengchuanmei* 風傳媒 [Storm Media], May 31, 2021, https://www.storm.mg/article/3717511.

40. Chung Jung-feng 鍾榮峰, "Guo Taiming: Yongling jiang shenqing 500 wan ji dezhi BNT zhiyun Taiwan" 郭台銘：永齡將申請500萬劑德製BNT疫苗直運台灣 [Terry Gou: Yungling will apply for 5 million doses of German-made BNT vaccines shipped directly to Taiwan], Zhongyang She 中央社 [Central News Agency], February 26, 2021, https://www.cna.com.tw/news/firstnews/202105295011.aspx.

41. Yang Ching-yuan 楊清緣, "Ri juan Tai 124 wan ji AZ yimiao. Jiang Qichen: Ying yi tongyang biaozhun kandai guonei minjian yimiao juanzeng" 日捐台124萬劑AZ疫苗 江啟臣：應以同樣標準看待國內民間疫苗捐贈 [Japan donates 1.24 million doses of AZ vaccine. Johnny Chiang: Should use the same standard for vaccine donations from domestic groups], *Xintouke* 新頭殼 [New Talk], June 3, 2021, https://newtalk.tw/news/view/2021-06-03/583934.

42. Liu Yuan-lin 劉宛琳, "Jiang Qichen xuanbu: Guomindang yu 4 xianshi lianhe caigou 500 wan ji BNT yimiao" 江啟臣宣布：國民黨與4縣市 聯合採購500萬劑BNT疫苗 [Johnny Chiang announces: KMT and 4 cities and counties will jointly purchase 5 million doses of BNT vaccine], *Lianhe Bao* 聯合報 [United Daily News], July 14, 2021, https://udn.com/news/story/122190/5601060.

43. Chou Yen-yu 周彥妤, "Cai Yingwen 8 xiaoshi weiji chuli! Huajie Guo Taiming yimiao fengbao. Lüwei: juti xingdong an guoren de xin" 蔡英文8小時危機處理！化解郭台銘疫苗風暴　綠委：具體行動安國人的心 [Tsai Ing-wen 8 hours of crisis management! Resolves the Terry Gou vaccine tempest. Green legislators: Concrete action calms people's mood] *Pingguo Ribao* 蘋果日報 [Apple Daily], June 19, 2021, https://tw.appledaily.com/politics/20210619/JVRWV2FHAJBB5BEL2KPIXL7JRI/.

44. Pan Wei-ting 潘維庭, "Pi lü da nei xuan gongji minjian yimiao taigui. Guomindang: weifubu 40 meiyuan cai shi 'da pan zai'" 批綠大內宣攻擊民間疫苗買太貴 國民黨：衛福部40美元才是「大盤仔」[Criticizing Green propaganda that private vaccines are too expensive. KMT: Health Ministry's $40 price is the real market manipulator], *Fengchuanmei* 風傳媒 [Storm Media], July 17, 2021, https://www.storm.mg/article/3820516.

45. Chien Li-hsin 簡立欣 and Huang Fu-chi 黃福其, "Zhengfu ka Guoguang, tuo Lianya, zhu Gaoduan qiang touxiang" 政府卡國光、拖聯亞 助高端搶頭香 [Government blocks Adimmune, Delays United Biomedical, helps Medigen finish first], *Zhongguo Shibao* 中國時報 [China Times], March 26, 2021, https://www.chinatimes.com/newspapers/20210326000503-260102?chdtv.

46. Liu Kuan-ting 劉冠廷, "Gaoduan erqi jiemang chenggong. Guomindang: heshi zuo sanqi yu huo guoji renzheng" 高端二期解盲成功 國民黨：何時做三期與獲國際認證 [Medigen unblinds successful Phase 2 results. KMT: When will it do Phase 3 tests and get international certification?], Zhongyang She 中央社 [Central News Agency], May 4, 2021, https://www.cna.com.tw/news/aipl/202106100363.aspx.

47. Chou Chih-hao 周志豪, "Gaoduan yimiao guo you wuxiao? Guomindangtuan: Guo sanqi shiyan caineng gei EUA" 高端疫苗貴又無效？國民黨團：過三期實驗才能給EUA [Medigen vaccine is both expensive and ineffective? KMT caucus: Must pass Phase 3 before getting EUA], *Lianhe Bao* 聯合報 [United Daily News], June 11, 2021, https://udn.com/news/story/122190/5526106.

48. Lee Chun-yi 李俊毅, "Gaoduan yimiao 4 da zhengyi puguang. Lanying chijing: Cai zhengfu lihai le" 高端疫苗4大爭議曝光 藍營吃驚：蔡政府厲害了 [Medigen vaccines 4 big controversies revealed. Shocked blue camp: Tsai government is too much], *Zhongguo Shibao* 中國時報 [China Times], July 23, 2021, https://www.chinatimes.com/realtimenews/20210723005777-260407?chdtv.

49. "Cheng yuan daitou da lu yimiao! Ding Shouzhong pu yida AZ" 稱願帶頭打陸疫苗！丁守中爆已打AZ [Claimed he would be first to get a Mainland vaccine! Ting Shou-chung revealed to have already gotten AZ], *Sanli Xinwenwang* 三立新聞網 [SET], June 23, 2021, https://tw.news.yahoo.com/稱願帶頭打陸疫苗-丁守中爆已打az-014507815.html; Hsieh Wen-che 謝文哲, "Yida 'wenxin wukui' ti Huang Zhaoshun, Zhang Xianyao leifan da yimiao. Weifubu kaifa jin'e puguang" 義大「問心無愧」替黃昭順、張顯耀累犯打疫苗 衛生局開罰金額曝光 [I-Da's "clear conscience," breaks rules again to give Huang Chao-shun and Chang Hsien-yao vaccines. Health Ministry's fines are revealed], *Jingzhoukan* 鏡週刊 [Mirror Media], June 26, 2021, https://www.mirrormedia.mg/story/20210626edi008/; Lee Cheng-ying 李承穎, "Lanying jielian pu tequan da yimiao. Minjindangtuan: Guomindang beihou you tao yinmou" 藍營接連爆特權打疫苗 民進黨團：國民黨背後有套陰謀 [Blue camp revealed to repeatedly use special privilege to get vaccines. DPP caucus: KMT has a hidden conspiracy], *Lianhe Bao* 聯合報 [United Daily News], June 26, 2021, https://udn.com/news/story/122190/5562648.

50. "Meilidao mindiao: 2021 nian 6 yue guozheng midiao" 美麗島民調：2021年6月國政民調 [Formosa Survey: June 2021 National Government Survey], *Meilidao Dianzi Bao* 美麗島電子報 [Formosa Online News], June 28, 2021, http://www.my-formosa.com/DOC_171709.htm.

51. United Kingdom 12 percent, Japan 15 percent, Singapore 15 percent, Germany 17 percent, Canada 18 percent, South Korea 22 percent, United States 28 percent, and Australia 30 percent.

52. Chen 2021.

53. As of February 25, 2022, 37,238,879 initial protocol doses had been administered. 40.7 percent were AZ, 33.1 percent were BNT, 21.9 percent were Moderna, and 4.3 percent were Medigen. See "Vaccines, February 25, 2022," Taiwan Center for Disease Control, https://www.cdc.gov.tw/File/Get/bSZ9lEUCqbeGSS4vKeRCzw.

54. See "Vaccines, February 25, 2022," Taiwan Center for Disease Control.

REFERENCES

Achen, Christopher H., and T. Y. Wang. 2017a. "The Taiwan Voter: An Introduction." In *The Taiwan Voter*, edited by Christopher H. Achen and T. Y. Wang. Ann Arbor: University of Michigan Press.

Achen, Christopher H., and T. Y. Wang. 2017b. "Conclusion: The Power of Identity in Taiwan." In *The Taiwan Voter*, edited by Christopher H. Achen and T. Y. Wang. Ann Arbor: University of Michigan Press.

Baker, William D., and John R. Oneal. 2001. "Patriotism or Opinion Leadership? The Nature and Origins of the 'Rally 'Round the Flag' Effect." *Journal of Conflict Resolution* 45 (5): 661–87. https://doi.org/10.1177/0022002701045005006.

Chen, Lu-huei. 2021. Taiwan's Election and Democratization Study, 2020–2024 (II): Telephone and Mobile Phone Interview Survey of the Presidential Satisfaction—The Thirty-Sixth Wave (TEDS2021_PA09). MOST 109-2740-H-004-004-SS4 (in Chinese). Taipei: Ministry of Science and Technology Research Project.

Groeling, Tim, and Matthew A. Baum. 2008. "Crossing the Water's Edge: Elite Rhetoric, Media Coverage, and the Rally-Round-the-Flag Phenomenon." *Journal of Politics* 70 (4): 1065–85. https://doi.org/10.1017/S0022381608081061.

Hsiao, Yi-ching, Su-feng Cheng, and Christopher H. Achen. 2017. "Political Left and Right in Taiwan." In *The Taiwan Voter*, edited by Christopher H. Achen and T. Y. Wang. Ann Arbor: University of Michigan Press.

Kavanagh, Matthew A., and Renu Singh. 2020. "Democracy, Capacity, and Coercion in Pandemic Response: Covid-19 in Comparative Political Perspective." *Journal of Health, Politics, Policy, and Law* 45 (6): 997–1012. https://doi.org/10.1215/03616878-8641530.

Kerr, John, Costas Panagopoulos, and Sander van der Linden. 2021. *Personality and Individual Differences* 179: 110892.https://doi.org/10.1016/j.paid.2021.110892.

Kritzinger, Sylvia, Martial Foucault, Romain Lachat, Julia Partheymuller, Carolina Plescia, and Sylvain Bouard. 2021. "'Rally Round the Flag': The Covid-19 Crisis and Trust in the National Government." *West European Politics* 44 (5–6): 1205–31. https://doi.org/10.1080/01402382.2021.1925017.

Mao, Yexin. 2021. "Political Institutions, State Capacity, and Crisis Management: A Comparison of China and South Korea." *International Political Science Review* 42 (3): 316–32. https://doi.org/10.1177/0192512121994026.

Sheng, Li. 2022. *How COVID-19 Reshapes New World Order: Political Economy Perspective*. Singapore: Springer.

Sheng, Shing-yuan, and Hsiao-chuan Liao. 2017. "Issues, Political Cleavages, and Party Competition in Taiwan." In *The Taiwan Voter*, edited by Christopher H. Achen and T. Y. Wang. Ann Arbor: University of Michigan Press.

Yam, Kai Chi, Joshua Conrad Jackson, Christopher M. Barnes, Jenson Lau, Xin Qin, and Hin Yeung Lee. 2020. "The Rise of COVID-19 Cases Is Associated with Support for World Leaders." *PNAS* 117 (41): 25429–33. https://doi.org/10.1073/pnas.2009252117.

4

Partisan Cues and Vaccine Hesitancy

Dennis Lu-Chung Weng, Chia-hung Tsai, and Yi-Ning Katherine Chen

INTRODUCTION

By the end of the first week of May 2021, with more than 157 million COVID-19 cases confirmed and almost 3.4 million COVID-19 confirmed deaths worldwide,[1] Taiwan seemed the heaven of peace and happiness outside of the world. With slightly over one thousand confirmed cases and twelve COVID-19 confirmed deaths, Taiwan enjoyed the normal way of living cautiously amid the global pandemic for over a year and a half. While the world sees the start of the clinical trial for COVID-19 vaccines as a beacon of hope for normal life to return, most people in Taiwan do not have to worry too much about the COVID-19 and therefore do not urgently see vaccination necessary. In fact, before the unprecedented "lockdown" in place to curb the pandemic spread in May 2021, many people in Taiwan were skeptical about the effect of the AstraZeneca (AZ) vaccine delivered from Japan in March and refused to be vaccinated. However, the COVID-19 virus swept through the island in mid-May, powered by the contagious alpha variant. It brought the daily confirmed cases from single digits to over hundreds of cases. The change forced the islanders to reconsider their attitude toward vaccination, but the hesitation about taking particular brands of vaccine became another issue in Taiwan as the shortage of vaccine supply further politicalized the hesitancy.

Unlike the vaccine hesitancy in other Asian democracies, such as Japan and Korea, where vaccine hesitancy is mainly due to the concern about the side effects, vaccination in Taiwan, and several other countries, is not simply a medical issue but a political one. Undoubtedly, the approval of the COVID-19 vaccines, such as AZ, Pfizer-BioNTech (BNT), Moderna, etc., sent waves of excitement and relief across the world. However, receiving a vaccine for COVID-19 is not as welcome as expected. Politicians politicalize vaccination for different purposes. For instance, President Trump in the United States and Prime Minister Boris Johnson of the United Kingdom hesitated to get vaccinated as they both did not view COVID-19 seriously until they got infected. Their hesitation drove supporters to refuse the vaccines as they believed that vaccination was just the opposition party's strategy against their leaders. On the other hand, politicians in countries that lack vaccines either accuse the government of not purchasing more vaccines in advance or blame the opposition party for exaggerating the vaccine's side effects to smear the incumbent government.

While politicalizing vaccination is believed to hinder the vaccine injection rate in Taiwan, there are very few studies on the effect of individuals' political preference on vaccine hesitancy. Also, not many studies aim to delineate the relationship between anxiety and COVID-19 in Taiwan, as the confirmed cases did not cause severe concerns in Taiwan before the outbreak. Previous studies demonstrated that vaccine hesitancy results from a complex decision-making process influenced by contextual, individual and group, and vaccine-specific factors (MacDonald et al. 2015). As various factors may impact the vaccine hesitancy in Taiwan, in this study, we contend that social media usage, social network, socioeconomic status, partisanship, and confidence in the government would be the potential determinants. Unlike previous studies that focus on countries with a large amount of COVID-19 confirmed cases, the current research aims to examine the factors that cause the vaccine hesitancy in Taiwan by collecting data after the first large outbreak in mid-May 2021. Ironically, this research may not be possible if Taiwan had never experienced the outbreak, which led to the natural fear of COVID-19.

As mentioned earlier, scholars worldwide have conducted ample research on vaccine acceptance and confidence in many countries; however, there is still an apparent lack of research attempting to explore the relationship between vaccine hesitancy and various indicators in Taiwan.

Specifically, this paper investigates why people in Taiwan are anxious about COVID-19 when there are only limited cases and why the islanders are reluctant to get the vaccine for COVID-19 when the cases soared. Also, we would like to see if individuals view the global pandemic through their partisan lens. This study on vaccine hesitancy in Taiwan primarily analyzes the various factors that may cause people to refuse the necessary vaccines. Our investigation is expected to provide a different perspective to understanding the attitude toward COVID-19 in Taiwan and the effect of politics on vaccination.

The remainder of this study is structured as follows. In section 2, we discuss the idea of vaccine hesitancy and the current literature on the relationship between vaccine hesitancy for COVID-19 and various driving factors. Section 3 details how we collect our data and conduct our research. In section 4, we present our empirical findings and interpret the influence of partisan support on vaccine injection. Finally, in section 5, we discuss the implications of our preliminary results and what steps can be taken to the next level on this topic.

VACCINE HESITANCY

Vaccine hesitancy is not a new phenomenon. As one can imagine, it is easy to allow people to choose a preferred vaccine if the vaccine is safe and the supply is not an issue. While COVID-19 is a new global pandemic and the vaccine was not available for the first year, previous epidemic experiences provide helpful information to us. For instance, the U.S. Centers for Disease Control and Prevention (CDC) reports that about half Americans did not get flu shots in 2020.[2] Many think getting a flu shot or not is a personal decision and there is no big deal. People view flu just like smallpox, yellow fever, and all the other previous epidemics that used to cause millions of deaths and illnesses in many parts of the world that are now no longer worrisome, largely thanks to vaccination. While vaccination for most existing epidemics is now viewed as a personal preference, having the same attitude toward the vaccination for the new COVID-19 global pandemic may be problematic.

Since the first case of COVID-19 was reported in Wuhan, China, at the end of 2019, the disease spread rapidly throughout China, after which it soon evolved into a global public health crisis. By the end of November 2021, the total number of confirmed cases globally exceeded 252 million, and the cumulative number of deaths was over 5 million, with a mortality rate of approximately 2 percent.[3] The rapid spread of COVID-19 has brought unprecedented challenges to the world in various aspects. To deal with the challenge, the world again finds vaccination is the most effective way to counter the global pandemic. While the Seventy-Third World Health Assembly (WHA) issued a resolution recognizing the vaccine is the solution,[4] various reasons drive the hesitation of getting the COVID-19 vaccine amid the global pandemic across countries. Also, from the WHO's exports, vaccine hesitancy is commonly defined as "a delay in acceptance or refusal of vaccination despite the availability of vaccination services."[5] It is not uncommon to see people are skeptical about any newly developed vaccines in the previous epidemics. Many countries have a long history of vaccine hesitancy due to the fear of getting unnecessary side effects—the potential side effects of the COVID vaccine concern the elderly. The reported cases about different side effects globally via news outlets and social media drove the high hesitancy despite the COVID infection number showing exponential growth in many countries.

While the stagnation in vaccine uptake was partially associated with vaccine hesitancy, it is also true that there was a real shortage of available vaccines. Ironically, it led to a scarcity mentality prevailing, especially among the elderly with less preexisting attitudes toward vaccination. Senior citizens saw how older people in other countries were dying, thus scrambling to get vaccinated before supplies ran low. When the elderly in some countries changed their minds due to the escalated fear, others decided not to be inoculated because vaccination was a political position. Specifically in Asian countries, like Japan and Korea, the fear of not getting vaccinated gradually exceeded the concern about side effects and drove the extremely high uptake rate among the elderly. Due to the vaccine availability, the sluggish vaccination rate also meant younger people had to wait and watch as hundreds of millions of people in other countries got shots without dramatic side effects. That reassured them the vaccines were safe and willing to get vaccine ramp-up.[6]

As most of these studies on COVID-19 vaccine hesitancy were conducted before October 2020, when the vaccine was still far away, we recognized that the discussion about hesitancy was based on hypothetical questions because the vaccines were not yet available. People may respond differently once the pandemic situation improves and the effective medical solutions are available. However, the current literature certainly helps us understand and provides suggestions to ensure future action to achieve vaccine coverage and allow herd immunity to be attained. Taiwan had a lower vaccine coverage than the world average for several vaccines when it faced the first outbreak in May 2021. Vaccination coverage is highly influenced by its acceptability and the overall perception of its benefit/safety profile. Vaccine hesitancy is a barrier to achieving high vaccination coverage against infectious diseases. Therefore, understanding its determinants is necessary to aid acceptability, tackle vaccine hesitancy, and achieve high coverage for this new vaccine. Hence, this study aims to assess and identify factors associated with COVID-19 vaccine hesitancy in Taiwan.

KEY TO VACCINE INJECTION: SOCIAL MEDIA AND PARTISAN CUE

As various vaccines launched their clinical trials in different countries in March 2020,[7] scholars also began to explore COVID-19 vaccine acceptance and their determinants. By conducting surveys in countries across continents, the preliminary findings implied that vaccination is again viewed as the most effective means to control the new global pandemic and indicated several influential factors associated with vaccine hesitancy (Harapan et al. 2020). A systematic review of how people view vaccines for COVID-19 showed that social demographic variables, such as age, income, and education levels, were correlated with the willingness to accept vaccines. Several of these studies indicated that older individuals and those with higher income and education levels were more likely to get a vaccine (Fisher et al. 2020; Reiter, Pennell, and Katz 2020; Head 2020; Mercadante and Law 2020; Khuchandani et al. 2021; Lin et al. 2020). Other factors associated with the intention of vaccination included higher trust in government decisions (Lazarus et al. 2020), having been vaccinated against the flu in the previous year (Reiter, Pennell, and Katz 2020; Mercadante and Law 2020), and knowing people who were COVID-19 infected (Reiter, Pennell, and Katz 2020; Mercadante and Law 2020). Although preliminary, the existing evidence suggests that some factors influence vaccination opinions and drive downstream vaccine hesitancy.

In addition to the factors mentioned earlier, the internet era makes the vaccine-related information perceived by individuals challenging to control. Previous research has demonstrated that the spread of fake news and misinformation on social media is considered the primary cause of vaccine hesitancy. During the COVID-19 pandemic, the WHO also warned that misinformation about vaccines has become one of the major threats to global health. This study would like to know whether persons who hesitated to take vaccines provided by the government selectively used social media to receive COVID-19-related information. According to the existing research, individuals with certain predispositions are prone to accept conspiracies (Bruder et al. 2013; Moscovici 1987), including those associated with the coronavirus pandemic (Uscinski et al. 2020). Furthermore, Uscinski et al. show that conspiracy theories are more likely to affect beliefs when the recipient is predisposed to conspiracy thinking (Uscinski et al. 2016). Enders et al. (2021) proposed a similar hypothesis that instead of social media causally promoting conspiracy beliefs, the association is conditional on the preexisting conspiracy belief of its users. In short, scholarly work implies that conspiratorial thinking encourages selective exposure to like-minded media whose content reinforces and facilitates the incorporation of conspiracy beliefs that reduce support for pandemic-preventive behavior. Selective exposure to information is well documented (Bakshy et al. 2015; Hart et al. 2009). In particular, partisan content attracts audiences with similar political preferences and, in the process, not only reinforces partisan differences but also insulates an audience from divergent information and opinions (Mitchell et al. 2014; Stroud 2011). However, others suggest that the extent of partisan selective exposure has been exaggerated (Eady et al. 2019). This argument provides an alternative suggestion that, because most people in democracies are exposed to various mainstream news sources, they should be able to receive different viewpoints (Allen et al. 2020; Guess 2021) and, as a result, may be buffered from distortive misinformation or conspiracy theorizing in partisan channels.

While exposure to mainstream media and alternative viewpoints may be widespread, conspiracy beliefs linked to the partisan position are a particularly troublesome form of misinformation during the pandemic. It is not only challenging to disconfirm but also to assert that sources of information that could undermine them are implicated in the conspiracy. That is to say, the information from experts (Sunstein and Vermeule 2009; Uscinski et al. 2016) is not to be trusted, except when the experts are affiliated with recipients' preferred party. In the United States, for instance, conservative media were especially likely to support conspiratorial claims made by President Trump regarding the pandemic (Evanega et al. n.d.; Summers 2020). President Trump suggested that efforts to provide accurate information about cures and prevention contradicted his opinions and were politically motivated (Associated Press 2020). The purpose of sharing information provided by the Democrats to "correct" his statements is to undermine his presidency for political gains (Herper and Florko 2020). Trump made two claims: China created the virus as a bioweapon. Another is that some government officials within the CDC exaggerated the severity of COVID-19 to undermine his presidency. Because Donald Trump made these claims, even if users of conservative media were not prone to conspiratorial thinking, they were likely to be influenced by these claims because they were offered by a leader with whom these individuals identified (Romer and Jamieson 2020, 2021).

Furthermore, previous research also confirmed that users' baseline personal values and biases before their exposure to social media content, and political beliefs in particular, may modulate their response to such posts (Jaones et al. 2012). This study assessed how information is conveyed, perceived, and altered between links and found that participants would vastly adjust messages to align with their baseline attitude. In addition, messages were perceived to be more convincing if they aligned with the individual's attitudes. Accordingly, one can imagine in a highly politically polarized society, a political party would play such an essential role in interpreting the necessity of vaccines to their followers. The previously mentioned situation illustrated that partisan bias would direct the individual to receive a specific perspective, where accuracy is not guaranteed or even not important. People can believe that only those with solid partisan identification would be influenced by misinformation. However, scholars demonstrated that the effect of media exposure on vaccine hesitancy is more crucial than previously expected. In comparing individuals' perceptions of vaccine risks among those exposed to control websites versus vaccine-critical websites, Betsch et al. found that even brief exposure—as little as five to ten minutes—to vaccine-critical websites increased the overall perception of vaccine risk in comparison to exposure to control websites (Betsch et al. 2010). Similarly, Ahmed et al. demonstrated that Twitter and Facebook as sources of health information and influenza knowledge have a significant inverse association with influenza vaccine uptake (Ahmed et al. 2018). Bhattacharyya et al. generated a social network simulation model in which the introduction of a perceived small vaccine adverse event had a pronounced impact on vaccine uptake (Bhattacharyya et al. 2019). The latest researches shows that individuals who received information from traditional media were more likely to accept the vaccine than social media users (Piltch-Loeb et al. 2021). In Taiwan, the relationship between social media and individuals' attitudes toward the pandemic and vaccines is particularly worth studying as most people use social media to get daily news. As social media in Taiwan is considered the primary source of daily information, one can imagine the risks may be overestimated and may seem more immediate and tangible than the more abstract potential benefits of disease prevention.

Based on the previous discussion, this study argues that social media and political preference, along with other conventional indicators, such as age, social status, gender, and education level, may influence vaccine decisions during the global pandemic in Taiwan. Given the discussion, we would like to examine whether vaccine hesitancy is determined by certain factors, political preference, and social media, in particular. Also, we want to know if the level of anxiety is associated with social media consumption and political preference. Several propositions derived from the previous discussion in this section are empirically tested. Specifically, we propose the following hypotheses regarding anxiety about the pandemic:

Hypothesis 1-1: Anxiety about the pandemic is positively associated with the trust in the government, the CDC director in particular. People with a higher level of confidence in the health minister are less anxious about the pandemic.

Hypothesis 1-2: Anxiety about the pandemic is positively associated with social media usage. People who receive more information from social media are more likely to get anxious.

If these two hypotheses hold up, we can confirm that social media and political trust are related to people's psychological status. To make sure that these relationships are not spurious, we not only control for gender, age, and education but also include an emotion indicator: peer pressure. If people feel isolated or marginalized from their friends during the pandemic, we assume that they tend to have anxiety about the pandemic.

Next, we want to test the following hypotheses about vaccine acceptance.

Hypothesis 2-1: Taiwan's vaccine acceptance of the COVID-19 vaccine is positively associated with incumbent party support. People with more positive evaluations of the incumbent party, DPP, are more likely to accept the vaccine.

Hypothesis 2-2: Taiwan's vaccine acceptance for the COVID-19 vaccine is positively associated with the fear of COVID-19. People with higher anxiety about COVID-19 are more likely to accept the vaccine.

In addition, we contend that several conventional factors, such as gender, education level, age, and partisanship, would present a similar impact on vaccine acceptance and the level of anxiety in Taiwan. This study will discuss the data and our preliminary results in the following sections.

DATA AND MEASUREMENT

Our data comes from two internet surveys. Chen (2020) conducted an internet survey between May 5 and 8, 2020. Respondents are drawn from the databank maintained by the Election Study Center, which asked respondents if they could leave their email addresses for future internet surveys during various telephone surveys. The central theme of this study is media consumption during the pandemic, and the number of completions is 803. We merge this dataset with that from the Association of Election Study Center Alumni (2021), which has 3,193 cases. In doing so, we can track 803 respondents that participated in both surveys.

The first dependent variable is anxiety about the pandemic. It is a four-point scale. The mean of this variable is 2.394, which implies the modest level of anxiety. The second dependent variable is demand for vaccine. In the second wave of our polls, we asked respondents where their demand for vaccine is located on a 0–10 scale. We treat both variables as continuous variables, so we are able to regress them on a battery of variables. The average demand for vaccine is 7.446, which indicates that respondents expressed a high level of request for vaccine. We construct the "peer pressure" indicator to capture people's feeling of their friends regarding the pandemic. It is supposed to trigger anxiety of the pandemic. In addition, people's attention to vaccine information was included in the model. According to hypothesis 2, attention to social media is associated with demand for the vaccine. For wording, operation, and descriptive statistics of each variable, please refer to table 4.1.

Table 4.1. Descriptive Statistics of Variables

Variables	*Wording*	*Descriptive Statistics*
Demand for Vaccine	On a 0–10 scale, where is your demand for vaccine located?	Mean=7.446, S.D.=2.579, Min.=0, Max.=10
Anxiety about Pandemic	For the past two weeks, do you feel anxious about the rising pandemic?	Mean=2.394, S.D.=0.795, Min.=1, Max.=4
Attention to Vaccine Information on	Do you pay attention to information regarding COVID-19 on:	
Facebook	Facebook	Mean=3.548, S.D.=1.153, Min.=1, Max.=5
LINE	LINE	Mean=3.447, S.D.=1.177, Min.=1, Max.=5
TV	TV	Mean=3.990, S.D.=0.953, Min.=1, Max.=5
News Website	News Website	Mean=3.631, S.D.=1.030, Min.=1, Max.=5
Internet	Internet	Mean=3.188, S.D.=1.1371.153, Min.=1, Max.=5

Peer group	*Factor score**	*Mean=0, S.D.=0.944, Min.= −1.578, Max.=3.481*
Approval on Health Minister	On a 0–10 scale, how are you satisfied with Minister Chen?	Mean=8.609, S.D.=1.846, Min.=0, Max.=10
Pan-blue	Identifiers of KMT, New Party, and People's First Party	Mean=8.609, S.D.=1.846, Min.=0, Max.=10
Pan-green	Identifiers of DPP, Taiwan State-Building Party, and New Power Party	Mean=27.646, S.D.=34.859, Min.=0, Max.=1
Taiwan People's Party	Identifiers of Taiwan People's Party	Mean=27.665, S.D.=34.845, Min.=0, Max.=1
Female		Mean=0.413, S.D.=0.493, Min.=0, Max.=1
36–50 years old		Mean=0.491, S.D.=0.498, Min.=0, Max.=1
51–65 years old		Mean=0.274, S.D.=0.446, Min.=0, Max.=1
66 years old and above		Mean=0.059, S.D.=0.235, Min.=0, Max.=1
College		Mean=0.778, S.D.=0.416, Min.=0, Max.=1

Factor score: We asked respondents if they agree or disagree with the following five statement: I feel anxious when my friends own more information about the pandemic; I feel anxious when my friends do not ask me to join their conversation about the pandemic; I feel anxious when my friends share some news about the pandemic; it is important to me to understand my friends' subject of talk; it is important to me to share my experience on Facebook regarding the COVID-19 pandemic. We use principal factor analysis to compute the factor score.

Data: Chen 2020; Association of Election Study Center Alumni 2021.

EMPIRICAL RESULTS

Table 4.2 shows the OLS estimates of the anxiety model. Peer pressure is positively related to anxiety. When people feel left out in the discussion of the pandemic, they may get anxious about the situation. Media consumption of news on the internet is also associated with anxiety. News on the internet often exaggerates this public health crisis, which may boost people's anxiety. On the contrary, satisfaction with the health minister is negatively related to anxiety. The higher one's satisfaction with the handling of the pandemic, the lower the level of anxiety is. Pan-blue identifiers were more

Table 4.2. OLS Model of Anxiety about the Pandemic (1–4 point)

	Coef.	*Std. Error*
Attention to Vaccine Information on		
Facebook	–0.007	0.033
LINE	0.005	0.032
TV	0.042	0.039
News Website	0.067$	0.038
Internet	0.093**	0.034
Peer group	0.094*	0.036
Approval on health minister	–0.077***	0.019
Pan-blue	0.421***	0.088
Pan-green	–0.056	0.245
Taiwan People's Party	–0.367	0.252
Female	0.090	0.067
36–50 years old	–0.019	0.090
51–65 years old	–0.043	0.105
66 years old and above	–0.084	0.157
College	0.047	0.084
Constant	2.516**	0.232
N	540	
R^2	0.137	
Adjusted R^2	0.112	
F statistics	5.548** (df = 15; 524)	

Note: $ *p*<0.1, * *p*<0.05, ** *p*<0.01, *** *p*<0.001

Data: Chen 2020; Association of Election Study Center Alumni 2021.

anxious about the pandemic than other respondents, which implies that partisan bias plays an important role in times of crisis.

Table 4.3 shows the OLS estimates of the acceptance of the vaccine. The level of anxiety is positively related to the demand for the vaccine. If people are anxious about the pandemic, they are eager for vaccine injections. Note that anxiety about the pandemic is associated with peer pressure, attention to news on the internet, and most importantly, satisfaction with the health minister. In this model, satisfaction with the health minister remains a significant predictor in the vaccine hesitancy model. The higher one's satisfaction with the head of the Ministry of Health and Welfare, the greater the demand for the COVID-19 vaccine is.

Table 4.3. OLS Model of Demand for the Vaccine (0–10 point)

	Coef.	*Std. Error*
Anxiety about Pandemic	0.804***	0.143
Attention to Vaccine Information on		
Facebook	0.130	0.111
LINE	–0.059	0.107
TV	–0.160	0.128
News Website	0.002	0.127
Internet	0.221$	0.112
Peer group	–0.124	0.121
Approval on health minister	0.147	0.065
Pan-blue	–0.130	0.295
Pan-green	1.511$	0.806
Taiwan People's Party	–1.384$	0.830
Female	–0.566*	0.221
36–50 years old	–0.512$	0.295
51–65 years old	–0.054	0.347
66 years old and above	0.570	0.517
College	0.263	0.276
Constant	3.800***	0.845
N	540	
R^2	0.117	
Adjusted R^2	0.090	
F statistics	4.349**	
	(df = 16; 523)	

Note: $ $p<0.1$, * $p<0.05$, ** $p<0.01$, *** $p<0.001$

Data: Chen 2020; Association of Election Study Center Alumni 2021.

CONCLUSION

After waiting for almost an entire year, the world finally found the effective means to handle the global COVID-19 pandemic at the end of 2020. While widespread vaccination is considered the inevitable solution for stopping the virus and returning to normal, vaccine hesitancy in many countries presents a persistent challenge. It hinders the vaccination level from getting higher. Unlike many other advanced countries where the vaccine is generally accessible and vaccine hesitancy is derived from the concern about side effects, the psychological mechanisms associated with vaccine hesitancy are not the same in Taiwan. Before the island's first COVID-19 outbreak in May 2020, the vaccine shortage in Taiwan did not generate a high level of anxiety but politicalizing the vaccination. From the debate about whether the vaccines from China are reliable to the concern that the AZ vaccine delivered from Japan is not safe, political parties took sides on each controverting. Therefore, it is worth discussing if vaccine hesitancy in Taiwan is correlated with partisanship instead of health concern. According to previous research and the disputes in Taiwan, we hypothesized that partisanship, social media usage, anxiety, and trust in government are four routes that can interactively affect vaccine hesitancy.

Our hypotheses were generally supported in the findings. Respondents' low trust in the government official, particularly the Minister of Health and Welfare Chen Shih Chung, was more concerned about the pandemic. However, they were low in demand for the vaccine provided by the government. Specifically speaking, with the low trust level among people who do not support the incumbent party, the anxiety does not help with the vaccine hesitancy in Taiwan. Similarly, while respondents with a higher stress level and receiving more information via the internet were more likely to accept vaccines, their partisanship drove them in the opposite direction. Many people in Taiwan indeed got the vaccine because they were highly concerned about the consequences of the pandemic (for themselves and others). Others were reluctant to do so because they did not trust the incumbent party and the sources from which the government received the vaccines. As can be seen in our research, those who, for whatever reasons, do not trust the ruling party about the virus are much likelier to be hesitant about vaccination, even if they are also very concerned. Vaccine hesitancy was higher among females and younger respondents. Also, social media users highly influenced higher levels of vaccine hesitancy among respondents who use the internet as their primary news source. Our findings imply that the psychological variable, partisanship, explained that the anxiety level is not purely about the perception of public health concerns but also the attitude toward the political figure in charge. Unlike conventional indicators, we contend that anxiety and vaccine hesitancy are subject to external influence and could be manipulated by politicians aiming to tackle other parties.

The strengths of the present research include the two waves of online survey data from Taiwan; the ability to examine political, psychological, social media, and demographic factors; and the timely collection right after the first outbreak. The survey data enabled us to properly distinguish demographic and psychological factors in vaccine hesitancy. This critical point allows enhances our confidence that the results are generalizable across different countries in the future, especially those within Asia. Levels of anxiety and trust in politics do differ by country. For example, Americans may not feel too concerned about the pandemic anymore as the variety of vaccines is easily accessible. In contrast, people in countries where the vaccine is still not available to everyone, the levels of anxiety may differ.

While we do not know if the effect of anxiety and partisanship on vaccine hesitancy is generalizable to other national contexts, nothing in the current literature suggests that traditional demographic differences would conclude the question. With the political behavior and communication literature, we are confident that our findings in Taiwan have a much wider generality. Nonetheless, further work would help to establish this conclusion more firmly. Furthermore, this research has clear implications for policy and vaccination campaigns globally. Higher political trust and concern about the pandemic are two factors that can independently motivate positive vaccination intentions, whereas the lack of both is associated with substantially greater hesitancy.

There are at least two ways to address vaccine hesitancy in Taiwan. A low level of anxiety could become a problem if everyone believes that the pandemic is nothing to worry about. Yet the government and the politicians need to be very careful about rising anxiety levels as the higher level of anxiety may invoke unnecessary worries. A balanced perception of a pandemic can be challenging to share information. Still, it is the way for Taiwan and other democracies to get out of the politicized vaccination dispute. The alternative option is to increase political trust, but this may not last long as the political trust is highly volatile. The political trust typically increases when the society experiences a common concern or crisis. But politicians may lose trust when the government action fails to meet citizens' expectations. By providing clear guides and maintaining transparent communication, politicians could be perceived as competent and trustworthy; therefore, society may be willing to comply with rules and regulations in the future. The level of vaccine hesitancy would be slashed, if not reduced to zero.

NOTES

1. https://ourworldindata.org/coronavirus-data.
2. https://www.cdc.gov/flu/fluvaxview/nifs-estimates-sept2020.htm.
3. https://www.who.int/emergencies/diseases/novel-coronavirus-2019/situation-reports.
4. WHO COVID-19 response: "The role of extensive immunization against COVID-19 as a global public good for health in preventing, containing and stopping transmission in order to bring the pandemic to an end, once safe, quality, efficacious, effective, accessible and affordable vaccines are available." Agenda item 3, WHA73, Seventy-Third World Health Assembly, May 19, 2020, accessed January 25, 2021, https://apps.who.int/gb/ebwha/pdf_files/WHA73/A73_R1-en.pdf.
5. MacDonald et al. 2015.
6. https://www.nytimes.com/2021/09/30/business/economy/asia-covid-vaccinations.html.
7. https://www.nih.gov/news-events/news-releases/nih-clinical-trial-investigational-vaccine-covid-19-begins.

REFERENCES

Ahmed, N., S. C. Quinn, G. R. Hancock, V. S. Freimuth, and A. Jamison. 2018. "Social Media Use and Influenza Vaccine Uptake among White and African American Adults." *Vaccine* 36 (49): 7556–61.

Allen, J., Howland, B., Mobius, M., Rothschild, D., & Watts, D. J. (2020). "Evaluating the Fake News Problem at the Scale of the Information Ecosystem." *Science advances* 6(14), eaay3539.

Associated Press. (2020). AP Fact Check: Trump Trashing Virus Science He Doesn't Like. WTTW Radio.

Association of Election Study Center Alumni. 2021. Internet Survey on COVID-19. May 20–25.

Bakshy, E., Messing, S., & Adamic, L. A. (2015). "Exposure to ideologically diverse news and opinion on Facebook." *Science* 348(6239), 1130–1132.

Betsch, C., N. T. Brewer, P. Brocard, P. Davies, W. Gaissmaier, N. Haase, J. Leask, F. Renkewitz, B. Renner, V. F. Reyna, and C. Rossmann. 2012. "Opportunities and Challenges of Web 2.0 for Vaccination Decisions." *Vaccine* 30 (25): 3727–33.

Betsch, C., F. Renkewitz, T. Betsch, and C. Ulshöfer. 2010. "The Influence of Vaccine-Critical Websites on Perceiving Vaccination Risks." *Journal of Health and Psycholology* 15 (3): 446–55. doi:10.1177/1359105309353647.

Bhattacharyya, S., A. Vutha, and C. T. Bauch. 2019. "The Impact of Rare but Severe Vaccine Adverse Events on Behaviour-Disease Dynamics: A Network Model." *Scientific Reports* 9 (1): 1–13.

Biasio, L. R., G. Bonaccorsi, C. Lorini, and S. Pecorelli. 2020. "Assessing COVID-19 Vaccine Literacy: A Preliminary Online Survey." *Hum. Vaccines Immunother*, 1–9.

Bruder, M., Haffke, P., Neave, N., Nouripanah, N., & Imhoff, R. (2013). "Measuring individual differences in generic beliefs in conspiracy theories across cultures: Conspiracy Mentality Questionnaire." *Frontiers in Psychology* 4, 225.

Buller, D. B., B. J. Walkosz, J. Berteletti, S. L. Pagoto, J. Bibeau, K. Baker, J. Hillhouse, and K. L. Henry. 2019. "Insights on HPV Vaccination in the United States from Mothers' Comments on Facebook Posts in a Randomized Trial." *Human Vaccines & Immunotherapeutics* 15 (7–8): 1479–87.

Chen, K. 2020. Study on COVID-19. May 5–8.

Eady, G., Nagler, J., Guess, A., Zilinsky, J., & Tucker, J. A. (2019). "How Many People Live in Political Bubbles on Social Media? Evidence from Linked Survey and Twitter Data." *Sage Open* 9(1), 2158244019832705.

Enders, A. M., J. E. Uscinski, M. I. Seelig, C. A. Klofstad, S. Wuchty, J. R. Funchion, M. N. Murthi, K. Premaratne, and J. Stoler. 2021. "The Relationship between Social Media Use and Beliefs in Conspiracy Theories and Misinformation." *Political Behavior*, 1–24.

Evanega, S., Lynas, M., Adams, J., Smolenyak, K., & Insights, C. G. (2020). "Coronavirus Misinformation: Quantifying Sources and Themes in the COVID-19 'Infodemic.'" *JMIR Preprints* 19(10), 2020.

Fisher, K. A., S. J. Bloomstone, J. Walder, S. Crawford, H. Fouayzi, and K. M. Mazor. 2020. "Attitudes Toward a Potential SARS-CoV-2 Vaccine: A Survey of U.S. Adults." *Ann. Intern. Med.* 173: 964–73.

Giese, H., H. Neth, M. Moussaïd, C. Betsch, and W. Gaissmaier. 2020. "The Echo in Flu-Vaccination Echo Chambers: Selective Attention Trumps Social Influence." *Vaccine* 38 (8): 2070–76.

Guess, A. M. (2021). (Almost) "Everything in Moderation: New Evidence on Americans' Online Media Diets." *American Journal of Political Science* 65(4), 1007–22.

Harapan, H., A. L. Wagner, A. Yufika, W. Winardi, S. Anwar, A. K. Gan, A. M. Setiawan, Y. Rajamoorthy, H. Sofyan, and M. Mudatsir. 2020. "Acceptance of a COVID-19 Vaccine in Southeast Asia: A Cross-Sectional Study in Indonesia." *Frontiers in Public Health*, 8.

Hart, W., Albarracín, D., Eagly, A. H., Brechan, I., Lindberg, M. J., & Merrill, L. (2009). "Feeling Validated Versus Being Correct: A Meta-analysis of Selective Exposure to Information." *Psychological Bulletin* 135(4), 555.

Head, K. J., M. L. Kasting, L. A. Sturm, J. A. Hartsock, and G. D. Zimet. 2020. "A National Survey Assessing SARS-CoV-2 Vaccination Intentions: Implications for Future Public Health Communication Efforts." *Sci. Commun.* 42: 698–723.

Herper, M., & Florko, N. (2020). Drug Makers Rebut Trump Tweet that FDA 'Deep State' is Delaying Covid-19 Vaccines and Drugs. STAT.

Jones, A. M., S. B. Omer, R. A. Bednarczyk, N. A. Halsey, L. H. Moulton, and D. A. Salmon. 2012. "Parents' Source of Vaccine Information and Impact on Vaccine Attitudes, Beliefs, and Nonmedical Exemptions." *Advances in Preventive Medicine.*

Jones, P. E., Hoffman, L. H., & Young, D. G. (2013). "Online Emotional Appeals and Political Participation: The Effect of Candidate Affect on Mass Behavior." *New Media & Society* 15(7), 1132–1150.

Khubchandani, J., S. Sharma, J. H. Price, M. J. Wiblishauser, M. Sharma, and F. J. Webb. 2021. "COVID-19 Vaccination Hesitancy in the United States: A Rapid National Assessment." *J. Community Health.*

Kortum, P., C. Edwards, and R. Richards-Kortum. 2008. "The Impact of Inaccurate Internet Health Information in a Secondary School Learning Environment." *Journal of Medical Internet Research* 10 (2): e986.

Lazarus, J. V., S. C. Ratzan, A. Palayew, L. O. Gostin, H. J. Larson, K. Rabin, S. Kimball, and A. El-Mohandes. 2020. "A Global Survey of Potential Acceptance of a COVID-19 Vaccine." *Nat. Med.*

Lin, Y., Z. Hu, Q. Zhao, H. Alias, M. Danaee, and L. P. Wong. 2020. "Understanding COVID-19 Vaccine Demand and Hesitancy: A Nationwide Online Survey in China." *PLoS Negl. Trop. Dis.* 14: e0008961.

Lin, C., P. Tu, and L. M. Beitsch. 2021. "Confidence and Receptivity for COVID-19 Vaccines: A Rapid Systematic Review." *Vaccines* 9: 1–41.

MacDonald, N. E., J. Eskola, X. Liang, M. Chaudhuri, E. Dube, and B. Gellin. 2015. "Vaccine Hesitancy: Definition, Scope and Determinants." *Vaccine* 33, 4161–64.

Mercadante, A. R., and A. V. Law. 2020. "Will They, or Won't They? Examining Patients' Vaccine Intention for Flu and COVID-19 Using the Health Belief Model." *Res. Soc. Adm. Pharm.*

Mitchell, A., Gottfried, J., Kiley, J., & Matsa, K. E. (2014). Political polarization & media habits. Pew Research Center.

Moscovici, S. (1987). The conspiracy mentality. In C. F. Graumann & S. Moscovici (Eds.) *Changing Conceptions of Conspiracy* (pp. 151–169). New York, NY: Springer. doi:10.1007/978-1-4612-4618-3_9

Murphy, J., F. Vallières, R. P. Bentall, M. Shevlin, O. Mcbride, T. K. Hartman, R. McKay, K. Bennett, L. Mason, J. Gibson-Miller, et al. 2021. "Psychological

Characteristics Associated with COVID-19 Vaccine Hesitancy and Resistance in Ireland and the United Kingdom." *Nat. Commun.* 12: 1–15.

Neumann-Böhme, S., N. E. Varghese, I. Sabat, P. P. Barros, W. Brouwer, and J. van Exel. 2020. "Once We Have It, Will We Use It? A European Survey on Willingness to Be Vaccinated against COVID-19." *Eur. J. Heal Econ.* 21: 977–82.

Nan, X., and K. Madden. 2012. "HPV Vaccine Information in the Blogosphere: How Positive and Negative Blogs Influence Vaccine-Related Risk Perceptions, Attitudes, and Behavioral Intentions." *Health Communication* 27 (8): 829–36.

Piltch-Loeb, R., E. Savoia, B. Goldberg, B. Hughes, T. Verhey, et al. 2021. "Examining the Effect of Information Channel on COVID-19 Vaccine Acceptance." *PLOS ONE* 16 (5): e0251095. https://doi.org/10.1371/journal.pone.0251095.

Sallam, M., D. Dababseh, H. Eid, K. Al-mahzoum, A. Al-haidar, and D. Taim. "High Rates of COVID-19 Vaccine Hesitancy and Its Association with Conspiracy Beliefs: A Study in Jordan and Kuwait among Other Arab Countries." *Vaccines* 19: 1–16.

Reiter, P. L., M. L. Pennell, and M. L. Katz. 2020. "Acceptability of a COVID-19 Vaccine among Adults in the United States: How Many People Would Get Vaccinated?" *Vaccine* 38: 6500–507.

Robichaud, P., S. Hawken, L. Beard, D. Morra, G. Tomlinson, K. Wilson, and J. Keelan. 2012. "Vaccine-Critical Videos on YouTube and Their Impact on Medical Students' Attitudes about Seasonal Influenza Immunization: A Pre and Post Study." *Vaccine* 30 (25): 3763–70.

Romer, D., & Jamieson, K. H. (2021). "Conspiratorial Thinking, Selective Exposure to Conservative Media, and Response to COVID-19 in the US." *Social Science & Medicine* 291, 114480.

Stroud, N. J. (2011). Niche news: The politics of news choice. Oxford University Press.

Summers, J. (2020). "Timeline: How Trump has Downplayed the Coronavirus Pandemic." *NPR News*, 2.

Sunstein, C. R., & Vermeule, A. (2009). "Conspiracy theories: Causes and Cures." *Journal of Political Philosophy* 17(2), 202–227.

Uscinski, J. E., Enders, A. M., Klofstad, C., Seelig, M., Funchion, J., Everett, C., ... & Murthi, M. (2020)." Why do people believe COVID-19 conspiracy theories?" *Harvard Kennedy School Misinformation Review* 1(3).

Uscinski, J. E., Klofstad, C., & Atkinson, M. D. (2016). "What drives conspiratorial beliefs? The role of informational cues and predispositions." *Political Research Quarterly* 69(1), 57–71.

Wang, J., R. Jing, X. Lai, H. Zhang, Y. Lyu, and M. D. Knoll. 2020. "Acceptance of Covid-19 Vaccination during the Covid-19 Pandemic in China." *Vaccines* 8: 482.

Williams, L., P. Flowers, J. Mcleod, D. Young, and L. Rollins. 2021. "The Catalyst Project Team. Social Patterning and Stability of Intention to Accept a COVID-19 Vaccine in Scotland: Will Those Most at Risk Accept a Vaccine?" *Vaccines* 9: 17.

Yoda, T., and H. Katsuyama. 2021. "Willingness to Receive COVID-19 Vaccination in Japan." *Vaccines* 9: 48.

5

Political Polarization and Attitudes toward Democracy

Ching-Hsing Wang

INTRODUCTION

Since the outbreak of Coronavirus Disease 2019 (COVID-19), it has been observed that countries' approaches to combating the spread of COVID-19 have varied, leading to debates over what factors influence the performance of countries in the fight against COVID-19. While some argue that countries led by women have fared better during the COVID-19 pandemic than those led by men, Windsor et al. find no supporting evidence to this proposition.[1] Furthermore, it has been debated whether democracy or authoritarianism is the best political system to fight against COVID-19 that has posed a serious threat to global public health. Given that leaders in democracies must take democratic principles into consideration to cope with a crisis, some question the ability of democracies to undertake timely measures to protect their citizens during the COVID-19 pandemic. By contrast, authoritarian governments may act faster and stronger and mobilize resources effectively to respond to a crisis without worrying about the public's dissatisfaction with their dramatic measures. Several studies have attempted to examine the relationships between political regimes and COVID-19 outcomes and there is mixed evidence with respect to performance of democracy in dealing with the COVID-19 pandemic.[2] However, instead of emphasizing the importance of the political regime, Fukuyama contends that state capacity, social trust, and leadership have played a pivotal role in successful pandemic responses.[3] Specifically, countries with high state capacity, trustful societies, and effective leaders are more likely to perform well in response to the COVID-19 pandemic. By contrast, countries with dysfunctional states, polarized societies, or poor leadership might suffer worse outcomes from COVID-19. According to Fukuyama,[4] regime type does not matter for the performance of a country to handle COVID-19.

Nonetheless, the COVID-19 pandemic might influence individual attitudes toward democracy. For instance, Bol et al. find that COVID-19 lockdowns could increase public satisfaction with democracy perhaps because people regard the government as making the effort to prioritize the health of vulnerable individuals over economic interests.[5] On the other hand, some studies have demonstrated that political polarization comes into play during the COVID-19 pandemic. For example, Jiang et al. show that political polarization plays a nonnegligible role in online conversations about COVID-19,[6] whereas Kerr et al. demonstrate that political polarization drive liberals and conservatives to have different patterns of health protective behaviors (for example, wearing face masks).[7] Given rising political polarization in Taiwan,[8] little scholarly effort has been made to understand the consequences of political polarization. As a result, this study aims to examine the relationship between political polarization and individual attitudes toward democracy in the fight against COVID-19, that is, whether political polarization would lead people to cast doubt on the democratic system in response to COVID-19. Overall, this study is expected to not only broaden our understanding of consequences of political polarization but also provide new insights into the role of political polarization during the COVID-19 pandemic.

The remainder of this paper is structured as follows. The second section would provide a theoretical framework for the relationship between political polarization and individual attitudes toward democracy to address COVID-19 and formulate the hypotheses for empirical analysis. The third section would describe the data, operationalization of variables, and statistical methods. The fourth section would report the empirical results for the effect of political polarization on individual support for democracy as the best political system to combat COVID-19. The last section would summarize the key findings of this study and discuss the implications of results.

THEORETICAL RELATIONSHIP BETWEEN POLITICAL POLARIZATION AND SUPPORT FOR DEMOCRACY IN RESPONSE TO COVID-19

It is observed that political polarization has grown in many democracies in the past decades. For instance, by using the data from the American National Election Studies and national exit polls, Abramowitz and Saunders provide evidence that since the 1970s, ideological polarization has increased dramatically among the mass public in the United States as well as among political elites.[9] While the majority of studies on political polarization have focused on the United States, political polarization is not a phenomenon specific to the United States and is tearing at the seams of democracies around the world, from Brazil and India to Poland and Turkey.[10] There is no exception for Taiwan that the two major political parties in Taiwan—the Democratic Progressive Party (DPP) and the Kuomintang (KMT)—have become increasingly polarized in bitter political conflict, especially in terms of the issues of national identity and cross-Strait relations.[11] Given rising political polarization around the world, a large number of studies have attempted to identify the factors leading to individual level of political polarization, such as social media use,[12] social trust, income inequality,[13] and so on.

On the other hand, tremendous effort has been made to look at the consequences of political polarization. On the whole, there are two distinct theoretical perspectives about the role of political polarization in politics. The first theoretical perspective contends that political polarization brings about adverse effects on individual political attitudes and behavior mainly because political polarization would affect how citizens perceive objective political and social facts, further leading them to produce political biases in the evaluation of various issues and have different behavioral patterns. For example, Stanig reveals that although political polarization does not influence economic evaluations of citizens of different ideological persuasions and partisan affiliations during economic downturns, economic evaluations are polarized along partisan and ideological lines during recoveries.[14] McCright et al. demonstrate that political polarization on environmental concern among elites would likely extend to the general public, which leads to significant partisan and ideological polarization on support for environmental spending since 1992 in the United States.[15] Similarly, several studies have indicated that political polarization exerts influence on individual attitudes and behavior toward various issues relevant to COVID-19. Bruine de Bruin et al. show that risk perceptions and preferences for risk mitigation vary by political inclinations in the United States.[16] That is, Democrats tend to perceive more risk associated with COVID-19 than Republicans, including for getting infected, being hospitalized, and dying if infected, as well as running out of money as a result of the COVID-19 pandemic. Moreover, Kerr et al. find that compared to conservatives, liberals are more likely to perceive higher risk, place less trust in politicians to deal with the COVID-19 pandemic, exhibit more trust in medical experts such as the WHO, and be more critical of the government response.[17] In addition, it is documented that news coverage is highly politicized during the COVID-19 pandemic, which then might have contributed to political polarization in individual attitudes toward COVID-19.[18] Because a public health crisis such as COVID-19 requires the government to act in an effective and efficient way to protect people's health and save their lives, political polarization could lead people in different political camps to make differentiated assessments of government responses during the COVID-19 pandemic. Specifically, people in the opposition camp tend to hold the government to a high standard during the COVID-19 pandemic and criticize the government for its COVID-19 policies. By contrast, people who support the incumbent government are inclined to regard criticism from the opposition camp as malicious and think that they intentionally impede the government from taking proper and timely actions through the COVID-19 crisis. In a nutshell, people in different political camps have become increasingly polarized and tend to view each other as lacking collaboration to address the major problems facing the country. Moreover, the ramifications of the COVID-19 pandemic have the potential to drastically reinforce such polarization,[19] which further causes people to lose confidence in democracy's capacity for coping with the COVID-19 pandemic. Accordingly, this study formulates the first hypothesis about the relationship between political polarization and individual attitudes toward democracy to fight against COVID-19 as follows:

Hypothesis 1: People with high levels of political polarization are less likely to support democracy as the best political system to combat COVID-19.

In contrast to the negative view of the influence of political polarization on politics, some argue that political polarization could have a positive effect on the functioning of democracy. In particular, political polarization could lead competing political parties or candidates to adopt clear and distinct policy positions so that people are able to easily distinguish between different political parties or candidates in terms of their positions on various policy issues and accordingly cast policy-oriented ballots.[20] Furthermore, previous studies have documented that political polarization is conducive to democracy. For instance, using the aggregate-level data from sixty-fix countries, Wang finds that party polarization is positively associated with the level of democracy in a country.[21] That is, countries with higher levels of party polarization tend to have higher levels of democracy. Besides, Brown et al. demonstrate that high levels of political polarization are associated with perceptions that corruption is under control, implying that corruption can be constrained by the opposition camp as long as it is given an institutional role.[22] When it comes to voting behavior, some studies have indicated that political polarization could increase voter turnout,[23] mainly because political polarization allows voters to better understand the costs and benefits of turning out to vote given clear and distinct policy positions of competing political parties and candidates. The previous evidence has clearly pointed out that political polarization can provide democracy with certain benefits. Specifically, this study argues that political polarization can enhance public confidence in democracy during the COVID-19 pandemic. There is no doubt that transparency is of significance to deal with a public health crisis, allowing the public to acquire accurate and up-to-date information and take necessary precautionary measures to reduce the risk of infection. Because governments might manipulate the information about COVID-19 and implement public health policies that are susceptible to human rights violations, it is required to supervise the behavior of governments during the COVID-19 pandemic. Given that ideologically opposed groups have greater incentives to disclose improper governmental activities than ideologically similar parties, it is inferred that people who are ideologically far from the government will serve as a strong check against government action. Furthermore, access to information is one of the keys to democracy, enabling people to obtain required information to hold the government accountable. As a result, this study recognizes that an alternative effect of political polarization on individual attitudes toward democracy to combat COVID-19 is possible and comes up with the following hypothesis:

Hypothesis 2: People with high levels of political polarization are more likely to support democracy as the best political system to combat COVID-19.

DATA, MEASUREMENT OF VARIABLES, AND MODEL SPECIFICATION

To test the previously mentioned competing hypotheses, this study employs the data from the 2021 Benchmark Survey of Taiwan's Election and Democratization Study (TEDS2021). TEDS is a continual large-scale survey research project and has been carried out to explore Taiwanese people's political attitudes and behavior since 2001.[24] TEDS2021 used address-based sampling to sample the target population, that is, individuals aged eighteen years or older in Taiwan and was fielded from January 10 through May 17, 2021, using face-to-face interviews. Survey fieldwork was ended earlier than the scheduled completion date due to the COVID-19 pandemic. While the number of completed respondents slightly falls short of the expected sample size (that is, 3,650), a total of 3,547 eligible respondents participated in the survey. However, due to observations with missing values, the effective number of observations for empirical analysis is 2,419. In addition, the weights from the ranking process according to the population distribution of gender, age, education, and residence area are used in the estimation and analysis. The operationalization of variables used in the empirical analysis is explained as follows.

The dependent variable in this study is individual attitude toward democracy as the best political system to combat COVID-19. To operationalize this variable, this study employs the single-item survey question asking the respondents to indicate the extent to which they agree with the following statement: "Some people say that when confronting the coronavirus pandemic, democracy is always preferable to any other kind of government." The respondents are asked to answer this question using a four-point scale ranging from "strongly disagree" to "strongly agree." Accordingly, this variable is treated as an ordinal variable, and a higher value indicates that the respondents are more supportive of democracy as the best political system to combat COVID-19. On the other hand, the key independent variable in this study is political polarization. This study follows previous research to use party feeling thermometers to operationalize individual levels of political polarization.[25] Specifically, given that the DPP and the KMT are major political parties dominating politics in Taiwan, this study mainly focuses on individual feelings toward the DPP and the KMT. Two survey questions are respectively used to ask the respondents to rate their liking of the DPP and the KMT using an eleven-point scale and a higher value signifies a more positive feeling. This study further calculates the absolute difference of both values for individual feelings toward the DPP and the KMT. Consequently, individual level of political polarization can be presented as follows:

$$Political\ polarization = |F_{DPP} - F_{KMT}|$$

where F_{DPP} is the respondent's positive feeling toward the DPP and F_{KMT} is the respondent's positive feeling toward the KMT. The value of zero means that the respondent has the same feeling about both the DPP and the KMT. By contrast, if the value is great than zero, it indicates that the respondent has a more favorable feeling toward one party than the other. In other words, as the value increases, people are expected to be more politically polarized.

To ensure that the relationship between the variables of interest is not spurious, this study controls for some variables that might influence individual attitudes toward democracy as the best political system to combat COVID-19. First of all, there is no doubt that COVID-19 has had an enormous impact on the economy and many people have suffered economic losses caused by COVID-19. Given the longstanding debate over the relationship between economy and support for democracy,[26] this study includes two variables—national and personal economic evaluations—as controls in the model. Specifically, the respondents are asked to evaluate how they think the COVID-19 pandemic affected Taiwan's overall economic situation and personal economic situation on a five-point scale, respectively. A higher value indicates that the respondent views the COVID-19 pandemic as bringing a more positive impact on Taiwan's economic situation. Second, government performance is regarded as a key determinant of support for democracy,[27] and thus it is required to consider individual evaluation of government performance in dealing with COVID-19 when it comes to support for democracy during the COVID-19 pandemic. One single survey question is used to ask the respondents to indicate the extent to which they are satisfied with President Tsai Ing-wen's performance in handling the COVID-19 pandemic on a four-point scale. A higher value signifies a higher level of satisfaction with President Tsai's performance. Third, if people are inclined to support democracy in principle, they are supposed to support democracy as the best political system to combat COVID-19. Therefore, this study includes an individual's overall support for democracy as a control variable that a higher value means a stronger overall support for democracy. Fourth, in view of the winner-loser gap in satisfaction with democracy,[28] this study controls for the variable of partisanship in the analysis. It is expected that people who support political parties belonging to the pan-green coalition are more likely to view democracy as the best political system to fight against COVID-19 given they are electoral winners. By contrast, those identifying with political parties in the pan-blue coalition are less likely to regard democracy as the best political system to combat COVID-19 because of their status as electoral losers. Therefore, this study creates two dummy variables respectively for the pan-blue and pan-green coalitions and treats the independents as the reference group.

Last, in terms of demographic variables, this study controls for such demographic characteristics as ethnicity, marital status, occupation, household income, education, age, and gender. Specifically, the respondents are classified into four ethnic groups: "Hakka," "Minnan," "Mainlander," and "Others," and "Hakka" is treated as the reference group when estimating the statistical model. Two dummy variables—"Single" and "Others"—are generated to measure the respondents' marital status, whereas the respondents who are married are treated as the reference group. In terms of occupation, three dummy variables are created respectively for "High- and middle-class white collar workers," "Lower-middle and low-class white collar workers," and "Agriculture, forestry, fishery, and animal husbandry." That is, blue collar workers are treated as the reference group. An interval variable is used to gauge the respondents' household income, and a higher value indicates a higher level of household income. One dummy variable, "College degree or above," is generated to measure the respondents' educational level with 1 for individuals who had completed a

Table 5.1. Descriptive Statistics of Variables

	Mean	*S.D.*	*Min.*	*Max.*
Democracy is the best political system to combat COVID-19	2.58	0.66	1	4
Political polarization	3.01	2.82	0	10
National economic evaluation	2.53	1.21	1	5
Personal economic evaluation	2.72	0.78	1	5
Performance evaluation	3.03	0.77	1	4
Overall support for democracy	2.79	0.67	1	4
Partisanship				
Independent	0.37	0.48	0	1
Pan-green	0.42	0.49	0	1
Pan-blue	0.20	0.40	0	1
Ethnicity				
Hakka	0.12	0.32	0	1
Minnan	0.76	0.43	0	1
Mainlander	0.10	0.30	0	1
Others	0.02	0.14	0	1
Marital status				
Married	0.56	0.50	0	1
Single	0.34	0.47	0	1
Others	0.11	0.31	0	1
Occupation				
High- and middle-class white collar workers	0.38	0.49	0	1
Lower-middle and low-class white collar workers	0.30	0.46	0	1
Agriculture, forestry, fishery, and animal husbandry	0.03	0.16	0	1
Blue collar workers	0.29	0.45	0	1
Household income	4.81	2.85	1	10
College degree or above	0.37	0.48	0	1
Age	45.99	15.98	18	95
Female	0.47	0.50	0	1
N		2,419		

Source: TEDS2021.

bachelor's or higher degree and 0 otherwise. Gender is a dummy variable coded as 1 if the respondent is female and 0 if the respondent is male, and age is measured by the number of years since birth. Table 5.1 reports the descriptive statistics of all variables used for empirical analysis.

With regard to model specification, given that the dependent variable is an ordinal variable, this study employs the ordered logit model to estimate the relationship between political polarization and individual attitudes toward democracy as the best political system to combat COVID-19. Specifically, the ordered logit model takes the form of

$$\ln(Y_j) = \ln\left(\frac{\pi_j(x)}{1 - \pi_j(x)}\right) = \alpha_j + \beta_1 X_1 + \beta_2 X_2 + \ldots + \beta_k X_k$$

where $\pi_j(x) = \pi(Y \leq j \mid X_1, X_2, \ldots, X_k)$, which is the probability of being at or below category j given a set of explanatory variables $j = 1, 2, 3$, α_j. are the cut points. $\beta_1, \beta_2, \ldots \beta_k$, are the logit coefficients, whereas $X_1, X_2, \ldots X_k$, are explanatory variables, including political polarization, national and personal economic evaluations, performance evaluation, overall support for democracy, partisanship, ethnicity, marital status, occupation, household income, education, age, and gender.

EMPIRICAL RESULTS

Before examining the relationship between political polarization and individual support for democracy as the best political system to combat COVID-19, this study takes a first look at the distributions of Taiwanese people's attitudes toward democracy. Figure 5.1 demonstrates individuals' overall support for democracy in Taiwan that approximately three-fifths (that is, 61.8% percent) of Taiwanese people either strongly agree or agree on democracy to be always preferable to any other kind of government under all circumstances. However, when it comes to the role of democracy in fighting against COVID-19, less than half (that is, 48.7 percent) of Taiwanese people either strongly agree or agree that democracy is always preferable to any other kind of government (see figure 5.2). Although the percentage of support for democracy in the fight against COVID-19 is still higher than that of opposition (that is, 41.8 percent), it seems that Taiwanese people are not so confident in democracy in response to a public health crisis such as COVID-19. This further justifies the investigation of this study into what factors influence individual attitudes toward democracy to combat COVID-19.

After describing the distributions of individual attitudes toward democracy in Taiwan, the next step is to examine the relationship between political polarization and support for democracy as the best political system in the fight against COVID-19. As demonstrated in table 5.2, this study finds that political polarization has a significant positive effect on

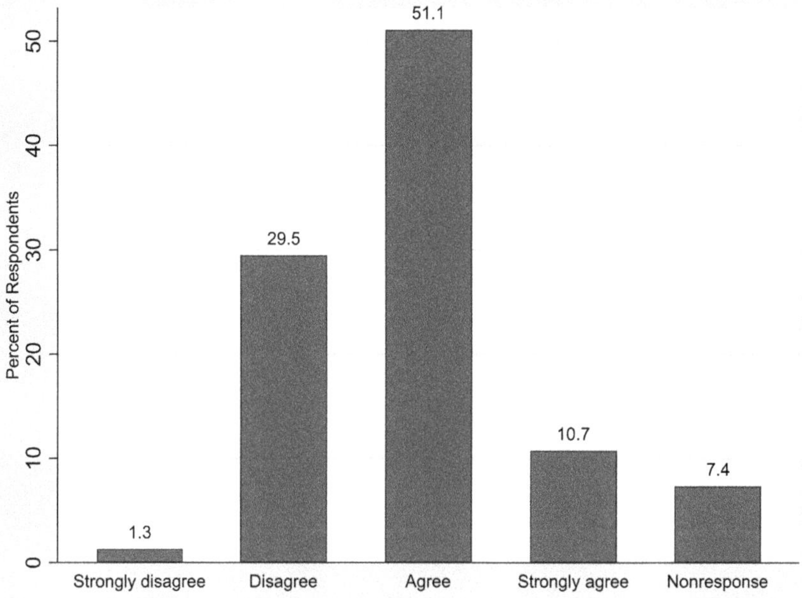

Figure 5.1. Overall Support for Democracy

Notes:

1. The number of observations is 3,547.
2. Nonresponse includes the answers such as "Don't know," "Refuse to answer," "It depends," and "No opinion."

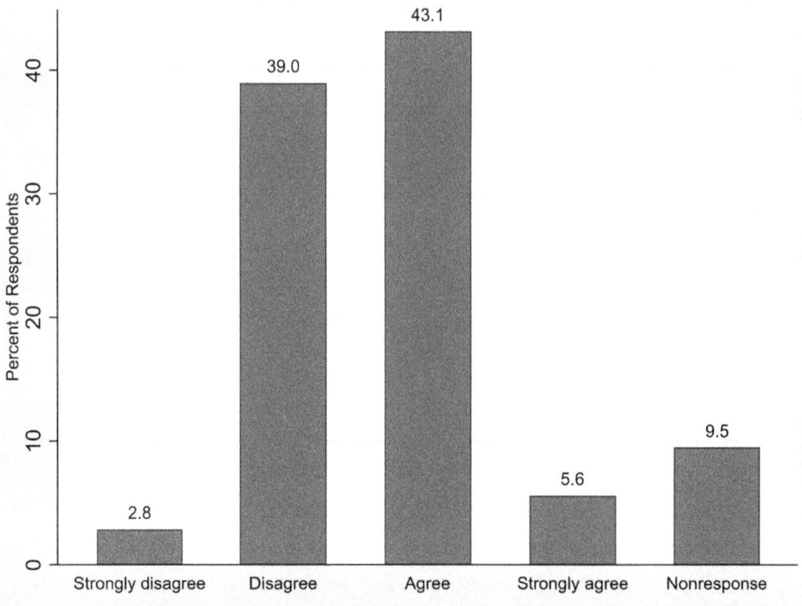

Figure 5.2. Support for Democracy as the Best Political System to Combat COVID-19

Notes:

1. The number of observations is 3,547.
2. Nonresponse includes the answers such as "Don't know," "Refuse to answer," "It depends," and "No opinion."

Table 5.2. Ordered Logit Analysis of Support for Democracy as the Best Political System to Combat COVID-19

	Coef.	*(S.E.)*	*O.R.*
Political polarization	0.051**	(0.018)	1.052
National economic evaluation	0.157***	(0.039)	1.170
Personal economic evaluation	–0.056	(0.060)	0.946
Performance evaluation	0.339***	(0.065)	1.403
Overall support for democracy	1.274***	(0.074)	3.576
Partisanship			
Pan-green	0.090	(0.112)	1.094
Pan-blue	–0.319*	(0.130)	0.727
Ethnicity			
Minnan	–0.230$	(0.129)	0.794
Mainlander	–0.598**	(0.185)	0.550
Others	–0.116	(0.308)	0.890
Marital status			
Single	0.268*	(0.112)	1.307
Others	0.004	(0.144)	1.004
Occupation			
High- and middle-class white collar workers	–0.339**	(0.109)	0.712
Lower-middle and low-class white collar workers	–0.246*	(0.116)	0.782
Agriculture, forestry, fishery, and animal husbandry	–0.326	(0.265)	0.722
Household income	–0.038*	(0.017)	0.963
College degree or above	–0.360***	(0.098)	0.698
Age	0.003	(0.004)	1.003
Female	0.211*	(0.085)	1.235
Cutpoint 1	0.522	(0.380)	
Cutpoint 2	4.266	(0.380)	
Cutpoint 3	7.672	(0.408)	
N	2,419		
Likelihood ratio test	655.15***		
Pseudo R^2	0.13		
–2× Log likelihood	4,220.65		

Notes:
1. ***: *p*<0.001; **: *p*<0.01; *: *p*<0.05; $: *p*<0.10.
2. Two-tailed test.
3. O.R: Odds ratio.

Source: TEDS2021.

individual support for democracy to combat COVID-19. Specifically, people with higher levels of political polarization are more likely to view democracy as the best political system to address the COVID-19 pandemic. The result lends support to the second hypothesis of this study regarding the beneficial effect of political polarization on individual attitudes toward democracy and refutes the negative view of political po-

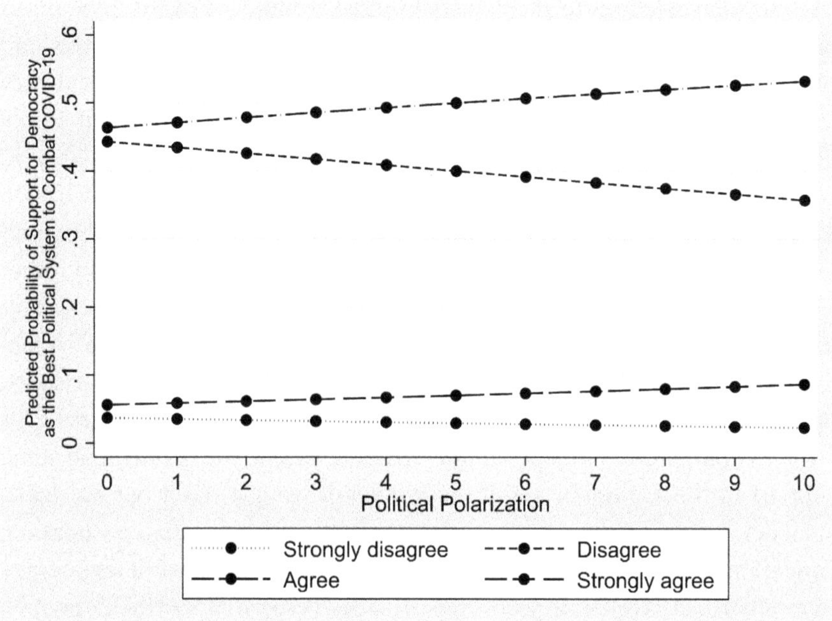

Figure 5.3. Effect of Political Polarization on Support for Democracy as the Best Political System to Combat COVID-19
Source: TEDS2021.

larization. To evaluate the substantive effect of political polarization, this study computes the predicted probability of support for democracy as the best political system to combat COVID-19. As displayed in figure 5.3, the predicted probability of support for democracy as the best political system to fight against COVID-19 increases as individual level of political polarization elevates. Specifically, the predicted probability increases from 46.7 percent to 53.2 percent. By contrast, the predicted probability of opposing democracy as the best political system to combat COVID-19 decreases from 44.3 percent to 35.7 percent. Overall, political polarization has a nontrivial effect on individual attitudes toward democracy in response to COVID-19.

In addition, this study also finds some factors that matter for individual attitudes toward democracy to combat COVID-19. First of all, when people perceive that the COVID-19 pandemic has a more positive impact on Taiwan's overall economic situation, they would tend to view democracy as the best political system to fight against COVID-19. However, whether the COVID-19 pandemic affects personal economic situation has nothing to do with individual attitudes toward democracy in response to COVID-19. Second, government performance comes into play when it comes to individual attitudes toward democracy to deal with COVID-19. That is, people who are more satisfied with President Tsai's performance in handling the COVID-19 pandemic are more likely to support democracy as the best political system to respond to COVID-19. Third, it is not surprising to find that people with higher levels of overall support for democracy are inclined to prefer democracy over any other kind of government to address COVID-19. Fourth, while there is no significant difference in support for democracy as the best political system to combat COVID-19 between pan-green identifiers and independents, pan-blue identifiers are less likely to buttress democracy to address COVID-19 compared to independents. To some extent, the results lend some support to the argument about the winner-loser gap. Last but not least, such demographic characteristics as ethnicity, marital status, occupation, education, and gender could affect individual attitudes toward democracy to combat COVID-19 as well. Specifically, compared to Hakka people, both Minnan people and Mainlanders are less likely to support democracy as the best political system to address COVID-19; single people are inclined to be in favor of democracy as the best political system in response to COVID-19 than those who are married; white collar workers are less likely to prefer democracy over any other kind of government to handle COVID-19 than blue collar workers; people with high household income and those with a college degree or above are less likely to support democracy as the best political system to deal with COVID-19; finally, women are more likely to regard democracy as the best political system to deal with COVID-19 than men.

The previous analysis has indicated a positive relationship between political polarization and individual attitudes toward democracy to fight against COVID-19. However, some might argue that in addition to the strength of political polarization used in the previous analysis, the direction of political polarization might also exert an influence on individual support for democracy to combat COVID-19. Therefore, this study further operationalizes political polarization by calculating the difference of both values for individual feelings toward the DPP and the KMT. Accordingly, the value for the direction of political polarization ranges from –10 to 10. A positive value means that the respondents have a strong liking for the

DPP, whereas a negative value signifies that the respondents have a strong liking for the KMT. Then this study estimates another model to investigate the relationship between the direction of political polarization and individual attitudes toward democracy to address COVID-10. As demonstrated in table 5.3, it is found that the direction of political polarization has a significant positive effect on individual support for democracy as

Table 5.3. Ordered Logit Analysis of Support for Democracy as the Best Political System to Combat COVID-19—Modified Model

	Coef.	*(S.E.)*	*O.R.*
Political polarization (DPP–KMT)	0.090***	(0.017)	1.094
National economic evaluation	0.148***	(0.039)	1.159
Personal economic evaluation	–0.050	(0.060)	0.952
Performance evaluation	0.226**	(0.069)	1.254
Overall support for democracy	1.265***	(0.074)	3.542
Partisanship			
Pan-green	–0.011	(0.110)	0.989
Pan-blue	0.083	(0.136)	1.086
Ethnicity			
Minnan	–0.232$	(0.130)	0.793
Mainlander	–0.562**	(0.186)	0.570
Others	–0.144	(0.308)	0.866
Marital status			
Single	0.268*	(0.112)	1.307
Others	–0.011	(0.144)	0.989
Occupation			
High- and middle-class white collar workers	–0.311**	(0.109)	0.733
Lower-middle and low-class white collar workers	–0.225$	(0.116)	0.798
Agriculture, forestry, fishery, and animal husbandry	–0.308	(0.265)	0.735
Household income	–0.037*	(0.017)	0.964
College degree or above	–0.355***	(0.098)	0.701
Age	0.003	(0.004)	1.003
Female	0.222**	(0.086)	1.249
Cutpoint 1	0.169	(0.388)	
Cutpoint 2	3.937	(0.387)	
Cutpoint 3	7.362	(0.413)	
N	2,419		
Likelihood ratio test	675.16***		
Pseudo R^2	0.14		
–2× Log likelihood	4,200.64		

Notes:

1. ***: *p*<0.001; **: *p*<0.01; *: *p*<0.05; $: *p*<0.10.
2. Two-tailed test.
3. O.R: Odds ratio.

Source: TEDS2021.

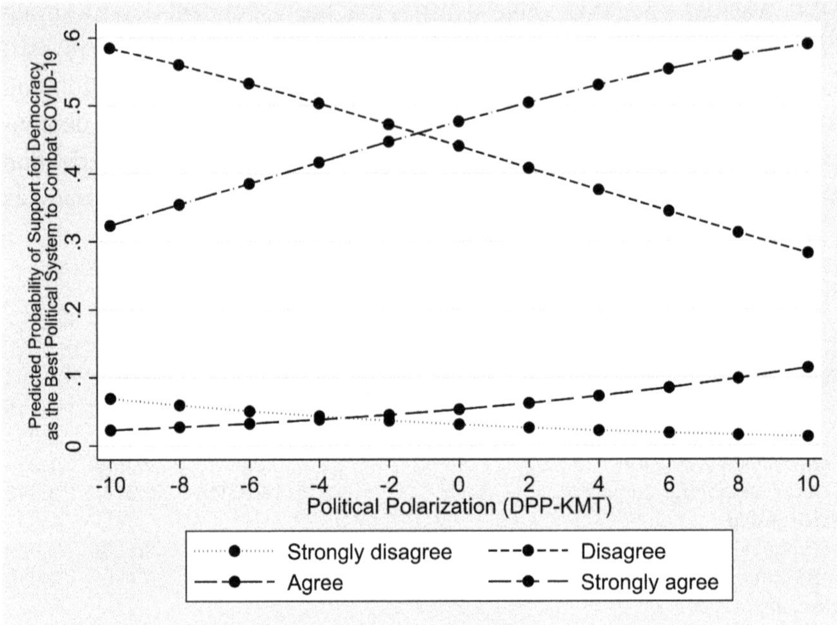

Figure 5.4. Effect of Political Polarization on Support for Democracy as the Best Political System to Combat COVID-19—Modified Model
Source: TEDS2021.

the best political system to fight against COVID-19. That is, people who have a more favorable feeling about the DPP are more likely to think of democracy as the best political system to combat COVID-19. Likewise, this study calculates the predicted probability of support for democracy as the best political system to combat COVID-19 to assess the substantive effect of the direction of political polarization. As seen in figure 5.4, the predicted probability of support for democracy as the best political system to combat COVID-19 increases as people have a more favorable feeling about the DPP. Specifically, the predicted probability increases from 32.3 percent to 59.0 percent. By contrast, the predicted probability of opposing democracy as the best political system to combat COVID-19 decreases from 58.5 percent to 28.3 percent. The result implies that there is a strong partisan divide apparent, as people who prefer the DPP over the KMT are more likely to support democracy as the best political system to address COVID-19. In addition, this study finds similar results as the previous analysis in terms of other control variables.

Finally, previous research has documented that Taiwanese people who have more diverse affects toward the two major parties are less supportive of the democratic system.[29] However, given that this study finds a positive relationship between political polarization and support for democracy as the best political system to combat COVID-19, it is worthwhile to explore whether political polarization indeed has a negative impact on overall support for democracy. As shown in table 5.4, in contradiction to previous

Table 5.4. Ordered Logit Analysis of Overall Support for Democracy

	Coef.	*(S.E.)*	*O.R.*
Political polarization	0.070***	(0.018)	1.073
National economic evaluation	–0.017	(0.037)	0.983
Personal economic evaluation	0.114*	(0.058)	1.120
Performance evaluation	0.658***	(0.064)	1.931
Partisanship			
Pan-green	0.400***	(0.110)	1.492
Pan-blue	–0.200	(0.126)	0.819
Ethnicity			
Minnan	0.221$	(0.126)	1.247
Mainlander	–0.019	(0.178)	0.981
Others	0.205	(0.302)	1.227
Marital status			
Single	0.176	(0.109)	1.192
Others	–0.077	(0.138)	0.926
Occupation			
High- and middle-class white collar workers	0.182$	(0.106)	1.200
Lower-middle and low-class white collar workers	0.158	(0.113)	1.171
Agriculture, forestry, fishery, and animal husbandry	0.549*	(0.265)	1.731
Household income	–0.012	(0.017)	0.988
College degree or above	0.089	(0.096)	1.093
Age	0.000	(0.004)	1.000
Female	–0.376***	(0.083)	0.687
Cutpoint 1	–1.861	(0.371)	
Cutpoint 2	1.886	(0.337)	
Cutpoint 3	4.909	(0.352)	
N	2,419		
Likelihood ratio test	368.0***		
Pseudo R^2	0.08		
–2× Log likelihood	4,522.80		

Notes:

1. ***: $p<0.001$; **: $p<0.01$; *: $p<0.05$; $: $p<0.10$.
2. Two-tailed test.
3. O.R: Odds ratio.

Source: TEDS2021.

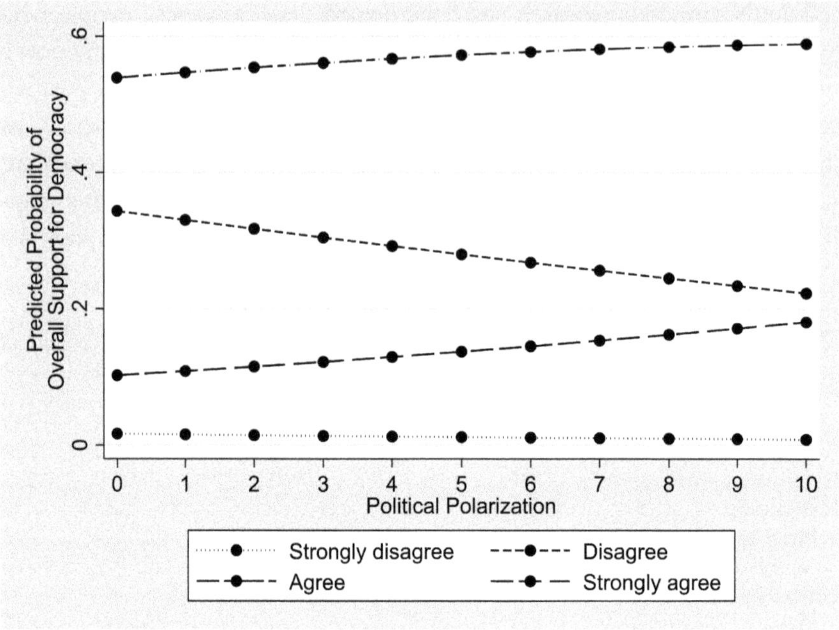

Figure 5.5. Effect of Political Polarization on Overall Support for Democracy
Source: TEDS2021.

research,[30] the results reveal that people with higher levels of political polarization are more likely to support democracy. This study also calculates the predicted probability of overall support for democracy to evaluate the substantive effect of political polarization. As illustrated in figure 5.5, the predicted probability of strong agreement that democracy is always preferable to any other kind of government increases as individual level of political polarization rises. Particularly, the predicted probability increases from 10.2 percent to 18.0 percent. By contrast, the predicted probability of disagreement that democracy is always preferable to any other kind of government decreases from 34.3 percent to 22.2 percent. The results imply that political polarization is not necessarily harmful to the functioning of democracy.

CONCLUSION

The COVID-19 pandemic has led to a dramatic impact on human life worldwide and presented an unprecedented challenge to public health.

Moreover, it has been debated on the merits of authoritarianism versus democracy to deal with the COVID-19 pandemic. Some might suspect whether democracy has the capacity to tackle the challenges caused by COVID-19 and even some public policies made in response to the COVID-19 pandemic would pose a serious threat to democracy because government may attempt to restrict democratic rules and human rights under the cover of pandemic management. Therefore, the key goal of this study is to contribute to a better understanding of how people perceive democracy during the COVID-19 pandemic and whether the public would lose confidence in democracy in the fight against COVID-19. On the one hand, this study finds that Taiwanese people indeed have a lower level of confidence in democracy to handle the COVID-19 pandemic. Specifically, although about three-fifths of the respondents agree that democracy is always preferable to any other kind of government under all circumstances, the percentage decreases to 48.7 percent when confronting the COVID-19 pandemic. To some extent, this reflects public concerns about the capacity of democracy to address the public health crisis. On the other hand, given rising political polarization in the past decade in Taiwan, this study examines the relationship between political polarization and support for democracy as the best political system to combat COVID-19. While previous research has mostly focused on the negative influence of political polarization on the health of democracy, the findings of this study demonstrate that political polarization is significantly positively associated with support for democracy as the best political system to deal with COVID-19. That is, people who have more polarized feelings about the DPP and the KMT are more likely to prefer democracy to any other kind of government to combat COVID-19. In view of growing political polarization in Taiwan, the results from this study might represent a positive signal that political polarization does not necessarily endanger democracy. Because democracy makes government information available to the public and people are endowed the rights to question the government, politically polarized people tend to think that in the democratic system, they can oversee government actions in response to the COVID-19 pandemic.

This study provides new insights into the role of political polarization in support for democracy. However, this study does not intend to argue that political polarization is bound to be beneficial to democracy. Given that political polarization would make political compromise more difficult, it might lead to political gridlock when the government and the opposition parties could not communicate with each other. It requires the government and the opposition parties to work together to address the global public health crisis such as COVID-19, but political polarization might rule out such a possibility of collaboration. Besides, although the results from this study demonstrate that people with higher levels of political polarization tend to support the democratic system during the COVID-19 pandemic, it does not necessarily mean that politically polarized people would be satisfied with democratic practices. As documented by previous studies,[31] political polarization has a negative effect on individual satisfaction with democracy. As a consequence, this study does not intend to overemphasize the positive impact of political polarization on individual attitudes toward democracy.

Last, it is acknowledged that the operationalization of political polarization in this study mainly focuses on the affective dimension and does not take issue or ideological polarization into consideration. Therefore, future research can be conducted to examine whether political polarization measured by issue or ideological position can still lead to support for democracy as the best political system to combat COVID-19.

NOTES

1. Windsor et al. 2020, e0244531.
2. Cassan and Steenvoort 2021, 100912; Karabulut et al. 2020, 109840.
3. Fukuyama 2020, 26–32.
4. Ibid.
5. Bol et al. 2021, 497–505.
6. Jiang et al. 2020, 200–211.
7. Kerr, Panagopoulos, and der Linden 2020, 110892.
8. Wang 2019, 275–87.
9. Abramowitz and Saunders 2018, 542–55.
10. Carothers and O'Donohue 2019, 1–4.
11. Clark and Tan 2012, 7–31.
12. Bail et al. 2018, 9216–21.
13. Grechyna 2016, 10–14.
14. Stanig 2013, 729–45.
15. McCright et al. 2014, 251–60.

16. Bruine de Bruin, Saw, and Goldman 2020, 177–94.
17. Kerr, Panagopoulos, and der Linden 2020, 110892.
18. Hart, Chinn, and Soroka 2020, 679–97.
19. Jungkunz 2021, 622512.
20. Levendusky 2010, 111–31.
21. Wang 2014, 687–99.
22. Brown, Touchton, and Whitford 2011, 1516–29.
23. Crepaz 1990, 183–205; Béjar, Moraes, and López-Cariboni 2020, 1–21.
24. More information about TEDS could be found at http://teds.nccu.edu.tw/main.php.
25. Hsiao 2014, 1–42.
26. Evans and Whitefield 1995, 485–514; Sing 2010, 175–205.
27. Magalhães 2014, 77–97.
28. Dahlberg and Linde 2017, 625–41.
29. Hsiao and Yu 2020, 1143–62.
30. Ibid.
31. Hoerner and Hobolt 2020, 1838–57; Hsiao and Yu 2020.

REFERENCES

Abramowitz, Alan I., and Kyle L. Saunders. 2008. "Is Polarization a Myth?" *The Journal of Politics* 70 (2): 542–55.

Bail, Christopher A., Lisa P. Argyle, Taylor W. Brown, John P. Bumpus, Haohan Chen, M. B. Fallin Hunzaker, Jaemin Lee, Marcus Mann, Friedolin Merhout, and Alexander Volfovsky. 2018. "Exposure to Opposing Views on Social Media Can Increase Political Polarization." *Proceedings of the National Academy of Sciences* 115 (37): 9216–21.

Béjar, Sergio, Juan A. Moraes, and Santiago López-Cariboni. 2020. "Elite Polarization and Voting Turnout in Latin America, 1993–2010." *Journal of Elections, Public Opinion and Parties* 30 (1): 1–21.

Bol, Damien, Marco Giani, André Blais, and Peter John Loewen. 2021. "The Effect of COVID-19 Lockdowns on Political Support: Some Good News for Democracy?" *European Journal of Political Research* 60 (2): 497–505.

Brown, David S., Michael Touchton, and Andrew B. Whitford. 2011. "Political Polarization as a Constraint on Government: Evidence from Corruption." *World Development* 39 (9): 1516–29.

Bruine de Bruin, Wändi, Htay-Wah Saw, and Dana P. Goldman. 2020. "Political Polarization in US Residents' COVID-19 Risk Perceptions, Policy Preferences, and Protective Behaviors." *Journal of Risk and Uncertainty* 61 (2): 177–94.

Carothers, Thomas, and Andrew O'Donohue, eds. 2019. *Democracies Divided: The Global Challenge of Political Polarization*. Washington, DC: Brookings Institution Press.

Cassan, Guilhem, and Milan Van Steenvoort. 2021. "Political Regime and COVID-19 Death Rate: Efficient, Biasing or Simply Different Autocracies? An Econometric Analysis." *SSM—Population Health* 16: 100912.

Clark, Cal, and Alexander C. Tan. 2012. "Political Polarization in Taiwan and the United States: A Growing Challenge to Catch-All Parties?" *Journal of Current Chinese Affairs* 41 (3): 7–31.

Crepaz, Markus M. L. 1990. "The Impact of Party Polarization and Postmaterialism on Voter Turnout." *European Journal of Political Research* 18 (2): 183–205.

Dahlberg, Stefan, and Jonas Linde. 2017. "The Dynamics of the Winner-Loser Gap in Satisfaction with Democracy: Evidence from a Swedish Citizen Panel." *International Political Science Review* 38 (5): 625–41.

Evans, Geoffrey, and Stephen Whitefield. 1995. "The Politics and Economics of Democratic Commitment: Support for Democracy in Transition Societies." *British Journal of Political Science* 25 (4): 485–514.

Fukuyama, Francis. 2020. "The Pandemic and Political Order." *Foreign Affairs* 99 (4): 26–32.

Grechyna, Daryna. 2016. "On the Determinants of Political Polarization." *Economics Letters* 144: 10–14.

Hart, P. Sol, Sedona Chinn, and Stuart Soroka. 2020. "Politicization and Polarization in COVID-19 News Coverage." *Science Communication* 42 (5): 679–97.

Hoerner, Julian M., and Sara B. Hobolt. 2020. "Unity in Diversity? Polarization, Issue Diversity and Satisfaction with Democracy." *Journal of European Public Policy* 27 (12): 1838–57.

Hsiao, Yi-Ching. 2014. "Political Polarization in Taiwan: An Analysis on Mass Feeling Thermometer toward Political Parties." *Journal of Electoral Studies* 21 (2): 1–42.

Hsiao, Yi-ching, and Eric Chen-hua Yu. 2020. "Polarization Perception and Support for Democracy: The Case of Taiwan." *Journal of Asian and African Studies* 55 (8): 1143–62.

Jiang, Julie, Emily Chen, Shen Yan, Kristina Lerman, and Emilio Ferrara. 2020. "Political Polarization Drives Online Conversations about COVID-19 in the United States." *Human Behavior and Emerging Technologies* 2 (3): 200–211.

Jungkunz, Sebastian. 2021. "Political Polarization During the COVID-19 Pandemic." *Frontiers in Political Science* 3: 622512.

Karabulut, Gokhan, Klaus F. Zimmermann, Mehmet Huseyin Bilgin, and Asli Cansin Doker. 2020. "Democracy and COVID-19 Outcomes." *Economics Letters* 203: 109840.

Kerr, John, Costas Panagopoulos, and Sandervan der Linden. 2021. "Political Polarization on COVID-19 Pandemic Response in the United States." *Personality and Individual Differences* 179: 110892.

Levendusky, Matthew S. 2010. "Clear Cues, More Consistent Voters: A Benefit of Elite Polarization." *Political Behavior* 32 (1): 111–31.

Magalhães, Pedro C. 2014. "Government Effectiveness and Support for Democracy." *European Journal of Political Research* 53 (12014): 77–97.

McCrighta, Aaron M., Chenyang Xiao, and Riley E. Dunlap. 2014. "Political Polarization on Support for Government Spending on Environmental Protection in the USA, 1974–2012." *Social Science Research* 48: 251–60.

Sing, Ming. 2010. "Explaining Mass Support for Democracy in Hong Kong." *Democratization* 17 (1): 175–205.

Stanig, Piero. 2013. "Political Polarization in Retrospective Economic Evaluations during Recessions and Recoveries." *Electoral Studies* 32 (4): 729–45.

Wang, Ching-Hsing. 2014. "The Effects of Party Fractionalization and Party Polarization on Democracy." *Party Politics* 20 (5): 687–99.

Wang, Austin Horng-En. 2019. "The Myth of Polarization Among Taiwanese Voters: The Missing Middle." *Journal of East Asian Studies* 19 (3): 275–87.

Windsor, Leah C., Gina Yannitell Reinhardt, Alistair J. Windsor, Robert Ostergard, Susan Allen, Courtney Burns, Jarod Giger, and Reed Wood. 2020. "Gender in the Time of COVID-19: Evaluating National Leadership and COVID-19 Fatalities." *PLoS ONE* 15 (12): e0244531.

6

Public Opinion toward U.S. Vaccine Diplomacy

George Yin, Chia-hung Tsai, and Iain Johnston

INTRODUCTION

Taiwan, lying roughly 100 miles (160 kilometers) off the coast of southeastern China, is dubbed the "most dangerous place on Earth" by *The Economist*. Since the end of civil war in 1949, the People's Republic of China (PRC) has long hoped to "reunify" with Taiwan even though today the Taiwanese public generally opposes unification with the PRC. Furthermore, the PRC has never ruled out the use of force to compel unification, and its ability to do so has increased as trends in relative material power capabilities increasingly favor the PRC.

Official U.S. policy has been aimed at maintaining peace and stability across the Taiwan Strait. Since the United States and China normalized relations, Washington has essentially adopted a policy of dual deterrence. On the one hand, the United States seeks to deter China from relying on military means to change the status quo across the Taiwan Strait. On the other hand, the United States has also sought to deter Taiwan from pursuing de jure independence, which could provoke China to use force. As the relative military power shifts in favor of China, some argue that deterring China from using force to invade Taiwan has become the primary concern (Haass and Sacks 2021).

Historically, the United States adopted a posture of strategic ambiguity about whether and how it might help Taiwan in the event of a Chinese attack. Ambiguity serves dual deterrence. Several analysts and policymakers, however, have started advocating for strategic clarity, arguing that such a policy will send a clear signal to Beijing that Washington, DC, will not tolerate a Chinese attack of Taiwan (Haass and Sacks 2021). Moreover, in principle, the more confidence Taiwan has that the United States will come to its aid in the event of a Chinese attack, the more Taiwan might also be encouraged to build up its own military, or at the very least not capitulate to PRC military and political pressure.[1] However, strategic clarity, from the U.S. perspective, comes with a cost. As Johnston, Tsai, Yin, and Goldstein (2021) find, public opinion polls suggest that strategic clarity could encourage the Taiwanese public to increase its support for de jure independence, which could destabilize cross-Strait relations. For Washington, this raises the issue of whether it can signal its commitment to Taiwan by going beyond the strategic clarity versus strategic ambiguity choice to include other domains of public policy.[2]

The COVID-19 pandemic provides a test of the idea of cross-domain signaling of commitment. The pandemic gave the United States an opportunity to boost Taiwan's confidence in the United States. Taiwan enjoyed an early success containing COVID-19 until May 2021, when the infectious British COVID-19 variant reached the island. Taiwan was taken by surprise—few people in Taiwan were vaccinated and Taiwan had not secured a supply line of vaccines sufficient for the entire population. This provided Beijing with an opportunity to further its objective of winning the "hearts and minds" of the Taiwanese people. Soon after the COVID-19 outbreak in Taiwan, China's Taiwan Affairs Office declared that China was open to donating Chinese vaccines to Taiwan. Beijing's "goodwill" put Taiwan in a difficult situation. Taiwan's acceptance of Chinese vaccines could undermine Taiwan's strategy of aligning with the United States to resist China. If China came to Taiwan's aid before the United States, Beijing could propagandize that the United States is an unreliable partner with neither the capabilities nor resolve to assist Taiwan in a timely fashion during a crisis (Sugimoto and Yin 2021). The Biden administration, to counter the Chinese vaccine diplomacy maneuver targeting Taiwan, quickly donated 2.5 million doses of Moderna vaccines to Taiwan in June 2021. The U.S. donation drive was announced with great publicity by Senators Tammy Duckworth, Dan Sullivan, and Chris Coons during a special visit to Taiwan. Subsequently, the United States sent another 1.5 million doses of Moderna vaccines to Taiwan in November

2021. It looked as though the United States had "stolen the march" on the PRC when it came to vaccine diplomacy.

Cross-domain signaling, however, is not easy. It requires that the targets of these signals think in fairly complex ways about how to draw inferences about the intentions of a signaler in one domain (military security) from actions taken in a very different domain (pandemic prevention). One can imagine, therefore, that the meaning and credibility of cross-domain signaling will differ depending on the cognitive or ideational traits of the target. To this point there is no evidence one way or the other as to whether the U.S. use of vaccine donations constituted a credible cross-domain commitment signal. How does the Taiwan public view the U.S. vaccine donation drive? Specifically, has the vaccination donation drive been successful in boosting Taiwan's confidence in the United States in the shadow of growing Chinese power? Are there any variations on how the public views the U.S. vaccination donation drive? If so, what are the factors driving how the Taiwanese public assesses this U.S. attempt at signaling its commitment? We present the first public opinion study to answer these questions, and we find that the efficacy of U.S. vaccine diplomacy is related to the public's prior images of the United States and China, to perceptions of identity, and levels of trust. Specifically, respondents often conflate capabilities with resolve ("if the United States is stronger than China, it should be more committed to Taiwan's security") and allow their pro-U.S./pro-China biases to color their assessment of U.S. credibility. In addition, those with strong Taiwanese identity and beliefs about shared values with the United States are also more likely to believe vaccine diplomacy is a signal of U.S. commitment. Finally, generalized trusters are also likely to make similar inferences about cross-domain commitments. Thus, respondents' cognitions and identities loom large in their assessment of the U.S. vaccine donation drive. This is not entirely surprising. As noted earlier, understanding cross-domain signaling for the target of signaling is difficult. This difficulty accentuates the roles preexisting beliefs play in how citizens—who often have limited time and energy to learn about foreign affairs—assess the connections between disparate foreign policy domains (in this case, global public health and great power politics).

The rest of the chapter is divided into the following sections. First, we provide a discussion of the background of the U.S. Moderna vaccination donation drive to Taiwan. Second, we develop a number of rationalist, psychological, and ideational hypotheses on how the public assesses cross-domain signals in the context of the U.S. Moderna vaccination donation drive to Taiwan. Third, we introduce our data from a representative survey administered in Taiwan in 2021, before outlining our empirical strategy. Fourth, we present our results. Fifth, we conclude and discuss avenues for further research.

THEORETICAL DISCUSSION

The COVID-19 pandemic expanded U.S.-China great power competition into a new domain, international public health.[3] Both the United States and China donated vaccines to various countries and regions to promote their agendas. Unsurprisingly, Taiwan too became enmeshed in U.S.-China great power politics, as discussed earlier. But did vaccine diplomacy work in Taiwan? Specifically, did U.S. vaccine donation to Taiwan boost the Taiwanese public's confidence in the United States as a geopolitical partner against China? There are different theoretical reasons to expect cross-domain commitment signals to be credible.

From a rationalist perspective, the average citizen is homo economicus, that is, an individual with coherent and transitive preferences and the ability to do cost-benefit calculations and to engage in Bayesian update (Elster 1986). In this context, the citizen should update his/her/their belief concerning the U.S. commitment to Taiwan if he/she/they believes that the U.S. vaccine donation to Taiwan is a costly demonstration of the U.S. commitment to Taiwan. Vaccine donation to Taiwan could be costly for the United States in two ways. First, donations to Taiwan attracted Beijing's ire. Indeed, the Chinese Foreign Ministry spokesperson Zhao Lijian criticized the United States after it sent 2.5 million doses of Moderna vaccines to Taiwan: "It is despicable that the U.S. makes an issue out of China whenever the topic of vaccines is brought up. It sets people wondering about U.S. true intention and motives."[4] While the United States considers the relationship with China to be highly competitive and adversarial already, it is trying to establish some limits or guardrails to this animosity.[5] A highly symbolic and sensitive act of support such as the vaccine donations to Taiwan, on the other hand, might reinforce Beijing's view that the United States is weakening its One China policy, thus worsening the U.S.-China relationship.

Second, given the global vaccine shortage at the time, the United States paid an opportunity cost for sending vaccines to Taiwan. In principle, the United States could have sent the vaccines to Vietnam, South Korea, India, or other U.S. partners to further consolidate relations and to help prevent the emergence of new COVID variants. Of course, eventually, the United States sent vaccines to more than one hundred nations, but some nations receive more vaccines than others in a timelier fashion.[6] It is perhaps not a coincidence that Taiwan received vaccines from the United States (and Japan, a key U.S. ally in the region) in less than a month after its COVID outbreak.

Importantly, the higher the perceived costs of U.S. vaccine donation, the more likely that an individual would update his/her/their belief about the U.S. commitment to Taiwan. The magnitude of the perceived costs, in turn, depend on an individual's assessment of the U.S.-China balance of power. From the rationalist perspective, an individual who believes that the United States is declining relative to China should be more likely to update upward his/her/their belief regarding U.S. resolve, for two reasons. First, Beijing's ire should be more concerning for the United States if one perceives China as the stronger power in the region. Second, if the United States is in decline relative to China, sending vaccines to Taiwan should make it more difficult for Washington, DC, to compete for influence with China elsewhere.

H1 (costly signaling): An individual is more likely to update upward his/her/their confidence in U.S. resolve to defend Taiwan after the U.S. vaccine donation if he/she/they believes that the United States is declining relative to China.

On the other hand, we might also expect the perception that U.S. domestic politics is beset by political polarization to reduce the signaling value of vaccine donation. Domestic political divisions can have foreign policy implications. An individual could reasonably question whether the costly signal truly reflects a U.S. consensus to help Taiwan if he/she/they believes that American political elites are often divided. For example, a signal of commitment from the executive branch might reflect pressure from the legislative opposition with different preferences trying to embarrass the top leadership. In this case the commitment would not represent a genuine consensus to support Taiwan; it would be a political act to reduce opposition pressure.[7] Indeed, the U.S. Congress is often seen as more "pro-Taiwan" compared to the executive branch, with several hawkish congressional members pushing the United States to modify its longstanding policy of strategy ambiguity.[8] In recent years, the U.S. Congress has passed several pieces of legislation—for example, the Asia Reassurance Initiative Act, the Taiwan Defense Assessment Commission Act, and the Taiwan Defense Act—to strengthen U.S.-Taiwan relations. H2 sums up this discussion.

> *H2 (political polarization): An individual is less likely to update upward his/her/their confidence in U.S. resolve to defend Taiwan after the U.S. vaccine donation if he/she/they believes that American foreign policy elites are divided.*

In contrast to these "simple" rationalist theories, psychological and ideational theories claim that individuals rely on cognitive heuristics and ideational orientations that bias judgments *ex ante* in particular directions (see, for example, Kahneman 2011). Here there might be several explanations for believing U.S. vaccine diplomacy constitutes a credible commitment to Taiwan.

First, the public, given China's reaction to the U.S. vaccine donation, might see it as a deliberate provocation aimed at China. This provocation implies that the United States does not care about Chinese reactions, which signals U.S. confidence in its ability to deal with China. This view is likely to be particularly prevalent among individuals who perceive the United States to be maintaining or increasing its power advantage over China. The public, importantly, could conflate capabilities with resolve and equate images of U.S. strength with U.S. resolve.[9] This conflation may be a product of attribute substitution, which occurs when individuals substitute a judgment that requires complex computation with another judgment that is more easily calculated (Kahneman and Frederick 2002). In this case, connecting U.S. vaccine donation with U.S. resolve to defend Taiwan requires the public to appreciate (1) the opportunity cost associated with U.S. vaccine donations to Taiwan (as discussed earlier) and

(2) and why the costliness of vaccine donation should increase as (perceived) U.S. power declines relative to China. Equating U.S. confidence with U.S. resolve is much more straightforward.

> *H3 (U.S. capabilities): An individual is more likely to update upward his/her/their confidence in U.S. resolve to defend Taiwan after the U.S. vaccine donation if he/she/they believes that the United States is maintaining or increasing its power advantage over China.*

A second nonrational explanation might be related to generalized trust, that is, a belief that most others will reciprocate cooperation. A generalized trusting individual is likely to expect friendly gestures from others and thus will interpret unreciprocal gestures of support as a natural indicator of future cooperation. General trust is an element in social capital and is therefore related to expectations of diffuse reciprocity and the relatively easy resolution of disputes (Rothstein and Stolle 2008). Thus, we expect that people who exhibit generalized trust might be more likely to interpret U.S. vaccine donation as indicative of the U.S. commitment to Taiwan. Importantly, however, this is a form of confirmation bias—the tendency to gather evidence that confirms preexisting expectations, typically by emphasizing or pursuing supporting evidence while dismissing or failing to seek contradictory evidence—triggered by a preexisting foreign policy belief (Nickerson 1998).

> *H4 (generalized trust): An individual is more likely to update upward his/her/their confidence in U.S. resolve to defend Taiwan after the U.S. vaccine donation if he/she/they exhibits generalized trust.*

Social psychology might suggest another possibility. For example, social identity theory (Tajfel and Turner 1979) posits that individuals tend to associate in-group members with positive traits (in-group favoritism) and tend to discount antigroup behavior as a mistake (or circumstances beyond one's control) rather than a predisposition. Consequently, individuals who perceive the United States as a member of an in-group that shares basic political, social, and economic norms and values should be more likely to associate the U.S. vaccine donation with U.S. trustworthiness, regardless of the "true" cost of the donations to the United States.

Social identity theory therefore also suggests that an individual who sees China—the U.S. competitor—as the in-group will tend to discount the signaling significance of U.S. vaccine donation. In the context of U.S.-China competition, individuals who have affinity toward China are likely to see the United States as the out-group and practice out-group denigration/discrimination, for example, discount evidence that would portray the United States in a positive light. As in the case of generalized trust, these tendencies are indicative of confirmation bias, but in this instance they are triggered by identity concerns.

Social identity theory, therefore, generates two more hypotheses.

H5 (U.S.-Taiwan values): An individual is more likely to update upward his/her/their confidence in U.S. resolve to defend Taiwan after the U.S. vaccine donation if he/she/they believes that Taiwan and the United States share basic social values.

H6 (China as in-group): An individual is less likely to update upward his/her/their confidence in U.S. resolve to defend Taiwan after the U.S. vaccine donation if he/she/they sees China as Taiwan's in-group.

DATA OPERATIONALIZATION AND EMPIRICAL STRATEGY

We designed an original survey to investigate cross-domain signaling in the context of the U.S. vaccine donation to Taiwan. The survey was conducted in Taiwan (by telephone) between November 24 and 29, 2021. Samples were randomly drawn from household telephone books. We stratified the samples in proportion to the size of landline telephone numbers of each county/city in Taiwan except for Penghu, Kinmen, and Matsu (following conventions of public opinion polling in Taiwan). Interviewers successfully completed 1,120 interviews. To ensure that the samples are representative of the Taiwanese population, we weighted the observations by gender, age, education, and residence area.

To measure the efficacy of cross-domain signaling in the context of U.S. vaccine diplomacy, we ask the respondents (q15) whether they agree with the statement "the U.S. has donated 4 million doses of Moderna vaccine to Taiwan, which demonstrates U.S. resolve to protect Taiwan" (有人說：「美國已經捐贈台灣400萬劑莫德納疫苗，證明美國有保

護台灣的決心」，請問您同不同意這個說法?), on a four-point scale: (1) strongly disagree; (2) disagree; (3) agree; and (4) strongly agree.

Our first independent variable is perception of U.S.-China balance of power in Asia. We know that individuals often make diverse assessments when it comes to international balances of power (Wohlforth 1993). We exploit this individual level variation to test H1 (costly signaling) and H3 (U.S. capabilities), two opposing hypotheses that both concern individual assessment of U.S.-China balance of power. We ask each respondent (q10) whether he/she/they believes that the United States or the China is more influential in Asia today. If H1 holds, respondents who believe that China is more influential in Asia today should be more likely to agree with the earlier statement on U.S. vaccine donation. If H3 holds, respondents who believe that China is more influential in Asia today should be less likely to agree with the earlier statement on U.S. vaccine donation.

To test H2 (political polarization), we proxy perception of divisions among U.S. foreign policy elites by asking respondents (q5) to assess whether the White House and the Congress exhibit different views on U.S.-Taiwan relations on a four-point scale (completely consistent views, partly consistent views, partly inconsistent views, and totally inconsistent views). If H2 holds, respondents should associate consistency with an increase in their confidence in the United States after the vaccine donation.

Turning to the effect of orientations toward intergroup relationships, H4 suggests that people who exhibits generalized trust are more likely to see U.S. vaccine diplomacy as a signal indicating U.S. support for Taiwan. To test H4, we ask respondents (q10a3–2) whether they believe that Taiwan should generally trust other foreign nations or act cautiously toward them (binary response).

H5 and H6 both draw on social identity theory. To test H5, we ask the respondents (q13) whether they believe that Taiwanese social values are consistent with U.S. social values on a four-point scale: (1) completely consistent; (2) partly consistent; (3) partly inconsistent; and (4) inconsistent). Respondents who believe that Taiwan and the United States share social values should be more likely to appreciate the signaling value of U.S. vaccine donation. We test H6, which concerns the respondents "Taiwanese-ness" vis-à-vis China, with two variables. First, we ask the respondents whether they identify as themselves as Taiwanese, Chinese, or both Taiwanese and Chinese (q1). We expect a higher likelihood for respondents who strongly identify as Taiwanese to associate vaccine donation with U.S. commitment toward Taiwan (compared to respondents who are only identified with China). Second, we ask the respondents to assess how similar Taiwanese culture is compared to Chinese culture on a four-point scale (q2): (1) completely the same; (2) mostly similar; (3) mostly dissimilar; and (4) completely different. We expect respondents who believe that Taiwanese and Chinese cultures are similar to discount the signaling value of U.S. vaccine donation.

To test our hypotheses, we estimate a series of ordered probit models:

$$y_i^* = x_i\beta + e_i$$

An ordered probit presumes a latent continuous metric y_i^* that corresponds to the ordinal responses observed; substantively, y_i^* is the estimated level of agreement/disagreement with the statement that U.S. vaccine donation constitutes a credible cross-domain signal. A large y_i^* indicates agreement, and a small y_i^* indicates disagreement. Thresholds partition the "real" latent metric into a series of regions that correspond to the ordinal categories (in our case, strongly agree, agree, disagree, and strongly disagree). We run ordered probit models because regular probit models overlook the ordering of the dependent variable while ordinal least squared (OLS) models assume that increments from one category to the next are the same and may produce predicted probabilities of less than 0 or greater than 1.

Probit estimators assume that y_i^* is represented by the cumulative normal distribution, and the predicted probability in ordered probit is $\text{Prob}(Y_{i=j}) = \Phi(\mu_j - x'\beta) - \Phi(\mu_{j-1} - x'\beta)$, where μ_j and μ_{j-1} denote the upper and lower threshold values for category j, x' denotes the matrix of independent variables, and β is the matrix of estimated coefficients. The ordered probit equation then computes the components of μ and β by maximum likelihood estimation.

The latent continuous variable, y*, is a linear combination of our explanatory variables and control variables (partisanship, gender, age, and education; all of them are dummy variables), x_i, plus a disturbance term that has a standard Normal distribution (Green and Hensher 2010). y_i, the observed ordinal variable, takes on values 0 through m according to the following scheme:

$$Y_{i=j} \Longleftrightarrow \mu_{j-1} < y_i^* \leq \mu_j ,$$

where j = 0, . . . , m. m is the number of partitions that defines the possible ordinal responses.

RESULTS

Figure 6.1 provides an overview of our respondents' assessments of the U.S. vaccine donation drive as a cross-domain signal. 38.8 percent of the respondents either agree or strongly agree that the U.S. vaccine donation is an indication that the United States is committed to Taiwan's security.

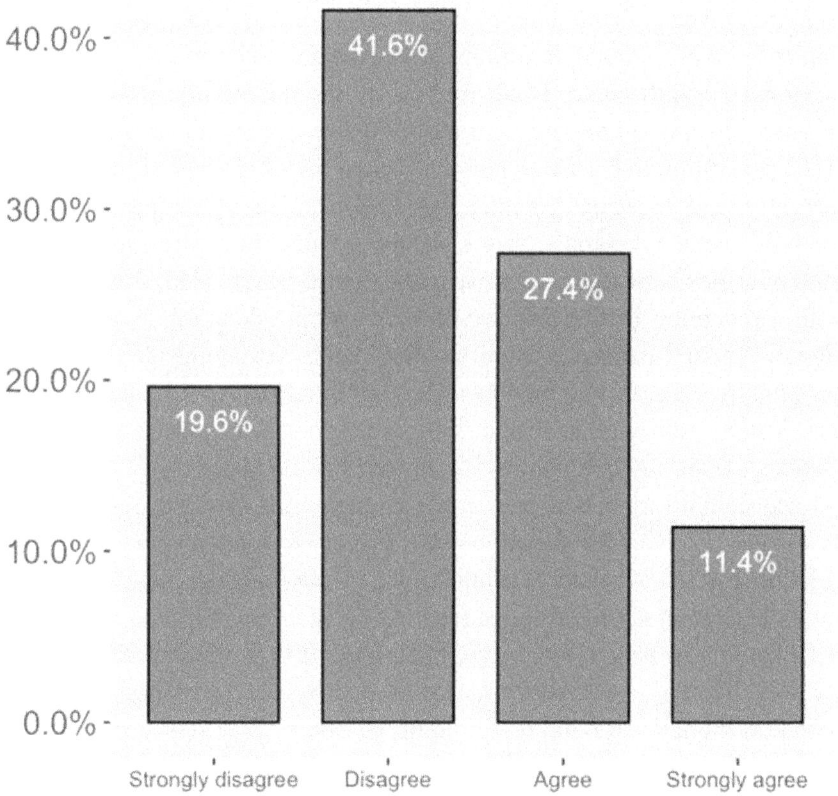

Figure 6.1. Relative Frequencies of U.S. Vaccine Donation as Commitment to Taiwan
Source: ESC-Fairbank Center Survey, 2021

On the other hand, 61.2 percent of the respondents either disagree or strongly disagree drawing a link between U.S. vaccine donation and U.S. commitment to Taiwan. As we expect, it is difficult for the public to draw connections between issues across different policy domains and appreciate how cross-domain signaling works.

Next, we investigate the factors driving our respondents' assessment of U.S. vaccine donation. Table 6.1 reports the results from a series of ordered probit regression analyses. Model 1 focuses on the rationalist hypotheses. It pits the costly signaling hypothesis (H1) against the U.S. capabilities hypothesis (H3), in addition to examining the political polarization hypothesis (H2). Model 1 supports H2: people that perceive political division in the United States would not consider the vaccine diplomacy as a credible signal of the U.S. commitment to Taiwan. On the other hand, model 1 rejects H1 in favor of H3: people who perceive the United States as more powerful than China in Asia would consider U.S. vaccine donation as an expression of commitment to Taiwan's security.

Model 2, on the other hand, focuses on the nonrationalist hypotheses (H4–6); it supports all the nonrationalist hypotheses. Generalized trust (H4), perception that Taiwan and the United States share basic social values (H5), and Taiwanese identity (H6) all correlate with a perception of the U.S. vaccine donation drive's signaling value. In contrast, perception of similarities between Taiwanese and Chinese culture (H6) is associated with a reduction in the efficacy of U.S. vaccine donation as a security signal. Model 3 examines all rationalist hypotheses alongside the nonrationalist hypotheses. Model 4 examines all hypotheses with full controls. The results from models 1 and 2 are consistent across models 3 and 4. Overall, images of U.S. and China power, beliefs about trust, and political and cultural identities are critical in explaining how our respondents assess the U.S. vaccine donation drive as a cross-domain signal.

To assess the substantive significance of our findings, we calculate a series of predicted probabilities (and confidence intervals) on whether a respondent will perceive the signaling value of U.S. vaccine donation as we vary our key explanatory variables one by one (all simulations are based on model 4 in table 6.1, holding all other covariates at their mean and median values).[10] Importantly, a one-unit change in any covariate will simultaneously affect the predicted probabilities for all categories—strongly agree/agree/disagree/strongly disagree that U.S. vaccine

Table 6.1. Determinants of U.S. Vaccine Donation as Commitment

Coefficients	*Model 1*	*Model 2*	*Model 3*	*Model 4*
U.S. power	0.409***		0.271***	0.238***
	(0.039)		(0.043)	(0.045)
President Congress Divided	–0.379***		–0.258***	–0.270***
	(0.041)		(0.047)	(0.049)
Generalized trust	—	0.169***	0.114*	0.121**
		(0.036)	(0.039)	(0.040)
U.S. value	—	0.328***	0.223**	0.198***
		(0.040)	(0.046)	(0.048)
Taiwan and China similar culture	—	–0.210***	–0.205**	–0.135*
		(0.040)	(0.044)	(0.046)
Taiwanese identity	—	0.488**	0.391*	0.511**
		(0.128)	(0.141)	(0.047)
Dual identity	—	0.157	0.146	0.325*
		(0.125)	(0.139)	(0.144)
Pan-blue	—	—		–0.058
				(0.047)
Pan-green	—	—		0.189**
				(0.046)
Taiwan People Party	—	—		–0.075
				(0.039)
Female	—	—	—	0.186**
				(0.042)
30–40 years old	—	—	—	0.034
				(0.041)
40–50 years old	—	—	—	–0.070
				(0.051)
50–60 years old	—	—	—	–0.208
				(0.142)
60 years old and more	—	—	—	0.057
				(0.075)
Middle school	—	—	—	–0.069
				(0.067)
High school			—	–0.274*
				(0.108)
Some college				–0.309*
				(0.094)
University				–0.440*
				(0.124)
Strongly disagree/Disagree	–0.997***	–0.955***	–1.024***	–1.195***
	(0.054)	(0.053)	(0.059)	(0.070)
Disagree/Agree	0.337***	0.439***	0.441***	0.381***
	(0.046)	(0.047)	(0.052)	(0.062)
Agree/Strongly agree	1.383***	1.525***	1.579***	1.610***
	(0.062)	(0.065)	(0.072)	(0.081)
n	844	862	758	758

Note: *$p<0.05$, **$p<0.01$, ***$p<0.001$

Source: ESC-Fairbank Center Survey 2021.

donation indicates a commitment to Taiwan—from our ordered probit model. The sum of the predicted probabilities for all four assessments of the cross-domain signal must add up to 100 percent for every category of respondents with a distinct attitude (for example, high level of generalized trust or belief that Taiwanese and Chinese cultures are completely identical). Figure 6.2 plots how the predicted probabilities change as we vary the key explanatory variables associated with H1–6.

Favorable assessment of U.S. power relative to China in Asia, levels of generalized trust, perception of U.S.-Taiwan similarities in social values, and Taiwanese identification are all associated with increases in the predicted probabilities for agreeing ("strongly agree" and "agree") that the United States demonstrates commitment to Taiwan with its vaccine donation drive. Belief that the U.S. Congress and president often disagree and the perception that China and Taiwan share much cultural values shared by China and Taiwan, in contrast, are associated with increases in the predicted probabilities for disagreeing ("strongly disagree" and "agree") that the United States demonstrates a commitment to Taiwan with its vaccine donation drive. For instance, the predicted probabilities of "strong disagreement"/"disagreement" decrease from 8.2 percent/49.2 percent to 0.9 percent/21.3 percent respectively as confidence in U.S. dominance over China in Asia increases from the fifth percentile to the ninety-fifth percentile. At the same time, the corresponding predicted probabilities of "strong agreement"/"agreement" increase from 7.8 percent/34.7 percent to 32 percent/45.6 percent across the same percentile changes in respondent assessment of U.S. power relative to China. On the other hand, when the perception of U.S. political polarization increases from the fifth percentile to the ninety-fifth percentile, the predicted probabilities of "strong disagreement"/"disagreement" increases from 18.8 percent/56.7 percent to 57.8 percent/38.3 percent while the predicted probabilities for "strong agreement"/"agreement" drop from 2.7 percent/21.6 percent to 0.1 percent/3.6 percent.

In terms of generalized trust, as we move from the fifth percentile of trustfulness to the ninety-fifth percentile of trustfulness, the predicted probabilities for "strong agreement"/"agreement" increase from 6.1 percent/21.6 percent to 14.5 percent/42.3 percent and the predicted probabilities for "strong disagreement"/"disagreement" decrease from 10.2 percent/51.9 percent to 3.5 percent/39.1 percent.

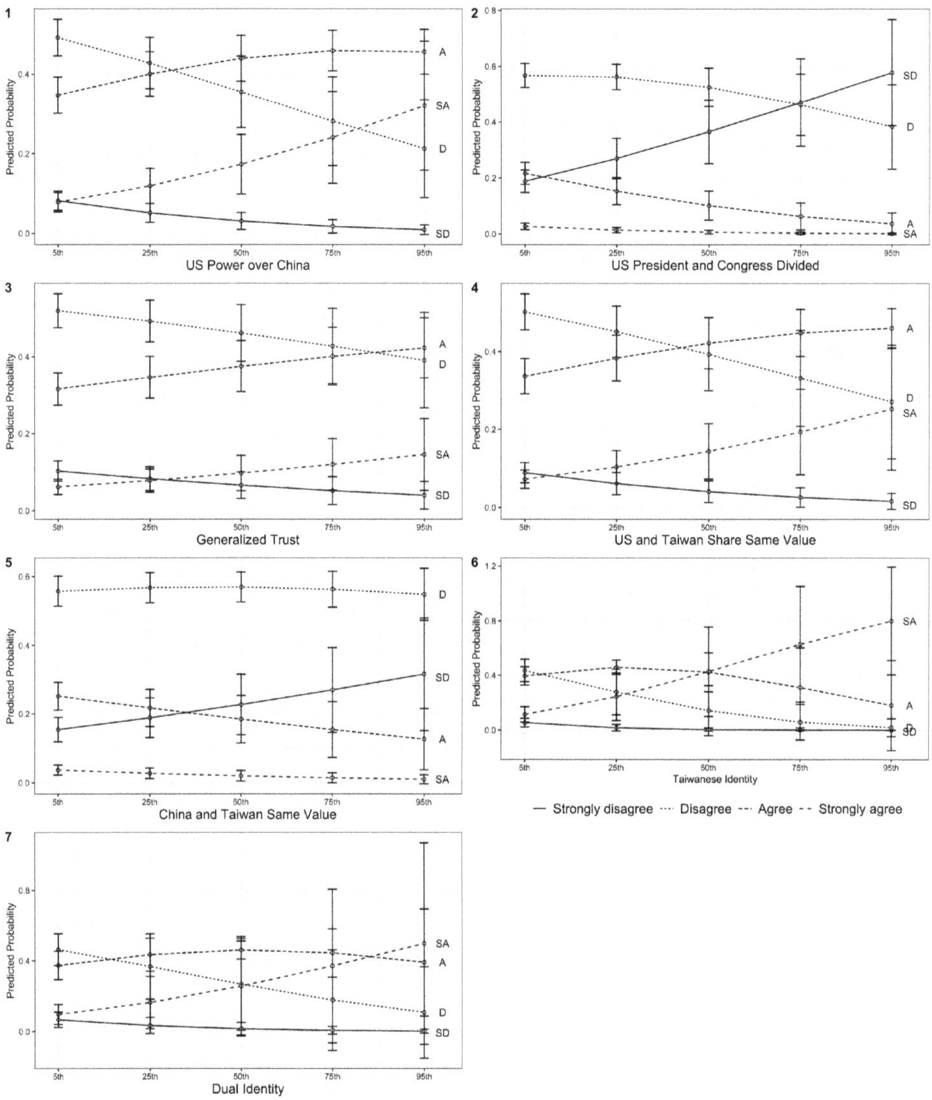

Figure 6.2. Predicted Probabilities based on Model 4 in Table 6.1

Source: ESC-Fairbank Center Survey, 2021

Turning to perceptions that the United States and Taiwan share social values, the predicted probabilities for "strong agreement"/"agreement" increase from 7.2 percent/33.6 percent to 25.2 percent/46 percent and the predicted probabilities for "strong disagreement"/"disagreement" decrease from 8.8 percent/50.2 percent to 1.6 percent/27.1 percent when perception of U.S.-Taiwan cultural affinity increases from the fifth percentile to the ninety-fifth percentile. Last, turning to the Taiwanese public's perception of China, the predicted probabilities for "strong agreement"/"agreement" increase from 6.1 percent/18.1 percent to 14.5 percent/39.5 percent and the predicted probabilities for "strong disagreement"/"disagreement" decrease from 5.4 percent/43.5 percent to 0 percent/1.9 percent when Taiwanese identification (as opposed to Chinese identification) moves from the fifth percentile to the ninety-fifth percentile. On the other hand, when perception of cultural affinity between Taiwan and China is fixed at the fifth percentile, the predicted probabilities for "strong agreement"/"agreement" are 3.6 percent and 12.6 percent, respectively. The predicted probabilities decrease to 1 percent/25.1 percent as we move to the ninety-fifth percentile perception of cultural affinity. In sum, the predicted probabilities show that images of China and U.S. power, generalized trust, and social identity concerns have very substantive effects on how our respondents assess the signaling value of the U.S. vaccine donation drive.

CONCLUSION

In this chapter, we have empirically demonstrated that the U.S. vaccine donation drive to Taiwan constitutes a cross-domain signal, and its efficacy rests on the respondents' images of the United States and China, generalized trust, and identity. Respondents who believe that the United States is more powerful than China in Asia and that the U.S. Congress and president work together are more likely to associate vaccine diplomacy with U.S. commitment to Taiwan. Respondents who trust other countries, identify as Taiwanese, and believe that Taiwan and the United States share many social values are also more likely to associate U.S. vaccine donation with U.S. commitment to Taiwan. On the other hand, people who think that China is more powerful than the United States, identify as

Chinese, and do not trust other countries tend to disagree that U.S. vaccine donation shows any commitment to Taiwan.

Our preliminary analysis confirms the role of nonrationalist hypotheses on cross-domain signaling about perceptions of shared culture and identity. Importantly, our results also have important policy implications. First, domestic political polarization—in Taiwan, driven by disagreement over Taiwan's identity—may also lead to polarization of the marketplace of ideas for foreign policy. In this study, we see a clear division between respondents who identify with the Taiwanese nation and the United States and respondents who identify with China in terms how they assess the U.S. vaccine donation drive. Domestic identity politics complicate international signaling. Second, Chinese criticisms of American and Japanese vaccine donations from the United States and Japan to Taiwan may remind the Taiwanese public of U.S.-China tensions and differences between Taiwan and China. These criticisms are therefore counterproductive—even from the Chinese perspective—as they could intensify dynamics of intergroup conflict, improve the efficacy U.S. cross-domain signaling, and drive the Taiwanese public further away from China.

NOTES

1. One might challenge this point by arguing that a strong U.S. commitment could encourage freeriding. See Olson and Zeckhauser 1966. But see also Alley 2021.

2. We draw on the idea of cross-domain signaling (Gartzke and Lindsay 2019) where policy in one domain (for example, public health) may serve communicative purposes in another domain (for example, international security). The concept of cross-domain signaling has been mainly applied to deterrence, and the domains concern land, sea, air, space, and cyberspace military operations.

3. In contrast, prior to 2020 the United States and China engaged in varying degrees of cooperative management of SARS after 2003, the 2014 Ebola outbreak in West Africa, HIV-AIDs in China, and various flu epidemics. See https://www.rand.org/content/dam/rand/pubs/testimonies/CT500/CT523/RAND_CT523.pdf; https://www.cartercenter.org/resources/pdfs/peace/china/trs-03-combating-ebola-breakout.pdf.

4. https://www.newsweek.com/china-accuses-biden-administration-suspicious-intentions-after-plan-donate-millions-covid-shots-1592506.

5. As Biden noted in his summit with Xi Jinping in November 2021, "It seems to me we need to establish some common-sense guardrails." https://www.nytimes.com/live/2021/11/15/world/biden-xi-summit.

6. https://www.usaid.gov/news-information/press-releases/oct-21-2021-commemorating-200-million-us- donated-covid-19-vaccines-successfully.

7. One might argue, in contrast, that this might be a case where a weak executive branch has its hands tied by a stronger legislature. This would mean that the U.S. commitment is especially credible because the executive is unable to resist congressional pressure (see Schultz 1998), which is for the foreseeable future to be hawkish and pro-Taiwan. We would argue, however, that rational Taiwanese respondents would see this commitment as unstable precisely because it rests on a shorter-term electoral cycle, the product of which could be a relatively stronger executive or a relatively weaker legislature.

8. See, for example, https://www.reuters.com/world/asia-pacific/pushing-against-china-us-lawmakers-plan-pro-taiwan-bill-2021-06-16/.

9. Equating capabilities with resolve is a tendency that even foreign policy analysts may sometimes exhibit (Kertzer 2016, 142).

10. We generate all predicted probabilities using the R package ggeffects. All numeric covariates are set to the mean, while all categorical covariates are set to their most common element (mode). Importantly, because the confidence intervals are link scale and not back transformed to response scale, the lower and upper bound of confidence intervals may be higher or smaller than predicted probabilities on the response scale. For more details, see https://cran.rproject.org/web/packages/ggeffects/ggeffects.pdf.

REFERENCES

Abdelal, Rawi, Mark Blyth, and Craig Parsons. 2010. "Introduction: Constructing the International Economy." In *Constructing the International Economy*, edited by Rawi Abdelal, Mark Blyth, and Craig Parsons, 1–19. Ithaca: Cornell University Press.

Alley, Joshua. 2021. "Reassessing the Public Goods Theory of Alliances." *Research and Politics* (January–March): 1–7.

Elster, Jon, ed. 1986. *Rational Choice*. New York: New York University Press.

Gartzke, Eric, and Jon Lindsay, eds. 2019. *Cross-Domain Deterrence: Strategy in an Era of Complexity*. Oxford: Oxford University Press.

Haass, Richard, and David Sacks. 2021. "The Growing Danger of U.S. Ambiguity on Taiwan." *Foreign Affairs*, December 13. https://www.foreignaffairs.com/articles/china/2021-12-13/growing-danger-us-ambiguity-taiwan.

Johnston, Alastair Iain, Tsai Chia-hung, George Yin, and Steven Goldstein. 2021. "The Ambiguity of Strategic Clarity." *War on the Rocks*, June 9. https://warontherocks.com/2021/06/the-ambiguity-of-strategic-clarity/.

Kahneman, Daniel. 2011. *Thinking, Fast and Slow*. New York: Farrar, Straus and Giroux.

Kahneman, Daniel, and Shane Frederick. 2002. "Representativeness Revisited: Attribute Substitution in Intuitive Judgment." In *Heuristics and Biases: The Psychology of Intuitive Judgment*, edited by T. Gilovich, D. Griffin, and D. Kahneman, 49–81. Oxford: Oxford University Press.

Kertzer, Joshua D. 2016. *Resolve in International Politics*. Princeton, NJ: Princeton University Press.

Nickerson, Raymond S. 1998. "Confirmation Bias: A Ubiquitous Phenomenon in Many Guises." *Review of General Psychology* 2 (2): 175–220.

Olson, Mancur, and Richard Zeckhauser. 1966. "An Economic Theory of Alliances." *The Review of Economics and Statistics* 48 (3): 266–79.

Rothstein, Bo, and Dietlind Stolle. 2008. "The State and Social Capital: An Institutional Theory of Generalized Trust." *Comparative Politics* 40 (4): 441–59.

Schultz, Kenneth A. 1998. "Domestic Opposition and Signaling in International Crises." *The American Political Science Review* 92 (4): 829–44.

Sugimoto, Koji, and George Yin. 2021. "With Vaccine Diplomacy to Taiwan, U.S. and Japan Steal March on China." *The National Interest*, June 28. https://nationalinterest.org/blog/buzz/vaccine-diplomacy-taiwan-us-and-japan-steal-march-china-188739?utm_source=researcher_app&utm_medium=referral&utm_campaign=RESR_MRKT_Researcher_inbound.

Tajfel, Henri., and John C. Turner. 1979. "An Integrative Theory of Inter-Group Conflict." In *The Social Psychology of Inter-Group Relations*, edited by W. G. Austin and S. Worchel, 33–47. Monterey, CA: Brooks/Cole.

Wohlforth, William C. 1993. *The Elusive Balance: Power and Perceptions During the Cold War*. Ithaca, NY: Cornell University Press.

7

The COVID-19 Pandemic and Cross-Strait Relations

Fang-Yu Chen, Austin Wang,
Charles K. S. Wu, and Yao-Yuan Yeh

INTRODUCTION

This chapter reviews how cross-Strait relations evolved under the COVID-19 pandemic from 2020 to 2021. We first discuss various critical events in Taiwan and how the pandemic was employed as an information cue in framing cross-Strait relations, including the Taiwanese government's response to the onset of the COVID-19 pandemic toward China, Chinese information penetration through disinformation tools during the pandemic, and debates over validity and reliability of COVID-19 vaccines. Furthermore, we investigate whether the COVID-19 pandemic has changed the public perception/assessment of cross-Strait relations and which direction it has brought to the Taiwanese public.

THE COVID-19 PANDEMIC AND CROSS-STRAIT RELATIONS

Crises or natural disasters often provide an opportunity for people to shake hands and cooperate, but, unfortunately, the pandemic does not provide much thawing of cross-Strait relations. Since the beginning of the pandemic in early 2020, China has found ways to isolate Taiwan internationally, threaten Taiwan's security, and sow discord to increase polarization and dissent within Taiwan. For instance, during the pandemic, China has increased the frequency of intruding into Taiwan's

Air-Defense Identification Zone (ADIZ). In 2021 alone, there were 950 intrusions into Taiwan's ADIZ. Compared to 2020, the frequency increased by 60 percent.[1] Despite the overt threats from China, most citizens in Taiwan remain unfazed.

China also utilizes the pandemic to suppress Taiwan's international participation. The most iconic event revolves around Taiwan's bid to join the World Health Organization (WHO). Not being a member of the WHO was a critical reason why Taiwan was hit especially hard during SARS.[2] Consequently, since the inception of the pandemic, Taiwan has been striving to participate in the WHO. However, such aspirations eventually went nowhere due to Chinese pressure. For instance, Taiwan was not allowed to participate in the first WHO meeting on the virus on January 22, 2020. In subsequent interactions, the organization also rejected Taiwan from sharing its experience combating the pandemic with the international community. Facing criticisms about excluding Taiwan from the organization and giving in to Chinese pressure, Director General Tedros Adhanom accused Taiwan of staging a smear campaign against him.

In addition to blocking Taiwan from joining the WHO, China also actively endangered public health in Taiwan by blocking the government's endeavors to purchase vaccines. For instance, Taiwan once reached an agreement to purchase vaccines directly from the German firm BioNTech. However, the purchase was never filled as it was later revealed due to an existing agreement between the German firm and China, Taiwan, in reality, would have to go through China and cannot directly receive vaccines from the firm.[3] In other situations, throughout the pandemic, China tried to poach Taiwan's diplomatic allies by engaging in "vaccine diplomacy," using vaccines as a quid pro quo arraignment to encourage those allies to sever ties with Taiwan.[4] The lack of vaccines endangered Taiwan's public security at the onset of COVID to a great extent.

Another incident that drew the ire of the public in Taiwan has to do with the transportation of Taiwanese citizens from the Mainland back to Taiwan at the early stage of the pandemic. The Mainland at that time already showed warning signs of a wide pandemic, whereas the situation in Taiwan was quite well under control. Thus, the government in Taiwan took cautionary steps to prevent the spread of the virus to Taiwan. During initial negotiations with China, both sides agreed that a clear list of passengers on board would be provided to help track and monitor infected individuals. To make the trip possible, the authorities in Taipei eventually gave in to China's request that the flight must be provided by the PRC's China Eastern Airlines. However, China did not live up to the agreement, as it was later found out that numerous seats were given to Taiwanese businesspeople who should not be prioritized. Worse, one within the group tested positive for COVID-19 upon landing in Taiwan. The mishap created much burden on the quarantine system and anger among the citizens in Taiwan toward the PRC.[5]

The repercussions of the previous incidents increased political polarization in Taiwan and divergent attitudes toward public health policies. For instance, the fallout of purchasing vaccines from BioNTech became a point of criticism for the KMT, who argued that the delay in purchase, coupled with the AstraZeneca vaccines considered ineffective or even dangerous, exposed citizens in Taiwan to higher risks.[6] The KMT also framed the delay in purchasing the BioNTech vaccines as a way for the Tsai administration to promote their homegrown vaccines.[7] The partisan difference is clearly visible in public opinion polls. It is thus no little surprise that in an August 2020 poll, DPP's (the incumbent party) supporters chose Medigen (Taiwan's homegrown vaccines) as their second choice for vaccination, whereas KMT supporters regarded it as their last (fourth) choice.[8]

Disinformation Came to the Forefront

Alongside flying warplanes into Taiwan's airspace and limiting Taiwan's international participation, during the pandemic, China also infiltrated Taiwan's society with disinformation campaigns. It is well known that China has been staging those attacks for years, and the pandemic and the resulting fears and anxiety among citizens created an ideal environment for such malign campaigns to take place. These attacks contributed to the polarization and cleavages inside the Taiwanese society and reduction in trust in the government.[9] A good example of such an attack occurred prior to the 2020 presidential election in Taiwan. Before the day of the presidential election in January 2020, rumors started to flow on social media sites that there were confirmed COVID cases in Taiwan and cautioned the citizens to wear masks when voting tomorrow. At such an early stage of the pandemic, such false information hoped to elicit public memories of

SARS and uncertainties of the new virus. The intent is clear—to discourage and suppress the turnout rate for the election. Fortunately, authorities and relevant NGOs quickly caught and disabused the information.[10] Unfortunately, such malign activities only continued to exacerbate during COVID in Taiwan.

Granted that disinformation and misinformation by the CCP is often not as obvious or visible as other threatening behaviors from China, such efforts to retake Taiwan with cognitive warfare could be traced back to the early 2000s. In 2008, a pro-China businessman purchased China Times Group (a newspaper company in Taiwan) and subsequently turned the newspaper and TV channels into a CCP mouthpiece. This incident is only the tip of the iceberg, as more cases were revealed in their investigations by local NGOs and the government that showed these companies' connections to the CCP. According to a report by Reuters, China paid at least five Taiwanese media companies to run certain stories in various publications and on a television channel. In one specific case, the Taiwan Affairs Office paid about $4,300 to have a pro-China news story appear in Taiwanese media outlets.[11]

Chinese efforts to influence Taiwan with misinformation showed no signs of abating during COVID. According to the Taiwan-based research group Information Operations Research Group (IORG), between January and May 2020, in one of the popular social media apps, Line, 70 percent of the 2,800 disinformation messages contained pro-China sentiment.[12] Starting in late January, when Taiwan decided not to offer masks made in China, Chinese netzines started a campaign by fabricating a Taiwanese government announcement that every citizen in Taiwan could receive ten masks immediately from medical facilities, hoping to incite anger among citizens toward the government when they do not receive masks as (falsely) promised. In order to increase the credibility of their posts, the creators of misinformation included logos and photos of real Taiwanese news outlets in their posts. According to Taiwan's Justice Investigation Bureau, there were already over four hundred cases under investigation in February, the second month when COVID became a major public concern in Taiwan.[13] In March 2020, China broadened its reach in spreading disinformation on major social media sites such as Facebook, Twitter, and YouTube to claim the Taiwanese government was intentionally hiding COVID cases and information about the deceased in the pandemic.[14]

In addition to wreaking havoc in Taiwanese society, China also attempted to misattribute the source of the pandemic in Taiwan. For instance, in early March, citizens started to receive information in Line, one of the most popular private social media messenger applications in Taiwan, that accused the United States of being the origin of the coronavirus and that 1,4000 citizens had died. In another case, when Taiwan's bid to join the WHO was struck down and citizens turned their anger toward the director-general Tedros Adhanom Ghebreyesus, messages started to float in Taiwan that focused on his personal achievements to weaken any criticisms and concerns about him.[15]

DO CHINA'S ACTIONS TOWARD TAIWAN CHANGE POLITICAL ATTITUDES IN TAIWAN?

There is some evidence to show that China's disinformation and other malign activities surrounding the pandemic worked, at least temporarily, to reduce Taiwanese's willingness to receive the vaccination. Figure 7.1 shows that public willingness to receive vaccinations dropped to around 34 percent after citizens had been bombarded with misinformation campaigns

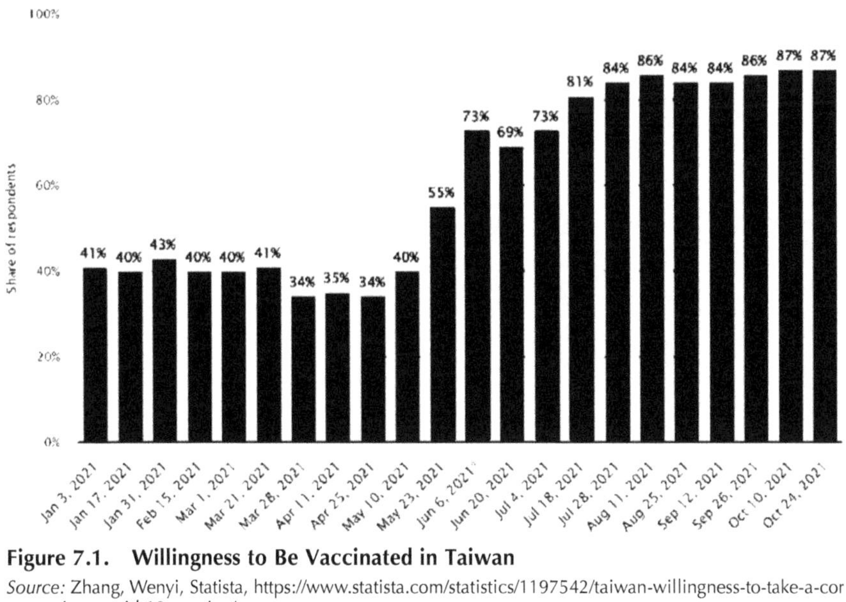

Figure 7.1. Willingness to Be Vaccinated in Taiwan

Source: Zhang, Wenyi, Statista, https://www.statista.com/statistics/1197542/taiwan-willingness-to-take-a-coronavirus-covid-19-vaccine/.

during the pandemic and that the government encountered difficulties purchasing vaccines. However, the effect is transient, as public willingness quickly recuperated to above 70 percent in just a matter of three months.

With respect to public approval of the president, we concluded that China's campaigns did little to reduce public support for the president. Numerous studies have attested to the fact that Tsai has clearly benefited from the rallying effect during the pandemic (for example, Wang and Cheng 2021). Figure 7.2 showed the results from a survey conducted by National Cheng-Chi University in Taiwan (NCCU). From the figure, we could state that Tsai's approval rate shot to 61 percent after the pandemic started in March 2020 and has remained around 50 percent since then. Such a record is impressive considering that Tsai only had 41 percent before the reelection. Interestingly, the rallying effect seems to come mostly not from Tsai's party supporters but from the opposition. In the two surveys conducted by Wang and Cheng in Taiwan in January and June 2021, 30 percent of opposition supporters and 28 percent of independents switched from disapproving to supporting the president.[16] In the same figure, we could also tell that the public became more distrusting of China, and the trajectory matched well with the increase of China's disinformation campaigns.

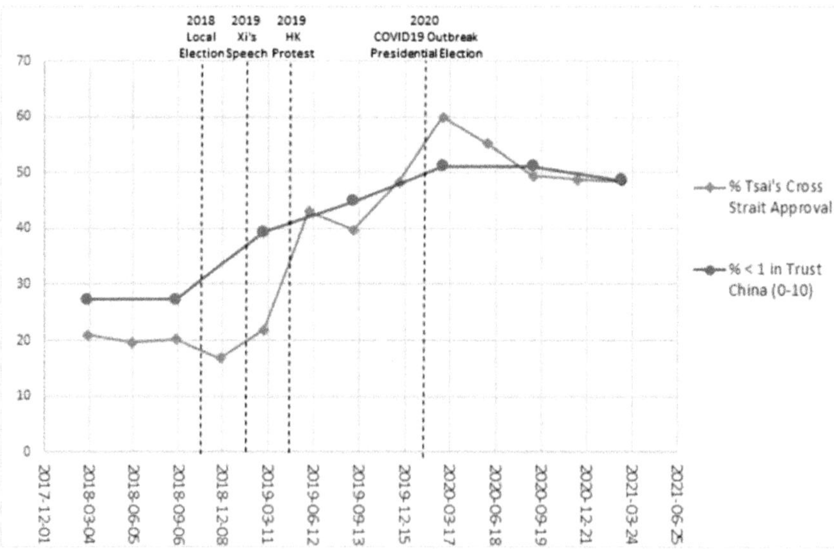

Figure 7.2. Presidential Approval and Mistrust toward China
Source: TEDS 2017PA12-2021PA06.

Independence and Identity

Does the pandemic create changes in Taiwanese citizens' views about independence and identity? On views toward the country's political future, figure 7.3 revealed a number of insights about the dynamics of public opinion from 2019 to 2020. First, there was a significant increase in public support for the stance of "maintain status quo, move toward independence" (from 21.8 percent to 25.5 percent). Figure 7.4, based on the results from TEDS, showed a similar trend: support for independence grew around 18 percent in March 2020 compared to a year ago. Second, Taiwan's sharp increase in support for eventual independence also translated into corresponding changes in identity as well. Figure 7.5 showed that from 2019 to 2020, those that chose the option that their identity is "Taiwanese only" increased from 58.5 percent to 64.3 percent, whereas those that identified as "both Taiwanese and Chinese" dropped from 34.7 percent to 29.9 percent.

The explanations for this sharp increase in support for independence and Taiwanese identity are twofold. First, the society in Taiwan closely watched how the protests in Hong Kong transpired from 2019 to 2020.

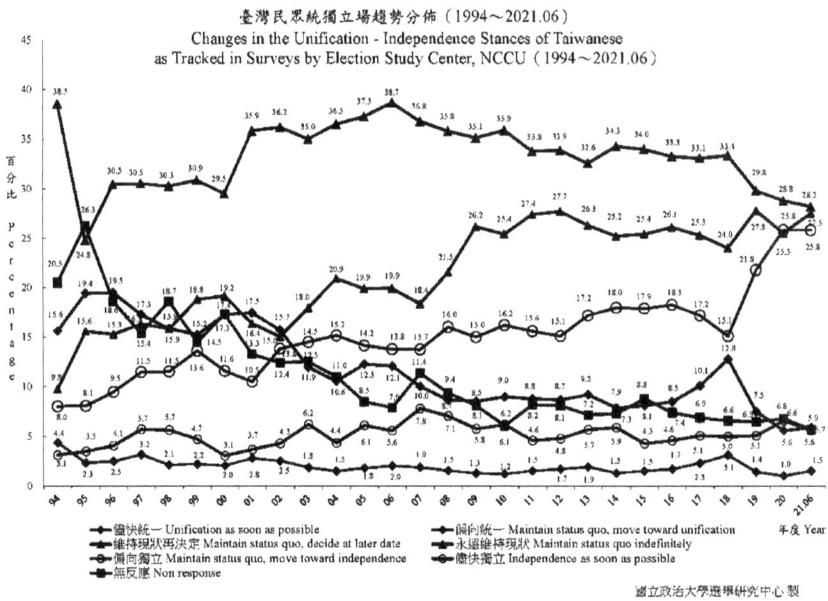

Figure 7.3. Attitude toward China-Taiwan Relationship in Taiwan
Source: NCCU-ESC, 1994–2021.

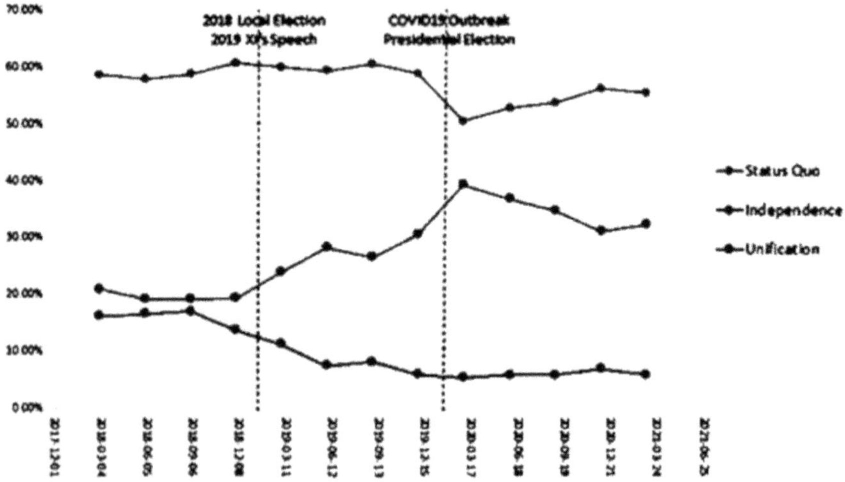

Figure 7.4. Attitude toward China-Taiwan Relationship in Taiwan
Source: TEDS 2017PA12-2021PA06.

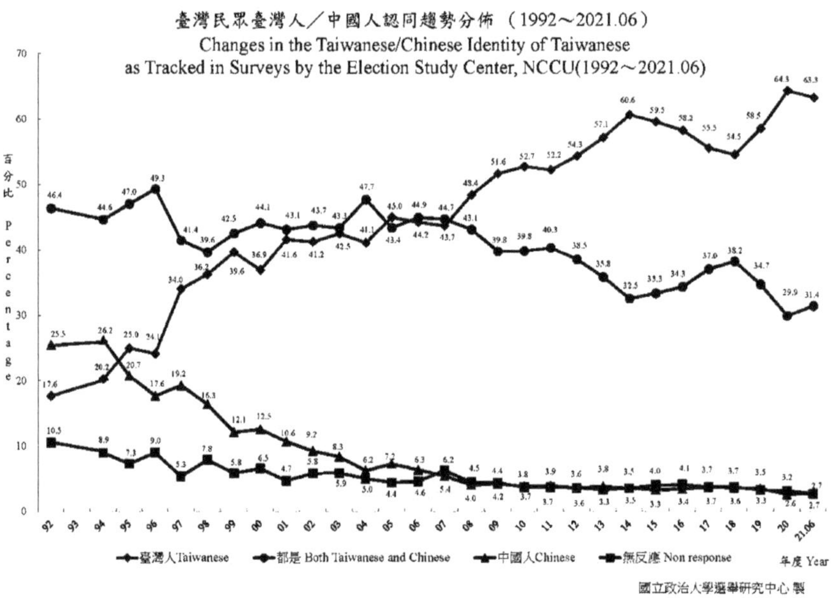

Figure 7.5. Change of National Identity in Taiwan
Source: NCCU-ESC, 1994–2021.

Beijing's severe crackdowns on protestors and civilians crashed any lingering hopes among citizens in Taiwan of the "one country, two systems" proposal and contributed to Tsai's landslide in her reelection in 2020.[17] The Hong Kong protest for many was an awakening call that only independence could preserve the island's democratic way of life. Another factor was Xi Jinping's speech on January 2, 2019, in which he proclaimed that "reunification is the historical trend and the right path, Taiwan independence is . . . a dead end" and "we make no promise to renounce the use of force and reserve the option of taking all necessary means."[18] The messages and the content were not new, and it only reinforced negative public perception in Taiwan toward the regime.

Public Willingness for Self-Defense

The pandemic coincided with some reports indicating that China could use force against Taiwan as early as 2025.[19] The worries also promoted inquiries within academia and policy circles into citizens' willingness to defend themselves should China attack.[20] Admittedly, many observers were pessimistic about Taiwanese citizens' willingness for self-defense, for reasons such as the country has greatly reduced the duration of mandatory conscription to just four months. However, the evidence we presented here contradicted such thinking—the public in Taiwan consistently demonstrated a high level of willingness to defend themselves.

As early as 2018, citizens were asked the following question by the Taiwan Foundation of Democracy: "Would you fight for Taiwan if Taiwan formally announces independence that causes Mainland China to use force against Taiwan?" The majority of respondents (55 percent) gave an affirmative answer.[21] Because most in Taiwan know that declaring independence is tantamount to provoking a war with China, the position, fight for Taiwan's independence, has not been the majority preference among the citizenry in Taiwan. Thus, we can imagine that in other scenarios where the conflict is not provoked by the Taiwan side (such as Taiwan maintaining the status quo but being attacked by China), the willingness for self-defense could be higher. And there was evidence to support such a conjecture. In 2021, the Taiwan New Constitution Foundation asked respondents if they would be willing to go to the battlefield if China invaded Taiwan: 65 percent said yes.[22] Another survey asking a similar question by the Taiwan International Strategic Study Society in 2020 showed a whopping 77.6 percent.[23]

The most recent polls, conducted after Russia invaded Ukraine, reflected an even higher level of willingness for self-defense among citizens in Taiwan. A poll by the Taiwan International Strategic Study Society and Taiwan International Studies Association reached several critical conclusions. First, the majority of citizens in Taiwan disagreed with the viewpoint that "today's Ukraine is tomorrow Taiwan," a defeatist slogan that started to appear after the war started. Concerning self-defense, over 70 percent of citizens expressed willingness to defend Taiwan if a war breaks out, reaffirming what we knew from previous polls. Another important finding was that citizens in urban areas, such as Taipei and Kaohsiung, showed a much higher willingness for self-defense.[24] In another survey conducted shortly after the onset of the Russo-Ukrainian War, the majority (48.9 percent) in Taiwan agreed with the statement, "some claim that in order to protect Taiwan's sovereignty from the PRC, we also need to do whatever it takes, even our own life."[25] Certainly, partisanship should influence one's willingness for self-defense, with DPP supporters being more supportive of defending Taiwan's sovereignty than KMT supporters. Nevertheless, even when the partnership was taken into consideration, the interpretations did not vary greatly. For instance, in a survey by a pan-blue think tank, over 40 percent of respondents opined that they would support the Taiwanese government in such an armed conflict, while only 7 percent expressed their willingness to leave Taiwan when conflicts occur.[26] At any rate, there was a sizable population in Taiwan that was willing to defend themselves.

In addition to willingness for self-defense, other polls tapped into citizens' expectations of the likelihood that a conflict will break out, especially after Russia invaded Ukraine. A poll by Formosa News asked Taiwanese citizens the following: "The Russo-Ukrainian War has drawn much international attention. In light of the current cross-Strait relations, do you think it is possible that China would invade Taiwan?" 37.4 percent of respondents said it was possible, while the majority (55 percent) dismissed such a possibility. The same survey also asked, "Some say that to resolve the long-lasting political dispute across the Strait, a war across the Strait is inevitable, do you agree or disagree with such a viewpoint?" Most citizens rejected such a viewpoint (56 percent). It is worth noting that most (over 60 percent) supporters from both major parties rejected such an idea, but the younger generations and those with higher education tended to believe that war was inevitable.[27]

Views on Conscription

Suffice it to say that the military in Taiwan has not been highly regarded for decades, and many citizens that go through conscription often complain about their experience. While some support the country's full transition into an all-voluntary force and the shortening of conscription to four months, others have dobuts of those plans and believe that the country should revert to the conscription system.

One reason proponents think it is necessary to move back to the one-year conscription is that the all-voluntary system has failed to meet its recruitment goals. In 2021, it was 7,000 short of the government's goal of 169,000. The shortage could potentially get worse as Taiwan continues to face a low birth rate and an aging population. Additionally, the new voluntary system also has a retention challenge. Every year, around 20 percent of recruits drops out, incurring unnecessary costs of training. Relatedly, the lack of supply of soldiers makes it difficult to sustain or expand elite divisions or units that require more long-term training. Despite these shortcomings, the Ministry of Defense in Taiwan defends the system by stating any voluntary soldier would serve at least four years under their contract, so in the end, they will be more combat ready than those who only have a four-month training.[28]

Reverting back to the one-year conscription also seems politically unappealing, as the current administration often counts on the younger generations for electoral support in the upcoming mayoral and presidential elections. Enforcing the change runs the risk of antagonizing this group. Here, public opinion polls could provide evidence to see if such electoral concerns are warranted. Overall, multiple polls suggested reverting to previous longer periods did have strong backing. For example, in 2020, the Taiwan National Security Survey concluded that 75 percent of the citizens in Taiwan considered the current conscription "too short." In the longstanding China Impact Survey by the Sociology Institute at Academia Sinica in Taiwan, the percentage of citizens that wanted the government to revive the conscription system increased from 60 percent in 2015 to

86 percent in 2017.[29] After the Russo-Ukrainian war started, a poll by Taiwan's International Strategic Study Society and Taiwan International Studies Association reached an identical conclusion—close to 70 percent of citizens support prolonging the current four-month period.[30]

While discussions for potential changes are still in the air, in early March 2022, the government has rolled out a new system of military leave that asks citizens to come back to the military for a short-term period of training. The change was proposed and adopted last year in 2021, and the Russo-Ukrainian war inadvertently created much attention for this new program. The new system is different from the original plan in important ways. The training period has been extended to two weeks, whereas the old system only required five days. The training also emphasized combat and shooting exercises, and reservists were assigned to areas close to where they lived.[31]

TRAJECTORIES OF CROSS-STRAIT RELATIONS

For Taiwan, the pandemic and worsening Sino-U.S. relations have attracted more attention and support from the international community. In addition to the vocal support from various governments around the world to support Taiwan's international participation, polls in many countries have also started to exhibit trends that support Taiwan among its citizenry. Public support and attention from other citizens will create impetus, legitimacy, and motivation for politicians to enact policies beneficial for Taiwan.

For instance, multiple polls in Japan in March 2022 indicated that the majority of citizens were worried that China would imitate Russia to invade Taiwan. For instance, when the Mainichi newspaper and Saitama University's Social Survey Research Center jointly conducted a poll, the results showed that nine out of ten Japanese citizens were afraid of such a possibility.[32] In preparation for a potential conflict across the Strait, Japan has also started to reevaluate its defense strategy and posture. Comments from officials in Japan documented these policy changes. In 2021, Japan's defense white paper referred to Taiwan as "important for Japan's security and the stability of the international community." The intention to support Taiwan was echoed by statements made by the defense minister, who maintained that "the peace and stability of Taiwan is directly connected to Japan" in an interview with Reuters.[33] Concomitantly, in 2021, for the first time in several decades, both the United States and Japan emphasized the importance of peace and security in the Taiwan Strait in an official bilateral meeting.[34] These changes of mindsets in Japan lead us to foresee potential changes to Japan's article 9 in its constitution. The constitution went through some changes in 2015 to allow Japan a list of options to increase their influence in the Taiwan Strait. Going forward, it remains to be seen if such involvements will be made more explicit and its scale and magnitude will be magnified.[35]

In terms of U.S.-Taiwan relations, several developments will benefit Taiwan's security. First, support for helping Taiwan among Americans has come to an all-time high. In the annual survey by the Chicago Council of Global Affairs, 2021 was the first time in decades that the majority of Americans (52 percent) supported using troops to defend Taiwan facing China's invasion. Just a year ago, the support rate was only 41 percent.[36] In another survey of elites and the public by Center for Strategic and International Studies in 2020, the results showed that both groups were prepared to take a considerable risk to defend Taiwan. On a scale of 1–10, where "10" means "worth taking a significant risk," Taiwan scored almost 8 in the leaders group and almost 7 among the public.[37]

In addition to public support, there are other movements in terms of legislations that are worth watching. For instance, several congressional leaders have started to push for reforms of the Taiwan Relations Act to allow the president to react more swiftly to contingencies in the Taiwan Strait. Currently, the act requires the president to seek congressional approval before intervening militarily should China invade Taiwan, a process that could easily take months and waste crucial moments for an early response. China could also be embolden knowing the lengthiness the process could take. The new bills propose solutions from alleviating the president of the burden to allowing the president to send in the military if China makes a direct attack on Taiwan.[38]

Another area to watch for U.S. policy toward Taiwan is the convergence of opinions for the United States to move away from its current strategic ambiguity policy toward Taiwan. Whereas some agree that it is necessary for the United States to keep this policy, we could see a gradual change in the number of supporting altering the policy. Most notably, the former Japanese prime minister Shinzo Abe commented in public in early 2022 that the United States should abandon such a policy.[39] The core of the strategic ambiguity rests on a key belief, that is, the United States will continue to be able to deter an increasingly assertive China with growing military capabilities.[40] However, as China continues to increase its military power by creating military installments in the South China Sea, for instance, most scholars do not have confidence in the vitality of this belief.

In reality, it could be argued that the policy is limiting Taiwan's security. Most citizens in Taiwan have mistaken the strategic ambiguity to be a security guarantee from the United States to protect them. Without a significant policy change, most in Taiwan will continue to be believe that the United States would come to Taiwan's defense, under all circumstances, in the event of a war with China. The belief is an important reason why military preparations have slacked off in Taiwan, underserving what the policy is for in the first place.[41] Clearly, a reassessment and reevaluation of the strategic ambiguity policy is necessary.

NOTES

1. ANI Asia 2021.
2. Chiou 2020.
3. Davidson 2021.
4. BBC 2021.
5. Lee, Wu, and Chung 2020; Yang and Hetherington 2020.
6. Chen 2021.
7. Hioe 2021.
8. Luo 2021.
9. Harold, Beauchamp-Mustafaga, and Hornung 2021.
10. Taiwan FactCheck Center 2020.
11. Lee and Cheng 2019.
12. Wang 2020.
13. TNL News 2020..
14. Monaco 2020.
15. Wang 2020.
16. Wang and Cheng 2021.
17. Bernstein 2020.
18. Griffiths 2019.
19. Davidson and Borger 2021.

20. Yeh and Wu 2021; Wu, Chen, Horng-En, and Yeh 2022; Wang et al. 2023.
21. Lin 2018.
22. Teon 2021.
23. Wu 2020.
24. Radio Free Asia 2022.
25. Formosa 2022.
26. Li 2021.
27. Ibid.
28. DW 2022.
29. Institute of Sociology n.d.
30. Tan Yingying 2022.
31. Blanchard 2022.
32. Nakamichi 2022.
33. Reuters 2021.
34. Ashley 2021.
35. Bosack 2021.
36. Smeltz and Kafura 2021.
37. "Mapping the Future of U.S. China Policy," CSIS, https://chinasurvey.csis.org/about/.
38. Doornbos 2022.
39. Moriyasu 2022.
40. Bandow 2021.
41. Wu et al. 2021.

REFERENCES

ANI Asia. 2021. "3 Chinese Warplanes Enter Taiwan Air Defense Zone, 23rd Intrusion of Month." *Business Standard*, December 31. Accessed February 10, 2023. https://www.business-standard.com/article/international/3-chinese-warplanes-enter-taiwan-air-defence-zone-23rd-intrusion-of-month-121123100517_1.html#:~:text=Taiwan%20on%20Thursday%20said%20it,increase%20from%20the%20previous%20year.

Ashley, Ryan. 2021. "Japan's Revolution on Taiwan Affairs." *Texas National Security Review*, November 23. Accessed February 13, 2023. https://warontherocks.com/2021/11/japans-revolution-on-taiwan-affairs/.

Bandow, Doug. 2021. "It's Time to End 'Strategic Ambiguity.'" CATO Institute, December 16. https://www.cato.org/commentary/its-time-end-strategic-ambiguity.

BBC. 2021. "Taiwan Accuses China of 'Vaccine Diplomacy' in Paraguay." April 7. Accessed February 10, 2023. https://www.bbc.com/news/world-asia-56661303.

Bernstein, Rachel. 2020. "The Impact of the Hong Kong Protests on the Election in Taiwan." The National Bureau of Asian Research, January 23. https://www.nbr.org/publication/the-impact-of-the-hong-kong-protests-on-the-election-in-taiwan/.

Blanchard, Ben. 2022. "Ukraine War Gives Taiwan's Military Reservist Reform New Impetus." *Reuters*, March 12. Accessed February 13, 2023. https://www.reuters.com/world/asia-pacific/ukraine-war-gives-taiwans-military-reservist-reform-new-impetus-2022-03-12/.

Bosack, Michael Macarthur. 2021. "What Can Japan Do in a Taiwan-China Clash?" *The Japan Times*, March 24. Accessed February 13, 2023. https://www.japantimes.co.jp/opinion/2021/03/24/commentary/japan-commentary/taiwan-self-defense-forces-china-u-s-defense/.

Chen, Kelvin. 2021. "Taiwan Ruling Party Calls Out Opposition's Vaccine Hypocrisy." *Taiwan News*, June 28. Accessed February 10, 2023. https://www.taiwannews.com.tw/en/news/4234523.

Institute of Sociology. N.d. "China Impact Survey." Academic Sinica. Accessed November 1, 2021. https://efenci.srda.sinica.edu.tw/webview/index.jsp?object=https://efenci.srda.sinica.edu.tw:80/obj/fCatalog/Catalog18.

Chiou, Katie. 2020. "China's Taiwan Policy Hurts World Health." *World Street Journal*, February 13. Accessed February 10, 2023. https://www.wsj.com/articles/chinas-taiwan-policy-hurts-world-health-11581618021.

Davidson, Helen. 2021. "Taiwan Accuses China of Interfering with Covid Vaccine Deals." *The Guardian*, May 27. Accessed February 10, 2023. https://www.theguardian.com/world/2021/may/27/taiwan-president-accuses-china-interfering-covid-vaccine-deals.

Davidson, Helen, and Julian Borger. 2021. "China Could Mount Full-Scale Invasion by 2025, Taiwan Defense Minister Says." *The Guardian*, October 6. Accessed February 12, 2023. https://www.theguardian.com/world/2021/oct/06/biden-says-he-and-chinas-xi-have-agreed-to-abide-by-taiwan-agreement.

Doornbos, Caitlin. 2022. "House Lawmaker Calls for Legislation to Allow a Faster US Military Response Should China Invade Taiwan." *Star and Stripes*, January 12. Accessed February 13, 2023. https://www.stripes.com/theaters/us/2022-01-12/taiwan-china-invasion-navy-legislation-ships-luria-biden-4272849.html.

DW 德國之聲. 2022. "Yanzhang yiwu bingyi? Taiwan guofang mianlinde shizilukou" 延長義務兵役？台灣國防面臨的十字路口 [Prolonging conscription, cross-roads for Taiwan's defense]. March 17. Accessed February 13, 2023. https://bit.ly/36rnbPI.

Formosa 美麗島電子報. 2022. "Meilidaomindiao: 2022nian 3yue guozheng mindiao" 美麗島民調：2022年3月國政民調 [Formosa polls: 2022 March national sentiments]. March 28. Accessed February 13, 2023. http://my-formosa.com/DOC_181756.htm.

Griffiths, James. 2019. "Xi Jinping Warns Taiwan Independence Is 'a Dead End.'" *CNN*, January 2. Accessed February 12, 2023. https://www.cnn.com/2019/01/02/asia/xi-jinping-taiwan-tsai-intl/index.html.

Harold, Scott W., Nathan Beauchamp-Mustafaga, and Jeffrey W. Hornung. 2021. "Chinese Disinformation Efforts on Social Media." RAND. https://apps.dtic.mil/sti/pdfs/AD1142311.pdf.

Hioe, Brian. 2021. "The Politics of Taiwan's Covid-19 Response." *The Diplomat*, September 10. Accessed February 10, 2023. https://thediplomat.com/2021/09/the-politics-of-taiwans-covid-19-response/.

Lee, I-Chia, Liang-yi Wu, and Li-hua Chung. 2020. "Wuhan Flight Passenger List Rumors Ignite Furor." *Taipei Times*, February 6. https://www.taipeitimes.com/News/front/archives/2020/02/06/2003730449.

Lee, Yimou, and I-hwa Cheng. 2019. "Paid 'News': China Using Taiwan Media to Win Hearts and Minds on Island—Sources." *Reuters*, August 9. Accessed February 10, 2023. https://www.reuters.com/article/us-taiwan-china-media-insight/paid-news-china-using-taiwan-media-to-win-hearts-and-minds-on-island-sources-idUSKCN1UZ0I4.

Li, Tzu-Yin. 2021. "What Would Citizens Do If Taiwan and China Go to War? Results Are Surprising." *China Times*, September 29. Accessed February 13, 2023. https://www.chinatimes.com/realtimenews/20210929002379-263101?chdtv&fbclid=IwAR1r-55GpMZQtHAYM9CjxPV7qBukfF1N4XKnJ4zHhZK0Z0skQO3GNdrM7qk.

Lin, Sean. 2018. "Taiwanese Willing to Fight China." *Taipei Times*, April 20. Accessed February 12, 2023. https://www.taipeitimes.com/News/front/archives/2018/04/20/2003691661.

Luo, Li-Bang 羅立邦. 2021. "Taiwan Mingyi Jijinhui Mindiao" 台灣民意基金會民調 [TPOF polls—favor Medigan over AZ; citizens preferences on vaccines revealed]. *Fengchuanmei* 風傳媒, August 24. Accessed February 10, 2023. https://www.storm.mg/article/3897422.

Monaco, Nick. 2020. "No Rest for the Sick: Coronavirus Disinformation from Chinese Users Targets Taiwan." Digital Intelligence Lab, March 5. Accessed February 10, 2023. https://medium.com/digintel/china-coronavirus-disinfo-targets-taiwan-2490d99ce6a9.

Moriyasu, Ken. 2022. "U.S. Should Abandon Ambiguity on Taiwan Defense: Japan's Abe." *Nikkei Asia*, February 27. Accessed February 13, 2023. https://asia.nikkei.com/Politics/U.S.-should-abandon-ambiguity-on-Taiwan-defense-Japan-s-Abe.

Nakamichi, Takashi. 2022. "Majority of Japanese Worry China May Invade Taiwan: Polls." *Bloomberg*, March 19. Accessed February 13, 2023. https://www.bloomberg.com/news/articles/2022-03-20/majority-of-japanese-worry-china-may-invade-taiwan-poll-shows.

Radio Free Asia 自由亞洲電台. 2022. "Taiwan qicheng minzhon yuanyi weitai erzhan bingliting yanzhang guojun yiwuyiqi" 臺灣七成民衆願意爲臺而戰併力挺延長國軍義務役期 [70% of citizens support defending Taiwan and prolonging conscription]. March 15. Accessed February 13, 2023. https://www.rfa.org/mandarin/yataibaodao/gangtai/hcm2-03152022082446.html.

Reuters. 2021. "Tokyo Says Taiwan Security Directly Connected to Japan—Bloomberg." June 24. Accessed February 13, 2023. https://www.reuters.com/article/japan-taiwan-china-security/tokyo-says-taiwan-security-directly-connected-to-japan-bloomberg-idUSL3N2O64E5.

Smeltz, Dina, and Craig Kafura. 2021. "For First Time, Half of Americans Favor Defending Taiwan If China Invades." Chicago Council on Global Affairs, August 26. https://www.thechicagocouncil.org/research/public-opinion-survey/first-time-half-americans-favor-defending-taiwan-if-china-invades.

Taiwan FactCheck Center 台灣事實查核中心. 2020. "Wan cheng dajia toupiao dantian jide yidingyao dai kouzhao . . . wu han nabien di buming feiyan . . . taiwan ye you chuizhengbingli?" 網傳大家投票當天記得一定要戴口罩哦 . . . 武漢 那邊的不明肺炎 . . . 臺灣也有確診病例? [Internet rumor. Everyone must remember to wear a mask during the election day . . . unverified pneumonia in Wuhan . . . Taiwan has confirmed cases?]. January 10. Accessed February 10, 2023. https://tfc-taiwan.org. tw/articles/1955.

Tan Yingying 譚英瑛. 2022. "【taiwan guoji zhanrue xiehui mindiao】70%yuanweibao Taiwan erzhan, 77% panliangan heping, Taiwanren henmaodun" 【台灣國際戰略學會民調】70%願為保台而戰、77%盼兩岸和平 台灣人很矛盾 [Taiwan International Strategic Study Society poll: 70% willing to fight for Taiwan; 77% hoping for peace. Taiwanese face a dilemma]. March 15. Accessed February 13, 2023. https://polls.com.tw/14205/.

Teon, Aris. 2021. "64% of Taiwanese Willing to Fight If China Attacked, Poll Shows." *The Greater China Journal*, August 12. Accessed February 12, 2023. https://china-journal.org/2021/08/12/64-of-taiwanese-willing-to-fight-if-china-attacked-poll-shows/.

TNL News 關鍵評論. 2020. "Taiwan minyi jijinhui mindiao" 台灣疫情失控, 每人可領10片口罩 [Taiwan pandemic losing control; every citizen could claim

10 masks]. February 28. Accessed February 10, 2023. https://www.thenewslens.com/article/131849.

Wang, Austin Horng-En, Charles K. S. Wu, Fang-Yu Chen, and Yao-Yuan Yeh. 2023. "High-Level Visit and National Security Policy: Evidence from a Quasi-Experiment in Taiwan." *International Interactions*.

Wang, Shi 王希. 2020. "Taiwan yiqing yueyanzhong, LINE qunzu qu qinzhong bushi zhixunxi yue fanlan jian" 台灣疫情越嚴重, LINE 群組親中不實訊息越氾濫 [Taiwan pandemic worsens, coupled with pro-China propaganda on Line]. IORG, July 9. Accessed February 10, 2023. https://iorg.tw/_en/a/pro-china-line-messages.

Wang, T. Y., and Su-Feng Cheng. 2021. "COVID-19 and the Anatomy of the Rally Effect in Taiwan." *Asian Survey* 61 (3): 388–410.

Wu, Charles K. S., Fang-Yu Chen, Austin Horng-En, and Yao-Yuan Yeh. 2022. "Public Support for the Use of Force in Non-Western and Non-Major Powers: The Case of a China–Taiwan War." *International Political Science Review*.

Wu, Charles K. S., Yao-Yuan Yeh, Fang-Yu Chen, and Austin Horng-En Wang. 2021. "Why the US Should Ditch Strategic Ambiguity Toward Taiwan." *The Defense Post*, December 1. Accessed February 13, 2023. https://www.thedefensepost.com/2021/12/01/us-strategic-ambiguity-taiwan/.

Wu, Su-Wei. 2020. "More than 77 Percent Willing to Fight in the Event of an Invasion by China: Poll." *Taipei Times*, October 25. Accessed February 13, 2023. https://www.taipeitimes.com/News/taiwan/archives/2020/10/25/2003745764.

Yang, Chun-hui, and William Hetherington. 2020. "Virus Outbreak: China Meddles with Evacuation Flights." *Taipei Times*, March 12. Accessed February 10, 2023. https://www.taipeitimes.com/News/front/archives/2020/03/12/2003732531.

Yeh, Yao-Yuan, and Charles K. S. Wu. 2021. "When War Hits Home: Taiwanese Public Support for War of Necessity." *International Relations of the Asia-Pacific* 21 (2): 265–93.

8

The Effectiveness of the COVID-19 Pandemic Policy in China

Hsuan-Yu Shane Lin, Charles K. S. Wu, Yao-Yuan Yeh

INTRODUCTION

Does regime type matter for fighting the pandemic? This is the question that numerous works on COVID grapple with, but a consensus has yet to be formed. The situations in the United States and China are often drawn as a comparison.[1] Figure 8.1 shows the United States and China's daily new COVID-19 cases from January 2020 to November 2021. As of November 2021, China has effectively curbed the number of new cases despite being a country with a vast territory and population, while the situation for the United States is much direr. Although numerous scholarly works such as Cepaluni, Dorsch, and Branyiczki (2020);[2] Piazza and Stronko (2020);[3] and Bunyavejchewina and Sirichuanjunb (2021)[4] have argued that authoritarian regimes are more effective at combating the pandemic, others disagree. Work by Frey, Chen, and Presidente (2021)[5] points out that although autocracies can rule out more stringent policies than democracies, the latter is significantly more effective (20 percent) in reducing geographic mobility among citizens, a key factor to ensuring that policies as social distancing can be successful. Last, work by Kleinfeld (2020) suggests that neither regime type is better at fighting the pandemic.[6]

On the surface, the disparity could be attributed to different policies. The United States takes a laissez-faire attitude to coexist with the virus, with policies including opening its borders, wearing masks, and increas-

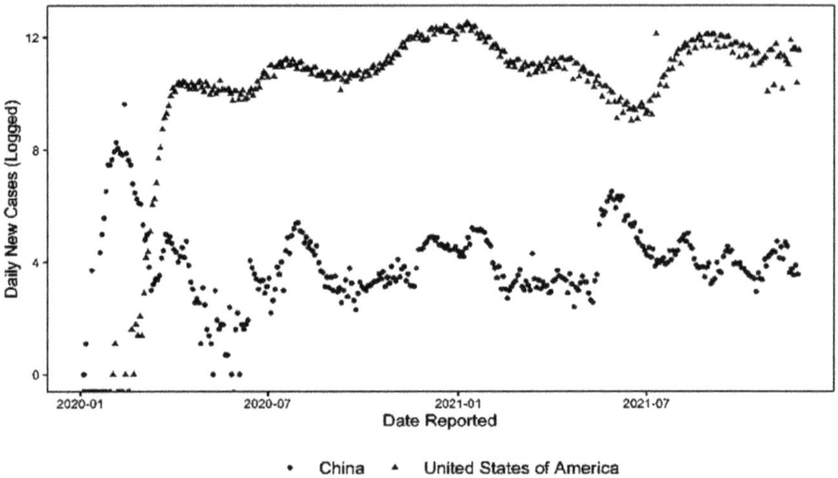

Figure 8.1. United States and China's Daily New COVID-19 Cases, January 4, 2020, to November 22, 2021

Source: The World Health Organization COVID-19 Dashboard.

ing the vaccination rate. This living-with-the-virus strategy, while it cannot eliminate the spread of the virus, allows society to go mostly back to normal, including resuming travel, social interactions, and business activities. On the other hand, China employed the zero-COVID strategy to eliminate the coronavirus within its borders. The strategy includes draconian measures, including month-long quarantine regulations for international and intraprovincial travelers, extensive testing, contact tracing, and community lockdowns if there are confirmed cases. As new virus variants continue to appear, even the *Washington Post* believes China's zero-COVID strategy is more appropriate.[7]

Although it is still early to tell which policy is superior and ascertain the criteria for making that decision, not everyone agrees that China has the upper hand in dealing with COVID. To begin with, some speculate on the accuracy of the case report. Authoritarian regimes like China tend to underreport COVID cases so that it could mislead the international society about the severity of the pandemic inside their country. Analyses by Kapoor et al. (2020)[8] and Adiguzel et al. (2020)[9] suggest that China's reported deaths do not exhibit characteristics of naturally produced data.

Others suggest no significant relationship exists between regime type and casualties of COVID. When researchers consider the transparency of reporting, there ceased to be any relationship between regime type and

COVID deaths.[10] The disparity and unresolved inquiry lead us to wonder: To what extent does the nature of the autocratic regime contribute to their superior performance, and how does the regime type influence the design, execution, and effectiveness of COVID-19 policies?

In this chapter, we argue that overemphasizing the factor of the regime type neglects critical nuances that could reveal important insights about how countries deal with the pandemic. For instance, in addition to a country's regime, the society's willingness to cooperate with its government's professional public health guidelines and its willingness to sacrifice personal freedom temporarily are also key factors. In this view, democracy can still implement effective[11] COVID-19 policies if citizens are willing to cooperate. In other words, autocratic institutions are not the only reason for China to contain COVID. Furthermore, the harsh policies imposed by autocratic institutions could actually incur backlash or draw unintended consequences, ultimately weakening the effectiveness of such policies.

We begin by reviewing extant scholarly work on the influence of regime types on combating the COVID-19 pandemic. And then, we zoom into China's policy responses to the COVID-19 pandemic, with more emphasis on research in political science than public health. In other words, we will not render judgment as to whether a specific COVID-19 policy helps contain the spread of the virus. In the end, based on China's responses to the COVID-19 pandemic, we discuss what we can learn from China's reactions and their implications for the world. This chapter provides insights into the core elements leading to China's seemingly successful COVID-19 policies and contributes to the ongoing debate about the influence of regime type on combating COVID-19.

CHINA'S RESPONSES TO THE EARLY OUTBREAK OF COVID-19 IN CHINA

Before we discuss some of the factors that motivate democracies and autocracies to respond to the pandemic differently, we first review the early timeline of the coronavirus outbreak in China to have a clearer sense of how the Chinese government responded to the outbreak. We will focus on China's "zero-COVID" strategy and explore the relationship between the "zero-COVID" strategy and the nature of autocracy.

China's Early Response

COVID-19, first identified in Wuhan, China, in late 2019, became a global pandemic.[12] In late December, hospitals in Wuhan started to discover novel cases of pneumonia. The Wuhan Municipal Health Commission released "urgent notices" to local hospitals about unknown diseases linked to the Huanan Seafood Wholesale Market in Wuhan. The notices were leaked online, and some local medical workers, including ophthalmologist Li Wenliang, who was posthumously labeled as a whistleblower of COVID-19, exchanged messages about this unknown disease online. Chinese and Taiwanese netizens widely shared the message.

On December 31, 2019, the Wuhan Municipal Health Commission issued a public statement on the outbreak, admitting that there had been twenty-seven cases. The next day, authorities shut down the city's wholesale seafood market. On the same day, the city's Public Security Bureau announced the investigation of eight citizens for "spreading rumors" about the virus. Dr. Li Wenliang was also reprimanded for spreading allegedly false statements about the outbreak online. The week after, a research team at Fudan University in Shanghai sequenced the novel coronavirus genome and deposited the genome in the U.S. National Institutes of Health's GenBank database of publicly available DNA sequences. Two days after, the Chinese Center for Disease Control and Prevention (China CDC) released a report sequencing the genome of the novel coronavirus. On January 12, Dr. Li Wenliang was hospitalized because of the coronavirus and passed away on February 7.

In late January, the Chinese government confirmed that the coronavirus could transmit from person to person. Soon, Wuhan established an epidemic prevention and control command center. China declared this disease a statutory notifiable infectious disease under the PRC Law on the Prevention and Treatment of Infectious Diseases and infectious disease for the purposes of the PRC Health and Quarantine Law; since then, the Chinese government has provided the legal foundation for local officials to conduct mandatory public health policies, such as mandatory quarantines and lockdowns. On the same day, almost one month after the outbreak in Wuhan, Chinese President Xi Jinping issued an "important instruction" to prioritize epidemic prevention and control work and orders "timely issuance of epidemic information and deepening of international cooperation."

On January 23, Wuhan's epidemic command center issued its first order, suspending public transportation and locking down the whole Wuhan city. On the next day, additional cities in the Hubei Province, where Wuhan is in, also imposed travel and transport restrictions on their residents. On January 25, China's seven-man Communist Party Politburo Standing Committee, the Chinese Communist Party's most senior and powerful decision-making body, met and, for the first time, put the COVID-19 issue into its agenda.

China's "Zero-COVID" Policy

Since the outbreak, China has adopted a series of policies to contain the spread of the virus, such as border control, strict quarantine rules, mass testing, contact tracing, and regional lockdowns. The major goal of these strict policies is to cut virus transmission chains, preventing more people from being infected. These measures are consistent with what public health experts suggested to adopt during the outbreak and were later followed by many other states. However, after the appearance of vaccines, several countries, such as the United States and Japan, adjusted their policies; they opened their borders and schools incrementally and resumed economic activities.

Although the pandemic has been controlled to a certain extent, the Chinese government still decided to enforce most of these strict policies. The decision to continue these strict measures to eliminate the existence of COVID-19 within its borders reflected the idea of "zero-tolerance." News media use the "zero-COVID" strategy or policy to refer to a government's continuation of conducting strict COVID-19 policies aiming to make the coronavirus disappear in its territories.

Under this principle, the Chinese government has been conducting serious contact tracing and requires their close contacts to quarantine and receive the polymerase chain reaction (PCR) test to the source of contagion. In practice, the government often enforced a regional lockdown when a group could be exposed to the virus or had contact with confirmed cases—the lockdown of Shanghai's Disneyland was an example. On October 31, 2021, Shanghai Disneyland announced the closure of their park as city healthcare workers conducted mass testing of all the visitors.[13] The action originated from a confirmed case in the nearby city of Hangzhou, which had visited Disneyland Park the day before the lockdown. Tens of thousands of families and visitors received the testing and waited for the testing result in the park and were permitted to leave if the result was negative.

The Disneyland lockdown is one of the many cases illustrating the Chinese government's "zero-COVID" policy. The government mobilizes its sources, including staff and society, to cut the virus' transmission chain as quickly as possible. However, it is worth discussing whether China's continuing "zero-COVID" policy is proportionately effective and the extent to which the policy's continuation and its seemingly "success" reflect the nature of autocracy.

HOW DEMOCRACIES AND AUTOCRACIES RESPOND TO COVID-19 DIFFERENTLY

The rapid response from China created a sharp contrast with the policies and responses from democracies. Democracies are often lauded for their successes in improving public health compared to autocracies in areas such as infant mortality, life expectancy, and mortality from noncommunicable diseases (McGuire 2013; Wigley and Akkoyunlu-Wigley 2011; Bollyky et al. 2019). So what challenges do democracies face that prevent them from handling the pandemic as swiftly as authoritarian regimes?

The first reason is politicization, defined as how certain facts or ideas are being interpreted politically and consequently become the subject of contestation surrounding this pandemic.[14] Political discussions on COVID, as their predecessors, are politicized and polarized.[15] For instance, in Italy, the media's COVID-19-related narratives focused more on politics than science.[16] The situation in the United States is no different—Box-Steffensmeier and Moses find clear partisan differences in the tone of congressional members in social media messages from members of the U.S. Congress related to the COVID-19 pandemic.[17]

Green et al. found evidence to suggest that both parties talk about COVID-19 differently on social media.[18] On Twitter, Democratic congressional members mentioned the pandemic more often than their GOP counterparts. In addition to talking about the pandemic more frequently, Democratic leaders focused more on the threat of the pandemic on public health and U.S. workers, while GOP members focused more on the culpability of China in spreading the virus and the negative economic impact on businesses. Clearly, the divergent and partisan-divided elite cues impacted how the public reacted to the pandemic. It is possible that GOP supporters, receiving the cues from their leaders, became less aware of the threat of COVID-19 to their own health to focus more on the economy and the China issue.

Comparatively, autocracies are less likely to be hindered by politicization concerns as their government holds a tight grip on their media. State-owned media in autocracies are mouthpieces of their government. Molter and DiResta outline three recurring behaviors during the outbreak of the pandemic of Chinese state media: sharing positive stories and promoting the party's response, rewriting recent history in a manner favorable to the Chinese Communist Party, and using targeted ads to spread preferred messages.[19] These efforts make the public in autocracies less likely to receive "politicized" and politically polarized messages about the pandemic than the public in democracies.

The second challenge that delays the response of democracies in this public health crisis is misinformation (and disinformation). Misinformation refers to false or inaccurate information, regardless of an intent to deceive, spreading among a targeted society.[20] Disinformation is a subset of misinformation that is intentionally false and intended to deceive or mislead.[21] The openness of the internet environment in most democracies makes it difficult to stop the spread of misinformation.

When misinformation about COVID-19 vaccines surfaced, it reduced some citizens' willingness to receive vaccination, undermining their government's effort to combat the pandemic. Take Taiwan as an example. Disinformation about the serious side effects of AZ vaccines and the fatal consequences of receiving Moderna mRNA vaccines may have scared certain Taiwanese citizens away from receiving the shot.[22] Likewise, the Russian antivaccine disinformation campaign targeted at Western countries also reduced citizens' willingness to vaccinate.[23]

Misinformation undermines not only the effectiveness of democratic governments' COVID-19 policies but also citizens' perceptions of their own or other governments. On December 2021, Meta Platforms Inc., formerly known as Facebook Inc., removed more than five hundred

China-based Facebook accounts that sought to push a false narrative about the U.S. government's attempts to blame the Chinese government for the pandemic. These fake accounts, along with some Chinese state-controlled media, broadcasted the story on social media platforms.[24] The story may change how people in the United States or other countries view the U.S. and Chinese governments during the pandemic and may increase people's negative perceptions of the U.S. government. Arguably, increasing negative perceptions of the U.S. government may undermine the solidarity of the U.S. society and the democratic world in combating the pandemic. Of course, the target is mainly non-Chinese citizens because several mainstream Western-based social media platforms are banned in China. The spread of misinformation about COVID-19 and democracies' relative internet openness together, to some extent, reduce the effectiveness of democracies' COVID-19 policies.

In autocracies like China, information is highly controlled and monitored by the Chinese government.[25] If the government notices any misinformation that it believes may disrupt its COVID-19 policy enforcement or touch upon politically sensitive issues such as the Tiananmen Square Incident, the government can immediately "remove" the information before it reaches citizens. Democratic governments cannot censure information like that. Even when the information directly threatens national security, democratic governments still have to tread carefully to justify their actions to censor and limit the spread of such information.[26]

The third challenge is from the public. Citizens in democracies often voice their dissent against government policies: freedom of speech and movement are core elements of a democracy. It is natural that public preferences do not always align with guidelines by public health professionals. This pressure from the public may impede the progress and efficiency of democratic governments in implementing public health protocols. Strong public opposition can be an essential reason why democracies often take harsh measures at a slower pace.[27]

Choosing between a lockdown or allowing economic activities to continue was the dilemma many democracies faced at the height of the pandemic. Democratic governments, however, often encounter strong opposition from citizens. For example, in late November 2021, the Netherlands decided to reimpose some lockdown measures due to a resurgence of coronavirus cases. Displeased by the lockdown measures, thousands of citizens went onto the streets to protest, eventually leading to riots and gunfire exchanges.[28] Public protests against COVID-19 restrictions also broke out in other European democracies such as Belgium, Austria, Croatia, and Italy.[29] In July 2020, at the peak of the pandemic outbreak, there were numerous antimask rallies in several U.S. states, such as Florida and Utah, although 3.5 million had already contracted the virus, and the health community strongly backed such a policy.[30] These protests highlight the fact that democratic governments have to respond to challenges from the virus and pressure from the public, which, if neglected, can dim their political future.

AUTOCRATIC NATURE AND CHINA'S "ZERO-COVID" STRATEGY

Aside from the reasons that prevent democracies from reacting sooner, what explains China's iron-fist efforts to contain the spread of the virus in their governing area? One possible explanation is a concern for their own political career. Chinese officials are fearful that the pandemic would jeopardize their political careers if left uncontrolled. Even when some local officials took a more lenient approach to deal with the pandemic, pressure from the central government often forced them to change their course of action. For instance, some Chinese officials were removed from their positions or punished over accusations of failing to respond properly to the pandemic.[31] Four officials in Manzhouli, a border city in northern China, were disciplined for failing to stop the disease from spreading as the city reported thirty new delta variant cases.[32] Fear of punishment motivated Chinese officials to take drastic measures to contain the virus. This motivation can explain why officials in Shanghai were willing to lock down the whole Disneyland Park and conduct mass testing when a confirmed case visited the park one day before. In the northern city of Heihe, local officials even declared a "people's war," providing up to $15,600 to reward residents for reporting illegal hunting, animal smuggling, or people crossing the border to fish. At the end of the day, incurring the public's wrath might still be preferable to being fired by their boss.[33]

Aside from obedience to higher authorities of local officials, the Communist Party also needs a "zero-COVID environment" to advance its political agenda or maintain its ruling legitimacy. The "zero-COVID" environment is propagandized as the Chinese government's achievement, creating an image that the regime cares deeply about its citizens. The policy also helped drum up national pride among citizens, allowing the regime to draw a sharp contrast between the United States and China in the number of COVID cases. "Community solidarity has been unprecedented during the COVID-19 outbreak in China."[34] Chinese media, such as the Xinhua News Agency, helped the regime's propaganda by making videos that suggest that the Chinese government's responses to the pandemic are superior to the U.S. government's.[35] Likewise, the editor-in-chief of the *Global Times*, a tabloid under the auspices of the Chinese Communist Party's official *People's Daily* newspaper, said that foreigners are jealous of China's virus-fighting record and criticized that the United States has eased pandemic controls because it values "money over life."[36] China's autocratic nature, for better or worse, "helps" the Chinese government to enforce these strict COVID-19 policies and mobilize the societal resources to combat the coronavirus.[37]

The central question is to what extent is China's "zero-COVID" strategy directly related to its autocratic nature? In reality, a zero-tolerance strategy is not exclusive to autocracies. While many democracies decided to gradually loosen the control and reopen society as their vaccination rate is rising, not all democracies are like that. Taiwan is one of the democratic cases that continues its "zero-COVID" strategy even when things were clearly better. Taiwan closed its borders from March 2020 to October 2022 and conducted very strict COVID-19 policies. Most residents in Taiwan showed a strong willingness to cooperate with the government. In other words, a strict strategy is not a policy China could implement. In addition to strict policies, it is also erroneous to suggest that democracies could not react swiftly. In the case of South Korea, two key reasons allowed the government to create a rapid response: close cooperation between the state and the private sector and the citizens' willingness to accept medical intervention.[38] Additionally, another faculty argument is that the sacrifices of political freedom and civil liberties by autocratic regimes are justifiable, as research shows that, three months into the pandemic, their records were no different from nondemocratic states.

We argue that the autocratic nature may be likely to impact the effectiveness of China's COVID-19 policies negatively. Because Chinese officials put their political careers ahead of people's well-being, they would not take into consideration whether these strict policies, such as sudden announcements of two-week lockdowns, may seriously hurt their people's economic, social, and psychological well-being. For the foreseeable future, Chinese officials will be rigid in adjusting their strict COVID-19 policies. The Xian lockdown from December 2021 to January 2022 is again a vivid case. Hospitals in this city rejected patients because the latter could not provide a COVID-19 negative result, leading to some Xian citizens dying or losing babies.[39]

The rigidity and lack of respect for public opinion would increase risks for an autocracy like China. Such policies would gradually sap people's patience and tolerance for the policy and the regime. Citizens would be increasingly tired of obeying the government's policies despite its propaganda about its COVID-19 achievement. The government may find it more difficult to enforce these strict policies. The tension between people and the government, at least at the local government level, may increase if the government does not adjust its policies with flexibility. Amid the tension, resentment, and tiredness, any small social issue, even non-COVID issues, may trigger conflicts between the government and society.

Historically, numerous incidents have suggested that the public reacts negatively to restrictions on their freedom. A strict quarantine measure also induced unintended consequences. For instance, citizens flocked to rural areas in India when the lockdown was announced, endangering local civilians that the policy should protect in the first place.[40] Protests against lockdown have also sparked protests worldwide, which elevated the potential for contagion among citizens. The Xian lockdown also caused tension between Chinese citizens and the local government. Xian residents complained that they did not have enough food and water, and the food price had become extremely expensive during the lockdown,[41] and the strict lockdown triggered an answer.[42]

Although it could seem too early to tell as new variants of the virus continue to surface, there are reasons to suggest that democracies could prevail against autocracies in handling a pandemic. First, compared to autocracies, democracies, in general, are also more receptive to open information than autocracies, so citizens in democracies will have more accurate, diverse, and timely information to safeguard their own interests. The informational advantage not only helps democracies design more effective policies that help their own citizens,[43] but authoritarian regimes often delay in providing solutions to major issues in their political systems.[44]

A democracy could also enforce a strict policy without the consequences of democratic backsliding. Taiwan, a democracy, conducts similar policies without pausing. Thus, a deciding factor for rolling out effective policies might not be regime type but state capacity. Scholars have found a relationship between state capacity, defined as the state's capacity to carry out its policies,[45] and its ability to design and implement policies to respond to natural disasters and pandemics.[46] Strong state capacity can positively help both democracies and nondemocratic regimes.[47] Democracies with strong capacities are certainly up for the task.

Allowing autocracies to continue to upload the sacrifices as a necessarily evil also would jeopardize the opportunities for the international society to react preemptively to the next pandemic. An often-neglected point in discussions of the pandemic is that, when it first originated in China, the civil society and local government had opportunities to distinguish it in the city. Unfortunately, as with how authoritarian regimes deal with controversial topics, information about the pandemic on social media was censored, and even a prominent physician's warning met punishment from relevant authorities. These mistakes prevent the international society from getting prepared and responding to COVID.

In conclusion, as an editor of the *Lancet* points out, achieving effective implementation of control measures for COVID-19 requires broad community engagement. The key is whether the public is willing to cooperate with their government, temporarily sacrificing their individual freedom. However, achieving collective solidarity arguably is a bit challenging for democratic societies, especially those highly polarized ones. Also, the openness of democracies may somehow delay the speed for the whole society to reach a consensus because of politicized public health issues and the spread of misinformation; this slowness in response may largely impact the effectiveness of democracies' COVID-19 policies. However, one thing is clear, improving the quality of democracy, rather than downgrading democracy, is the way to go for democracies and is what we learned from this global public health crisis.

NOTES

1. Dilip Hiro, "Comparing the US' and China's Response to Covid-19," *The Nation*, April 28, 2020, https://www.thenation.com/article/world/coronavirus-us-china-response/.
2. Cepaluni, Dorsch, and Branyiczki 2020.
3. Piazza and Stronko 2020.
4. Bunyavejchewin and Sirichuanjun 2021.
5. Frey, Chen, and Presidente 2020.
6. Kleinfeld 2020.
7. Christian Shepherd and Lyric Li, "As Omicron Variant Spreads, China Senses Vindication over 'Zero Covid' Strategy," *The Washington Post*, November 30, 2021, https://www.washingtonpost.com/world/asia_pacific/china-omicron-variant-coronavirus/2021/11/30/74e9788e-518d-11ec-83d2-d9dab0e23b7e_story.html.
8. Kapoor et al. 2020.
9. Fatih, Cansunar, and Corekcioglu 2020.
10. S. Annaka, "Political Regime, Data Transparency, and COVID-19 Death Cases," *SSM Popul. Health* 15 (2021): 100832.
11. By effective, we mean containing the spread of the virus within a country's borders.
12. The U.S. Congressional Research Service, a federal legislative branch agency answering requests from congressional members, published a report on COVID-19 and China, providing a clear timeline of the outbreak of the pandemic. The following description about the outbreak is cited from this report.
13. The Associated Press, "Shanghai Disneyland on Lockdown as Officials Test 30,000 Visitors," *NBC News*, November 1, 2021, https://www.nbcnews.com/news/world/shanghai-disneyland-lockdown-officials-test-30000-visitors-rcna4226.
14. Pillar 2010.
15. Greene 2022.
16. Stefano Crabu et al. 2021.
17. Box-Steffensmeier and Moses 2021.
18. Green et al. 2020.
19. Molter and DiResta 2020.
20. Meira Gebel, "Misinformation vs. Disinformation: What to Know About Each Form of False Information, and How to Spot Them Online," *Business Insider*, January 15, 2021, https://www.businessinsider.com/misinformation-vs-disinformation.

21. Ibid.

22. Taiwan FactCheck Center, https://tfc-taiwan.org.tw/articles/5135.

23. Jamie Dettmer, "Russian Anti-Vaccine Disinformation Campaign Backfires," Voice of America, November 18, 2021, https://www.voanews.com/a/russian-anti-vaccine-disinformation-campaign-backfires/6318536.html.

24. Naomi Nix, "Meta Removes China-Based Network Pushing Covid-19 Misinformation," *Bloomberg Technology*, December 1, 2021, https://www.bloomberg.com/news/articles/2021-12-01/meta-removes-china-based-network-pushing-covid-19-misinformation.

25. King, Pan, and Roberts 2017.

26. Note that we are not debating about whether democratic governments should obtain more information censoring power; instead, we want to point out the essential differences between democracy and autocracy and how these differences may impact the effectiveness of their COVID-19 policies.

27. A. Sebhatu, K. Wennberg, S. Arora-Jonsson, and S. I. Lindberg, "Explaining the Homogeneous Diffusion of Covid-19 Policies among Heterogeneous Countries," *PNAS* 117, (2020): 21201–8.

28. News Agencies, "COVID Protests in Netherlands Turn Violent for a Second Night," *Aljazeera*, November 21, 2021, https://www.aljazeera.com/news/2021/11/21/covid-protests-in-netherlands-turn-violent-for-second-night.

29. Daniel Michaels and Francis X. Rocca, "New Covid-19 Restrictions Spark Protests Across Europe," *Wall Street Journal*, November 20, 2021, https://www.wsj.com/articles/rioting-erupts-during-covid-19-rules-protest-in-the-netherlands-11637412545.

30. Tommy Beer, "Anti-Mask Rallies Continue in U.S. Amid Rising Coronavirus Cases And Death," *Forbes*, July 16, 2020, https://www.forbes.com/sites/tommybeer/2020/07/16/anti-mask-rallies-continue-in-us-amid-rising-coronavirus-cases-and-deaths/?sh=7e124c982246.

31. AP, "COVID-19: China Punishes 30 Officials for Pandemic Failing," *The Times of India*, August 9, 2021, https://timesofindia.indiatimes.com/world/china/covid-19-china-punishes-30-officials-for-pandemic-failing/articleshow/85168896.cms.

32. Amber Wang and Simone McCarthy, "Coronavirus: Officials Punished as China Races to Contain Inner Mongolia Outbreak," *South China Morning Post*, December 5, 2021, https://www.scmp.com/news/china/science/article/3158523/coronavirus-officials-punished-china-races-contain-inner?module=perpetual_scroll&pgtype=article&campaign=3158523.

33. Helen Davidson, "Chinese City Offers Cash for Clues as Covid Outbreak Declared a 'People's War,'" *The Guardian*, November 9, 2021, https://www.the

guardian.com/world/2021/nov/09/chinese-city-offers-cash-for-clues-as-covid-outbreak-declared-a-peoples-war.

34. The Lancet 2020.

35. Xinhua News Agency, October 28, 2021, http://news.xhby.net/tuijian/202110/t20211028_7289680.shtml.

36. The Economist, "Chaguan: China Will Stick to a Zero-Covid Policy, for Now," *The Economist*, November 13, 2021, https://www.economist.com/china/2021/11/12/china-will-stick-to-a-zero-covid-policy-for-now.

37. Nelson 2021.

38. https://www.washingtonpost.com/outlook/2020/04/10/south-korea-is-winning-fight-against-covid-19-us-is-failing/.

39. Phoebe Zhang, "Woman Says Father Died of Heart Attack After Being Denied Admission to Xian Hospital Amid Covid-19 Controls," *AsiaOne*, January 6, 2022, https://www.asiaone.com/china/woman-says-father-died-heart-attack-after-being-denied-admission-xian-hospital-amid-covid-19.

40. Mehta 2020.

41. Ken Moritsugu, "In Chinese City Locked Down Due to Coronavirus, Some Complain Food Hard to Find," *PBS News*, January 4, 2022, https://www.pbs.org/newshour/world/in-chinese-city-locked-down-due-to-coronavirus-some-complain-food-hard-to-find.

42. Saphora Smith, "Harsh Covid Lockdown in Chinese City Xi'an Triggers Online Anger," *NBC News*, January 7, 2022, https://www.nbcnews.com/news/world/xian-china-harsh-covid-lockdown-triggers-anger-coronavirus-rcna10989.

43. Baumgartner et al. 2017.

44. Chan and Zhao 2016.

45. Tilly 1985.

46. Kahn 2005; Raschky 2008; Lin 2015.

47. Hanson 2015; Knutsen 2013.

REFERENCES

Baumgartner, Frank R., et al. 2017. "Budgetary Change in Authoritarian and Democratic Regimes." *Journal of European Public Policy* 24 (6): 792–808.

Bollyky, Thomas J., Tara Templin, Matthew Cohen, Diana Schoder, Joseph L. Dieleman, and Simon Wigley. 2019. "The Relationships Between Democratic Experience, Adult Health, and Cause-Specific Mortality in 170 Countries Between 1980 and 2016: An Observational Analysis." *The Lancet* 393 (10181): 1628–40. https://doi.org/10.1016/S0140-6736(19)30235-1.

Box-Steffensmeier, Janet M., and Laura Moses. 2021. "Meaningful Messaging: Sentiment in Elite Social Media Communication with the Public on the Covid-19 Pandemic." *Science Advances* 7 (29): eabg2898. https://doi.org/10.1126/sciadv.abg2898.

Bunyavejchewinan, P., and K. Sirichuanjun. 2021. "How Regime Type and Governance Quality Affect Policy Responses to COVID-19: A Preliminary Analysis." *Heliyon* 7.

Cepaluni, G., M. Dorsch, and R. Branyiczki. 2020. *Political Regimes and Deaths in the Early Stages of the COVID-19 Pandemic*. Scholarly Paper ID 3586767, Social Science Research Network, Rochester, New York.

Chan, Kwan Nok, and Shuang Zhao. 2016. "Punctuated Equilibrium and the Information Disadvantage of Authoritarianism: Evidence from the People's Republic of China." *Policy Studies Journal* 44 (2): 134–55.

Crabu, Stefano, Paolo Giardullo, Andrea Sciandra, and Federico Neresini. 2021. "Politics Overwhelms Science in the Covid-19 Pandemic: Evidence from the Whole Coverage of the Italian Quality Newspapers." *PLOS ONE* 16 (5): e0252034. https://doi.org/10.1371/journal.pone.0252034.

Fatih, Serkant Adiguzel, Asli Cansunar, and Gozde Corekcioglu. 2020. "Truth or Dare? Detecting Systematic Manipulation of COVID-19 Statistics." *Journal of Political Institutions and Political Economy* 1 (4): 543–57.

Frey, C. B., C. Chen, and G. Presidente. 2020. "Democracy, Culture and Contagion: Political Regimes and Countries Responsiveness to Covid-19." Oxford Martin School, May 13. https://www.oxfordmartin.ox.ac.uk/publications/democracy-culture-and-contagion-political-regimes-and-countries-responsiveness-to-covid-19/.

Green, Jon, Jared Edgerton, Daniel Naftel, Kelsey Shoub, and Skyler J. Cranmer. 2020. "Elusive Consensus: Polarization in Elite Communication on the Covid-19 Pandemic." *Science Advances* 6 (28): eabc2717-eabc17. https://doi.org/10.1126/sciadv.abc2717. https://pubmed.ncbi.nlm.nih.gov/32923600.

Greene, Steven, Marc Hetherington, Rahsaan Maxwell, and Timothy J. Ryan. 2022. "Public Service Announcements and Promoting Face Masks During the Covid-19 Pandemic." *P.S.: Political Science & Politics* 55 (1): 7–12. https://doi.org/10.1017/S1049096521001086. https://www.cambridge.org/core/article/public-service-announcements-and-promoting-face-masks-during-the-covid19-pandemic/E39BBE374C492FB031348CBC8A0DA255.

Hanson, J. 2015. "Democracy and State Capacity: Complements or Substitutes?" *Studies in Comparative International Development* 50 (3): 304–30.

Kahn, M. E. 2005. "The Death Toll from Natural Disasters: The Role of Income, Geography, and Institutions." *Review of Economics and Statistics* 87 (2): 271–84.

Kapoor, M., A. Malani, S. Ravi, and A. Agrawal. N.d. "Authoritarian Governments Appear to Manipulate COVID Data." arXiv. Accessed January 15, 2022. https://arxiv.org/abs/2007.09566(2020/09/11.

King, Gary, Jennifer Pan, and Margaret E. Roberts. 2017. "How the Chinese Government Fabricates Social Media Posts for Strategic Distraction, Not Engaged Argument." *American Political Science Review* 111 (3): 484–501.

Kleinfeld, Rachel. 2020. "Do Authoritarian or Democratic Countries Handle Pandemics Better?" Carnegie Endowment for International Peace. Accessed January 15, 2022. https://carnegieendowment.org/2020/ 03/31/do- authoritarian-or-democraticcountries-handle-pandemics-betterpub-81404.

Knutsen, C. H. 2013. "Democracy, State Capacity, and Economic Growth." *World Development* 43: 1–18.

Lancet, The. 2020. "Covid-19 and China: Lessons and the Way Forward." *The Lancet* 396 (10246): 213–13. https://doi.org/10.1016/S0140-6736(20)31637-8.

Lawrence, Susan V. "Covid-19 and China: A Chronology of Events (December 2019–January 2020)." Congressional Research Service. Accessed January 15, 2022. https://crsreports.congress.gov/product/pdf/r/r46354.

Lin, T. 2015. "Governing Natural Disasters: State Capacity, Democracy, and Human Vulnerability." *Social Forces* 93 (3): 1267–300.

McGuire, Shelley. 2013. "Frayar, D.C., Ervin, R.B. Caloric Intake From Fast Food Among Adults: United States, 2007–2010. NCHS Data Brief, No. 114, February 2013. Hyattsville, MD: National Center for Health Statistics, 2013." *Advances in Nutrition* 4 (5): 578–578. https://doi.org/10.3945/an.113.003889.

Mehta, Manthank. 2020. "Covid-19: One Lakh Daily Wagers Flee Mumbai Ahead of Lockdown." *Times of India*, March 22. timesofindia.indiatimes.com/city/mumbai/covid-19-one-lakh-daily-wagers-flee-mumbai-ahead-of-lockdown/articleshow/74755595.cms.

Molter, Vanessa, and Renee DiResta. 2020. "Pandemics & Propaganda: How Chinese State Media Creates and Propagates CCP Coronavirus Narratives." *Harvard Kennedy School Misinformation Review* 1 (3).

Nelson, Michael A. 2021. "The Timing and Aggressiveness of Early Government Response to COVID-19: Political Systems, Societal Culture, and More." *World Development*: 146.

Piazza, K. S., and K. Stronko. 2020. "Democrats, Authoritarians, and the Coronavirus: Who Is Winning at Policy Efficacy? *Global Policy*, June 12. https://www.globalpolicyjournal.com/articles/health-and-social-policy/democrats-authoritarians-and-coronavirus-who-winning-policy.

Pillar, Paul R. 2010. "The Perils of Politicization." *The Oxford Handbook of National Security Intelligence*: 472–84.

Raschky, P. A. 2008. "Institutions and the Losses from Natural Disasters." *Natural Hazards and Earth System Sciences* 8 (4): 627–34.

Tilly, Charles. 1985. "War Making and State Making as Organized Crime." In *Bringing the State Back In*, edited by P. B. Evans, D. Rueschemeyer, and T. Skocpol. Cambridge: Cambridge University Press.

Stefano, Crabu, et al. 2021. "Politics Overwhelms Science in the Covid-19 Pandemic: Evidence from the Whole Coverage of the Italian Quality Newspapers." *PLOS ONE* 16 (5).

Wigley, Simon, and Arzu Akkoyunlu-Wigley. 2011. "The Impact of Regime Type on Health: Does Redistribution Explain Everything?" *World Politics* 63 (4): 647–77. https://doi.org/10.1017/S0043887111000177.

9

Pandemic Policy, Public Opinion, and Election in Japan

Koji Kagotani and Masahiro Yamada

INTRODUCTION

On December 31, 2019, an outbreak of pneumonia of unknown causes was reported in Wuhan, Hubei Province, China. On January 9, 2020, the Chinese authorities reported, via the media, that the viral pneumonia was confirmed to be caused by a novel coronavirus, unlike any other human coronavirus discovered in the past.[1] The coronavirus, so called the COVID-19, is highly contagious and can lead to death by making pneumonia more severe. The COVID-19 outbreak spread across the globe because many people could easily travel across borders in a globalized world. People everywhere confronted the global health threat associated with the COVID-19 outbreak. The COVID-19 pandemic forced politicians and policymakers to make the tough decisions of declaring a state of emergency and closing borders with the priority of protecting lives. Imposing restrictions on the movement of people has stalled economic activities, produced massive unemployment, and widened economic inequalities. Politicians and policymakers suffered from the tradeoff between saving lives and maintaining economic activities. Government policies on COVID-19 shaped public opinion in a variety of ways and generated different political outcomes.

The impact of the COVID-19 outbreak is not uniform around the world. In the early period, European countries and the United States were struggling with the COVID-19 pandemic, while East Asian countries were able to contain outbreaks. Particularly in severely affected European countries, policy responses to health threats shaped public opinion and yielded different political consequences. In some European countries, serious health threats encouraged the public to temporarily give positive evaluations to the government, the so-called a rally-around-the-flag phenomenon. In Denmark, unemployed Danes boosted their support for the administration in response to a social lockdown in Denmark (Bækgaard et al. 2020). In Austria, perceived health threats rather than perceived economic threats caused a strong but a short-term rally effect (Kritzinger et al. 2021). However, not all European governments increased their approval ratings with the spread of COVID-19. In Switzerland, the coronavirus pandemic generated negative emotions—fear and anger—with different consequences. Fear enhanced support for the government, while anger increased calls for the government to take responsibility for adverse circumstances (Erhardt et al. 2021). In Sweden, when the crisis of the coronavirus outbreak was no longer a matter of concern and government policy responses became an issue, the rally effect disappeared in a short period of time, with political ideologies shaping the public's support for the government (Johansson, Hopmann, and Shehata 2021). In France, the rally phenomenon did not emerge among the citizens in response to the spread of the coronavirus, leading to a strong partisan divide (Kritzinger et al. 2021). Therefore, global health threats do not uniformly shape the public opinion of countries and produce similar political consequences.

In this chapter, we address Japanese public opinion and the 2021 Lower House general election in the COVID-19 pandemic. The policy failure to deal with the COVID-19 pandemic forced Prime Minister Shinzo Abe to step down after more than seven years in office. Yoshihide Suga, chief cabinet secretary under the Abe administration, inaugurated a new government but was forced to step down after a year because his policies against the COVID-19 outbreak were not appreciated. In September 2020, Fumio Kishida won the LDP presidential election and inaugurated a new government. In October, Prime Minister Fumio Kishida dissolved the Lower House of the Diet and asked for the public's confidence in him, advocating a virtuous cycle of growth and distribution. In the 2021 Lower House general election, Japanese people voted for the reelection of the Liberal Democratic Party. The LDP secured 261 seats, despite losing 15 seats, and maintained its majority of seats. Why did Japanese citizens reelect the LDP and place their trust in the Kishida administration despite the fact that two prime ministers were forced to resign due to the policy failures against the COVID-19 pandemic?

To answer the puzzle, we will explore the relationship between Japanese public opinion during the COVID-19 pandemic from January 2020 to November 2021. In the following section, we review the Japanese government's policy response to the COVID-19 pandemic and examine trends in cabinet approval ratings over time. Because restrictions on the movement of people are at the sacrifice of economic activities, we will focus particularly on the impact of the declaration of the state of emergency. In the third section, we will present the results of the pre- and the postelection surveys. We will pay attention to the public's assessment of Prime Minister Suga's hosting of the Olympics and his rapid delivery of vaccinations. We also consider the strategic nature of campaigning with Kishida as the LDP leader, who advocates economic stimulus packages, in terms of both retrospective (Fiorina 1978) and prospective voting (Reed and Cho 1998; Hsieh, Lacy, and Niou 1998). Our concern is whether the LDP's victory in the 2021 Lower House general election is due to the public's appreciation of the LDP government's past policy responses to the COVID-19 pandemic or due to public expectations of the new Kishida administration. In the final section, we will discuss our findings and present the concluding remarks.

JAPANESE PUBLIC OPINION UNDER THE COVID-19 PANDEMIC

Japan confirmed its first case of COVID-19 in January 2020. While cases have risen since then, they remain far below the levels seen in Europe and North America. If this relatively low cumulative number of infections is due to Japan's infection control measures, the cabinet's approval rating is expected to remain high. However, after seven years and eight months, Prime Minister Abe was forced to resign, as was Prime Minister Suga. In October 2021, the LDP led by the new Kishida administration won a majority of seats in the general election for the House of Representatives. How did Japanese voters evaluate the government's measures against the spread of the virus and the restart of economic activities in the face of the outbreak? Figure 9.1 shows the cabinet approval ratings and the number

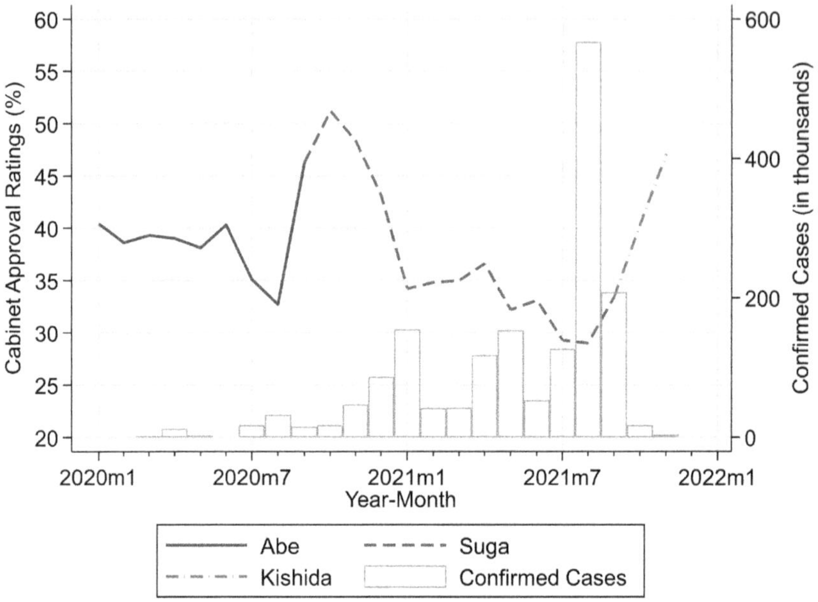

Figure 9.1. Cabinet Approval Ratings and Confirmed Cases

Source: Monthly Opinion Polls by Jiji Press for cabinet approval ratings andvhttps://info.vrs.digital.go.jp/dashboard/ for the number of infections.

of COVID-19 infections from January 2020 to November 2021.[2] When Japanese people were faced with the outbreak, their approval ratings for the cabinet declined, without causing a rally phenomenon. In the following, we examine the trends in the approval ratings of the Abe and Kan administrations, focusing on the government's efforts to combat the spread of the virus and resume economic activities.

The Abe Administration

On January 16, 2020, a man who returned from Wuhan City, Hubei Province, China, was confirmed as Japan's first case of COVID-19. A man among the passengers on the Diamond Princess cruise ship, which left the port of Yokohama on January 20, 2020, disembarked in Hong Kong on January 25, and tested positive for COVID-19.[3] The man had been in Mainland China on January 10 and had flown from Hong Kong to Tokyo on January 17.[4] After the Diamond Princess arrived in Yokohama on February 3, passengers were quarantined on board, and ten of them were confirmed to be positive for COVID-19 two days later. Two weeks later,

542 of the 3,711 passengers and crew on board were infected with the virus, raising questions about the infection control measures on board. Passengers who tested negative for the virus without a cough or fever were allowed to take public transport home but were later found to be infected. With passengers on the Diamond Princess coming from more than fifty countries, there were concerns that the virus could spread globally.[5]

The fact that passengers who tested negative for the virus were allowed to return home by public transportation, however, was not the only reason for Japan's first outbreak. The Chinese New Year holiday in 2020 was from January 24 to 30, and despite the Chinese government's ban on overseas group travel from January 27 to prevent the spread of COVID-19, the number of Chinese visitors to Japan during January was 924,700.[6] Because PM Abe gave priority to economic activities and did not impose entry restrictions on foreign visitors to Japan, Chinese tourists infected with COVID-19 stayed in Japan. Sanitary products like disposable masks and sanitizer sprays were in short supply in late January. These factors led to a steady increase in the number of COVID-19 infections in Japan.

The number of Infections in Japan rose steadily to 12 in January, 193 in February, and 1,930 in March. On February 27, Prime Minister Abe announced the nationwide closure of elementary, junior, and senior high schools from March 2 until the start of the spring holiday.[7] This decision not only failed to ensure adequate educational opportunities for children but also forced at least one parent to take care of them at home. Therefore, there was a widespread perception that the prolonged closure of schools would put pressure on households with children, making life difficult. On March 5, the Abe administration announced that it would push ahead with flexible border measures. On March 7, foreign nationals who had stayed in certain areas of North Gyeongsang Province in South Korea and in Qom Province in Iran, where the infection had been spreading, were newly subject to entry refusal under the Immigration Control Act. On March 9, the Abe administration attempted to control the number of arrivals by enforcing quarantine for arrivals from China and South Korea, limiting aircraft arrivals from both countries to Narita and Kansai airports, halting passenger transport by ship, and suspending the validity of issued primary and multiple visas, in addition to requiring two-week standby at designated locations.[8] On March 24, the Abe administration announced the postponement of the Olympics, which was expected to give a boost to the Japanese economy.[9]

The government's slow response to COVID-19 pushed the number of cases up to 12,889, and in April we saw the peak of the first wave of infections. On April 1, the Abe administration announced that it would distribute two reusable cloth masks per address to every household nationwide.[10] Then, on April 7, Prime Minister Abe declared a state of emergency for the first time, asking people to work and study at home, and trying to control the outbreak by imposing restrictions on the movement of people. On May 1, an online application for a single 100,000 yen benefit for all citizens was launched to help households under the coronavirus pandemic.[11] On May 4, Prime Minister Abe extended the state of emergency until May 31, and indicated that he would consider lifting the declaration before the deadline based on the infection situation and medical system on May 14.[12] On May 7, the Ministry of Health, Labour and Welfare granted special approval to a U.S. drug company for remdesivir as Japan's first treatment for COVID-19.[13] On May 14, the government decided to lift the state of emergency in thirty-nine prefectures, including thirteen prefectures on special alert.[14] On May 21, the government lifted the state of emergency in Hyogo, Kyoto, and Osaka prefectures,[15] and on May 25, the state of emergency was fully lifted.[16] The number of cases fell to 2,511 in May, and the first wave of COVID-19 infections was contained.

According to a public opinion poll conducted by the Jiji Press over the same period, the cabinet approval rating was 40.4 percent (January), 38.6 percent (February), and 39.3 percent (March), not conducted due to face-to-face surveys (April), and 38.1 percent (May). The public did not significantly change their evaluations of the Abe administration due to its policy responses to the spread of COVID-19. The public did not respond emotionally to the health threat posed by COVID-19 with a temporary boost in cabinet support. According to a labor force survey conducted in April, the number of nonregular employees fell by 970,000 from the same month a year earlier, and the declaration of a state of emergency had created social unrest by laying off nonregular workers ahead of the economic downturn as a means of adjusting employment.[17] Although Prime Minister Abe's cloth mask distribution cost a total of about 26 billion yen, the distribution of 120 million masks using Japan Post's system was completed around June 20, after the outbreak of infection was controlled and the shortage of masks was resolved.[18] Surprisingly, the harsh economic conditions and mismanagement of the distribution of masks did not affect the cabinet's approval rating.

On June 2, with signs of COVID-19's possible spread, Yuriko Koike of the Tokyo metropolitan government issued a "Tokyo Alert" warning against the spread of the virus. Koike was aware of signs of the spread of the virus, especially in nighttime entertainment districts and hospitals where patients had already been infected.[19] On June 13, Yasutoshi Nishimura, Minister for Economic Revitalization, issued guidelines on infection prevention measures for three types of businesses: restaurants, live houses, and nightclubs that provide entertainment.[20] While the need to restrict movement was reiterated, the government also sent a message urging economic activity to resume. On June 12, Kazuyoshi Akaba, Minister of Land, Infrastructure, Transport and Tourism, announced his intention to launch a "Go To Campaign" tourism program during summer vacation to help businesses hit by the COVID-19 outbreak.[21] On June 18, Prime Minister Abe stated that it would be possible to conduct professional sports without spectators, allowing free movement across prefectures and easing the maximum number of people allowed at events to one thousand.[22] Then society as a whole began gradually moving toward economic recovery. For example, on June 23, Oriental Land announced that Tokyo Disneyland and Tokyo Disney Sea would reopen on July 1.[23] The resumption of events and the reopening of amusement parks brought many people to one place, causing in a spread of infection in about two weeks.

On July 17, Akaba, Minister of Land, Infrastructure, Transport and Tourism, announced that the "Go Traveling" campaign, aimed at reinvigorating the travel industry and domestic travel that have suffered financial losses due to the COVID-19 outbreak, would be launched on July 22 and travel to and from Tokyo, where the spread of the disease is progressing, would not be included in the campaign.[24] The campaign, which was subsidized by the government to provide a 35 percent discount on the total cost of travel and a 15 percent regional coupon, helped spread the infection by encouraging citizens to travel across prefectural borders. On August 6, Prime Minister Abe attended a memorial ceremony for the victims of the atomic bombings and a prayer for peace in Hiroshima. "We are not in a position to declare a state of emergency," he said, indicating his intention to balance economic activities with preventing the spread of the virus.[25] Tokyo governor Yuriko Koike told a press conference that Tokyo residents should refrain from returning to their hometowns during the holiday season and from traveling during summer vacations to prevent the spread of the coronavirus.[26] On August 16, the Cabinet Office announced a preliminary report on gross domestic product (GDP, seasonally adjusted) for the April to June period of 2020, showing a decline of 7.8 percent in real terms excluding price fluctuations from the previous quarter, and a decline of 27.8 percent on an annualized basis assuming this pace continues for one year.[27] Personal consumption plunged due to the spread of COVID-19, surpassing the 17.8 percent annual decline in the January to March quarter of 2009 after the collapse of Lehman Brothers. On August 28, Prime Minister Abe, troubled by the recurrence of his chronic ulcerative colitis, announced his intention to resign and apologized for his resignation amid the spread of the COVID-19 infection, saying, "I sincerely apologize to the people."[28]

During this period, the number of infections rose from 1,747 (June) to 17,373 (July), 31,981 (August), and 15,045 (September), indicating that the Japanese people faced a second wave of infections. Meanwhile, the cabinet's approval rating remained at 40.3 percent (June), 35.1 percent (July), 32.7 percent (August), and 46.3 percent (September), showing that there was no rally in response to the spread of the disease. This means that the Japanese people strongly disapproved of the Abe administration's goal of simultaneously controlling the spread of the disease and restarting economic activities. And when Prime Minister Abe's intention to resign was announced at the end of August, expectations for the new government increased public support for the cabinet.

The Suga Administration

On September 16, 2020, Suga Yoshihide, the winner of the LDP presidential election, became prime minister. Prime Minister Suga, who took office under the slogan of "a cabinet working for the people," followed the Abe administration's COVID-19 policy, as he had served as chief cabinet secretary for seven years and eight months.[29] The Suga administration was busy fighting the spread of COVID-19. The economy-minded Suga government added arrivals and departures from Tokyo, the country's largest population, to the "Go Traveling" campaign on October 1.[30] This led to an increase in the number of infections. On November 24, the Suga administration temporarily removed Osaka and Sapporo from its "Go Traveling" campaign because of their concerns about the spread of the coronavirus.[31] The hotbed of infection was steadily spreading, until December when it became unmanageable and medical care was threatened by a shortage of hospital beds. In light of the outbreak, Prime Minister Suga finally announced on December 14 that the "Go Traveling" campaign would be suspended nationwide.[32] On the same night, however, Prime Minister Suga himself had a dinner with eight people, even as he urged the public to refrain from eating and drinking. Prime Minister Suga apologized, saying, "I regret it."[33] The lack of leadership sense of crisis surfaced here. On December 27, Yuichiro Haneda, an active Diet member, died after contracting COVID-19.[34] On December 31, the number of daily infections in Tokyo exceeded 1,300, sparking concern in Japan.[35]

Tokyo Governor Yuriko Koike and others asked the government to declare a state of emergency on January 2, 2021, and on January 7, Prime Minister Suga declared the state of emergency for the second time for four prefectures in the Tokyo metropolitan area (Chiba, Kanagawa, Saitama, and Tokyo).[36] On January 13, the state of emergency was expanded to cover eleven prefectures (adding Aichi, Fukuoka, Gifu, Hyogo, Kyoto, Osaka, and Tochigi), including Japan's industrial and economic hubs, such as the Tokyo metropolitan area, the Kansai area, and the Chubu region.[37] On January 4, Prime Minister Suga announced that vaccination would start by the end of February, with priority given to healthcare workers, the elderly, and workers in facilities for the elderly.[38] On January 18, Prime Minister Suga assigned Taro Kono, the minister in charge of regulatory reform, to serve concurrently as the minister in charge of vaccination promotion, and on January 22, signed a contract for a total of 314 million doses from Pfizer, Moderna, and AstraZeneca.[39] The Suga administration also called for measures to prevent infections, such as stopping the provision of alcohol at restaurants and shortening business hours. The declaration led to a contraction in demand for food services and undoubtedly had a serious impact on agriculture. Vegetables remained at low prices due to fluctuations in supply and demand, while stocks of staple food rice remained at an all-time high. In dairy products, butter stocks expanded due to sluggish demand at hotels and other businesses.[40] The restrictions at the expense of the economy worked, with cases peaking in January.

During this period, the number of infections stood at 15,045 (September), 17,529 (October), 47,158 (November), 86,541 (December), and 154,700 (January), indicating that Japanese people were facing a third wave of the pandemic. At the same time, the cabinet's approval rating remained at 46.3 percent (September), 51.2 percent (October), 48.3 percent (November), 43.1 percent (December), and 34.2 percent (January). The rally did not occur in response to the spread of the infection, and while the public increased their support by continuing the Suga government's "Go Traveling" campaign, support significantly decreased as the spread of the infection progressed. In January, the approval and disapproval ratings reversed, and the disapproval rating rose to 39.7 percent. As a result, it became clear that it would be extremely difficult to achieve a balance between curbing the spread of the infection and resuming economic activities, as the Suga administration's economy-oriented policies led to the spread of the disease and the failure to control the spread of the disease caused the cabinet's approval rating to decline.

On February 2, 2021, Prime Minister Suga lifted the state of emergency in Tochigi and extended it to March 7 for the remaining ten prefectures.[41] On February 3, the Diet passed a law that amends the Infectious Diseases Act and the Act on Special Measures Concerning Novel Influenza, etc. in a single package, and it will come into effect on the February 13. The revised Infectious Diseases Act (1) made active epidemiological surveys effective, (2) revised hospitalization measures, and (3) strengthened the authority of the Minister of Health, Labour and Welfare and prefectural governors. The revised Special Measures Law included (1) the introduction of a system of priority measures to prevent the spread of influenza, (2) orders to take measures against businesses that did not comply with the request for business self-restraint based on the declaration of an emergency, and (3) financial support for businesses affected by the pandemic influenza.[42] The declaration of a state of emergency is issued at a level equivalent to "Stage 4" among the four infection levels. The government designates the target at the prefectural level, orders restaurants to shorten their working hours and to close, and imposes a fine of up to 300,000 yen as a penalty for violation of the order. On the other hand, priority measures, such as measures to prevent the spread, are issued at the level equivalent to "Stage 3" out of the four infection levels. The prefectural governor can designate the target at the municipal level, issue orders and requests to restaurants for shorter hours, and impose a fine of up to 200,000 yen as a penalty for violation of the order. By introducing the latter, it was sought to realize flexible control of the spread of infection while maintaining economic activities.[43] The COVID-19 vaccine developed by U.S. pharmaceutical giant Pfizer was officially approved by the Ministry of Health and Welfare on February 14, and the vaccination of 40,000 healthcare beneficiaries started on February 17. On February 24, Prime Minister Suga announced that vaccinations for the elderly would begin on March 12. On February 26, Prime Minister Suga announced that the state of emergency in Aichi, Fukuoka, Gifu, Hyogo, Kyoto, and Osaka would be lifted on February 28.[44] However, in the four prefectures in the Tokyo metropolitan area, the number of confirmed cases has stopped falling and the situation has not improved. So, on March 5, Prime Minister Suga announced that the state of emergency in Chiba, Kanagawa, Saitama, and Tokyo would be postponed until March 21.[45] Finally, on March 18, Prime Minister Suga announced that the state of emergency would end on March 21.[46]

During this period, the number of infections declined significantly from January, with 41,838 in February and 42,300 in March. At the same time, the cabinet's approval rating stood at 34.8 percent in February and 35.0 percent in March. Despite the fact that the third wave of the pandemic was under control, the public did not show a significant increase in the approval rating of the Suga administration. The reason was that Tohoku Shinsha hosted senior officials of the Ministry of Internal Affairs and Communications, and eleven senior officials of the ministry were punished on February 26 for violating the National Public Service Ethics Code. Seigo Suga, Prime Minister Suga's son, was employed by Tohoku Shinsha and used Prime Minister Suga's influence to lobby the ministry for favors. On the same day, Tohoku Shinsha announced that it had punished Mr. Suga.[47] The issue made it clear that Suga would not investigate political corruption caused by his relatives, even though he pursued competition through regulatory reform. As a result, the cabinet's approval rating did not improve despite the fact that the third wave of infections was under control.

Even though the state of emergency was lifted on March 21, Prime Minister Suga had less than a month to declare a state of emergency in response to the surge in infection cases. The State of Emergency, which was declared on April 23, covers Hyogo, Kyoto, Osaka, and Tokyo.[48] On May 7, Aichi and Fukuoka were placed under the state of emergency, and the lifting of the state of emergency, scheduled for May 11, was postponed until May 31.[49] On May 14, Prime Minister Suga expanded the state of emergency declaration to include Hiroshima, Hokkaido, and Okayama,[50] and on May 21, it was extended to Okinawa.[51] On May 28, Prime Minister Suga announced that the lifting of the state of emergency in these ten prefectures would be extended until June 20.[52] On June 17, Prime Minister Suga announced that the state of emergency would be lifted for all prefectures except Okinawa on June 20, as scheduled, and extended for Okinawa until July 11. Seven prefectures, Aichi, Fukuoka, Hyogo, Hokkaido, Kyoto, Osaka, and Tokyo, were targeted for priority measures such as epidemic prevention.[53] In this way, the fourth wave of infection was contained.

Signs of the spread of the COVID-19 variant, however, were confirmed mainly in the Tokyo metropolitan area, and the infection situation in Okinawa did not improve. As a result, on July 8, Prime Minister Suga declared a state of emergency covering Tokyo and announced that the state of emergency in Okinawa would be extended, with plans to lift it on August 22. Prime Minister Suga decided to extend the priority measures to prevent epidemics in Chiba, Kanagawa, Osaka, and Saitama prefectures until August 22, and to end the priority measures to prevent epidemics in Aichi, Fukuoka, Hokkaido, Hyogo, and Kyoto prefectures on July 11.[54] On July 30, Prime Minister Suga declared a state of emergency in Chiba, Kanagawa, Osaka, and Saitama prefectures to contain the spread of the highly contagious delta variant and announced that Fukuoka, Hokkaido, Hyogo, Ishikawa, and Kyoto prefectures would be given priority measures to prevent the spread of the variant, which would be lifted on August 31.[55] On August 17, Prime Minister Suga declared states of emergency in Fukuoka, Gunma, Kyoto, Hyogo, Ibaraki, Shizuoka, and Tochigi and implemented priority measures to prevent outbreaks in Ehime, Gifu, Hiroshima, Kagawa, Kagoshima, Mie, Miyagi, Okayama, Toyama, and Yamanashi. The lifting of the measures, including those in the past, was scheduled for September 12.[56] On August 25, Prime Minister Suga expanded the scope of the state of emergency to include Aichi, Gifu, Hiroshima, Hokkaido, Mie, Miyagi, Okayama, and Shiga.[57] On September 9, Prime Minister Suga lifted the state of emergency in Miyagi and Okayama on September 12 and extended it to September 30 for the other nineteen prefectures.

The priority measures to prevent the spread of the disease were lifted in Ehime, Kochi, Nagasaki, Saga, Toyama, and Yamanashi prefectures, and the priority measures to prevent the spread of the disease were extended to September 30 by adding Miyagi and Okayama prefectures to the other six prefectures.[58] On September 28, Prime Minister Suga announced that the declaration of a state of emergency and all priority measures such as epidemic prevention in nineteen prefectures would be lifted on September 30.[59] In this way, the fifth wave of spread was contained.

During this period, the number of infections remained at 117,482 (April), 153,674 (May), and 52,977 (June), thereby suppressing the fourth wave of infection, and at 126,687 (July), 5675,72 (August), 208,174 (September), and 17,375 (October), thereby restraining the fifth wave of infection. Meanwhile, the cabinet's approval rating stood at 36.6 percent (April), 32.2 percent (May), 33.1 percent (June), 29.3 percent (July), 29.0 percent (August), 33.4 percent (September), and 40.3 percent (October). From April to September, the cabinet's approval rating remained low, partly because the infection continued to spread. On September 3, Prime Minister Suga announced his intention not to run for the LDP presidency in order to focus on tackling COVID-19.[60] And when Fumio Kishida, a proponent of economic growth, won the LDP presidential election and became prime minister, the cabinet's approval rating recovered to 40.3 percent. Therefore, when Japanese people were faced with the spread of COVID-19, their approval ratings for the Suga administration declined, and the rally phenomenon did not occur.

Prime Minister Suga not only declared a state of emergency and implemented priority measures to prevent the spread of COVID-19 but also actively promoted the spread of vaccination. Japan started the vaccination for people except for the medical worker on April 12, which was four months later than Europe and North America. The rate of second vaccine doses rose rapidly over a short period of time: 10.62 percent (June), 28.08 percent (July), 43.90 percent (August), 57.33 percent (September), and 69.16 percent (October).[61] While declaring a state of emergency, Prime Minister Suga also held the Tokyo Olympic Games (July 23 to August 8) and the Tokyo Paralympic Games (August 24 to September 5) while giving due consideration to infection control measures. Nevertheless, these policy choices did not increase positive evaluations of the Suga administration.

Summary

We have reviewed the Japanese government's policy response and public opinion during the COVID-19 pandemic and examined the public's assessment of politics in the face of health threats. Japanese citizens did not induce the rally phenomenon as observed in European countries and did not show an emotional response to the health threat posed by COVID-19. On the contrary, they tend to be calmer, view the spread of COVID-19 as mismanagement, and drop their support for the cabinet. Prime Minister Suga's policy choices, such as active vaccination and the Olympics, were not enough to improve his cabinet's approval rating. Failure to curb the spread of the COVID-19 epidemic would have caused both Prime Ministers Abe and Suga to lose their approval ratings and be forced to resign. Therefore, as of September 2021, political confidence in the LDP was not firmly established. Nevertheless, the LDP was able to secure a sole majority in the October 2021 Lower House general election. The reasons for this are explored in the next section using the results of recent opinion polls.

THE CHANGE OF THE PRIME MINISTER AND VOTING BEHAVIOR IN THE 2021 GENERAL ELECTION

Before the 2021 Lower House general election, there was a replacement of Japan's prime minister. On September 3, Prime Minister Suga announced his intention not to run in the next LDP presidential election to focus on tackling the COVID-19 crisis. Fumio Kishida won the LDP presidential election held on September 29 and was elected prime minister at the Diet on October 4. Prime Minister Kishida dissolved the Lower House on October 14 and held a general election on October 31 as a vote of confidence. The ruling coalition of the LDP and Komeito secured a majority of seats despite losing a few seats, while the main opposition Constitutional Democratic Party (CDP) failed to increase its number of seats (table 9.1).

We will explore how voters assessed the government performance. Specifically, by using panel data from online surveys conducted before and after the election, we will explore the determinants behind voting

Table 9.1. The Number of Seats Before and After the Election

	Parties	*Before*	*After*
Government	LDP	276	261
	Komeito	29	32
Opposition	CDP	109	96
	JCP	12	10
	JIP	11	41
	NDP	8	11
	ReiwaShinsengumi	1	3
	SDP	1	1
	NHKP	1	0
	Independents	12	10
	Others	1	0
Vacancy		4	0
Total		465	465

Source: https://www.soumu.go.jp/senkyo/senkyo_s/data/shugiin49/index.html and https://www.soumu.go.jp/main_content/000776967.xls.

behavior. The preelection survey was conducted from July 9 to 19, and the postelection survey was conducted from November 1 to 16.[62] As previously shown in figure 9.1, the approval rating of the Suga administration as of July 2021 was a low 29.3 percent, while that of the Kishida administration as of November 2021 was a very high 47.1 percent. What explains this change? We will address the key variables such as feeling thermometers to parties and the leaders, evaluations of government performance, voting intention (the preelection survey), and actual vote choice (the postelection survey). Exploring these variables will help us understand the logic of vote choice leading to LDP victory.

Evaluation to the Prime Ministers and Parties

Our pre- and post-election surveys measure feeling thermometers to parties and the leaders, with 11-points scaling (0 = "dislike," 5 = "neutral," and 10 = "like"). We begin by comparing these values before and after the election. Table 9.2 indicates descriptive statistics about feeling thermometers. The mean values of feeling thermometers toward the Japan Innovation Party (JIP) were the highest both in the pre- and postelection surveys, with 4.45 and 5.14, respectively. The mean values of feeling thermometers for the LDP was the second highest both in the pre- and

Table 9.2. Feeling Thermometers for Political Parties

	Pre-Election				Post-Election			
		Mean				Mean		
Party	*n*	*Value*	*St. Error*	*St. Dev.*	*n*	*Value*	*St. Error*	*St. Dev.*
LDP	3306	4.37	0.05	2.69	2210	4.80	0.06	2.83
CDP	3210	3.62	0.04	2.44	2129	3.57	0.06	2.56
Komeito	3229	3.19	0.04	2.43	2104	2.92	0.05	2.46
JCP	3188	3.15	0.04	2.48	2063	2.63	0.05	2.45
JIP	3172	4.45	0.04	2.37	2136	5.14	0.06	2.66
NDP	2917	3.62	0.04	2.11	1949	3.67	0.05	2.30
Reiwa Shinsengumi	2811	2.90	0.05	2.48	1959	2.63	0.06	2.54
SDP	2935	3.05	0.04	2.34	1936	2.45	0.05	2.27
StormParty-NHKP*	2344	2.32	0.05	2.33	1914	1.63	0.05	2.29

*Storm Party changed the name to 'The party fighting against NHK in the trial for violating Article 72 of the Attorney Act' from July 21, 2021, abbreviated as 'NHKP' here.

Source: The 2021 Panel Data for the Forty-Ninth General Election collected by Masahiro Yamada, Yukio Maeda, Airo Hino, and Tetsuya Mat.

postelection surveys, with 4.37 and 4.80, respectively. The postelection values look slightly better than the preelection values.

Table 9.3 displays descriptive statistics of feeling thermometers toward Prime Minister Suga, Prime Minister Kishida, and the LDP in the pre- and postelection surveys, showing the improvement of these evaluations from July to November. For example, the mean value of feeling thermometers toward the LDP rises from 4.37 to 4.80. More impressively, the post-

Table 9.3. Feeling Thermometers for the LDP and PMs

			Mean		
		n	*Value*	*St. Error.*	*St. Dev.*
Pre-Election	LDP	3306	4.37	0.05	2.69
	PM Suga	3374	3.68	0.04	2.52
Post-Election	LDP	2210	4.80	0.06	2.83
	PM Kishida	2180	4.67	0.05	2.35
	ex-PM Suga	2189	4.06	0.06	2.65
Difference	Post–Pre: LDP	2038	0.37	0.04	1.99
	Post (Kishida)–Pre (Suga)	2047	1.01	0.06	2.67
	Post–Pre: Suga	2064	0.39	0.05	2.08

Source: The 2021 Panel Data for the Forty-Ninth General Election.

Table 9.4. Feeling Thermometers for the CDP and Edano

			Mean		
		n	*Value*	*St. Error*	*St. Dev.*
Pre-Election	CDP	3210	3.62	0.04	2.44
	Edano	3252	3.46	0.04	2.44
Post-Election	CDP	2129	3.57	0.06	2.56
	Edano	2107	2.96	0.05	2.51
Difference	CDP	1935	–0.05	0.04	1.96
	Edano	1963	–0.52	0.04	1.87

Source: The 2021 Panel Data for the Forty-Ninth General Election.

election evaluation of Prime Minister Kishida exceeded the preelection evaluation of Prime Minister Suga by 1 point. Moreover, even feeling thermometers toward Prime Minister Suga increased by 0.4 point between the preelection and postelection period (from 3.68 to 4.06). Similar results were obtained when comparing only those who responded to both surveys. "Difference" represents the postelection value minus the preelection value for those who responded to both surveys.

Table 9.4 indicates descriptive statistics of feeling thermometers toward the CDP, and the CDP leader Yukio Edano in the pre- and postelection surveys, showing the decline of these evaluations from July to November. In the preelection survey, the CDP was not preferred over the LDP, and the CDP leader was not favored over the prime minister. Reputations of the CDP and the CDP leader Edano did not appear to improve in the postelection survey.

The previous simple analysis shows that the LDP was more preferred by voters before and after the election than other parties, and that its support recovered from pre- to postelection period. What improved support for the LDP and its leaders? We address voters' evaluations of individual government policies and explore the reasons for the recovery of the LDP popularity.

Evaluation of Government Performance and Votes for the LDP

The preelection survey includes a battery to ask the respondents' evaluation of the Suga administration's performance regarding fourteen policy

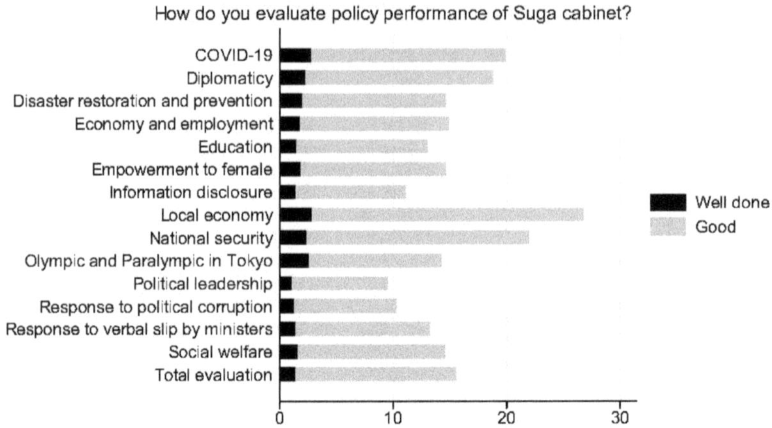

Figure 9.2. Policy Evaluations of the Suga cabinet (the Preelection Survey)
Source: The 2021 Panel Data for the Forty-Ninth General Election.

issues, including COVID-19 and total evaluation. Figure 9.2 shows the percentage of positive evaluation ("well done" or "good") of the Suga administration's policy performance. Respondents gave extremely poor ratings to the Suga administration. Even in the most positively rated policy area, local economy, the Suga administration managed to gain only 26.7 percent of support. Only 19.9 percent of respondents gave a positive assessment of COVID-19 measures. The worst performance was in leadership, implying a sign of Prime Minister Suga's resignation in the near future.

In the preelection and postelection surveys, we asked respondents about the performance of politicians and experts on infection control. Figure 9.3 shows that Prime Minister Suga received only 20.4 percent of the positive evaluations, while the ministers received fewer positive evaluations than the governors and mayors. On the other hand, primary doctors and nurses and the Self-Defense Forces received a huge support of 67.4 percent and 73.3 percent, respectively. However, as shown in figure 9.4, the public's assessment of Suga appears to have improved after his resignation. 48.6 percent of respondents in the postelection survey gave Suga positive ratings. The rapid rollout of vaccinations may have boosted Suga's popularity.[63]

Those who began to support the cabinet and former Prime Minister Suga during the survey period before and after the election may also give positive evaluations to the LDP. We estimated a regression model

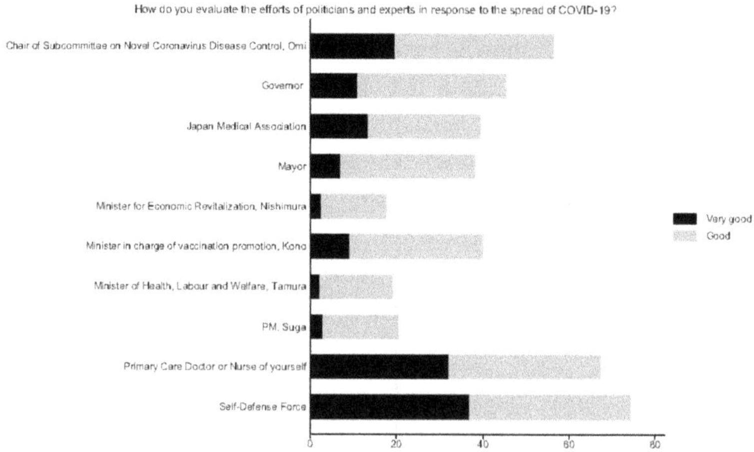

Figure 9.3. Evaluations of Politicians and Experts (the Preelection Survey)
Source: The 2021 Panel Data for the Forty-Ninth General Election.

to examine this scenario. The dependent variable is the change in feeling thermometers toward the LDP between preelection and postelection. The independent variables are the difference in feeling thermometers toward Prime Minister Suga before the election and Prime Minister Kishida after the election, and the change in feeling thermometers toward Suga between preelection and postelection. We also include possible control variables:

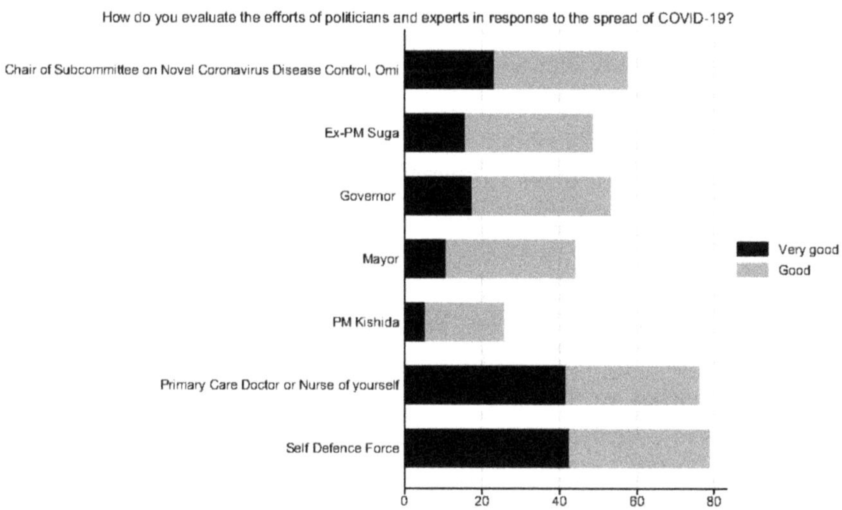

Figure 9.4. Evaluations of Politicians and Experts (the Postelection Survey)
Source: The 2021 Panel Data for the Forty-Ninth General Election.

evaluation of Tokyo Olympics,[64] change in threat perception of COVID-19 between preelection and postelection, sociotropic and pocketbook evaluations, expectations about the economy for the preelection period, respondents' socioeconomic variables (household income, age, gender, job, permanent employed status), and vaccination status.

Table 9.5 summarizes the estimated result. Only four variables had statistically significant effects at the 0.05 level and are shown in italics in the table. First, the difference in feeling thermometers toward Prime Minister Suga before the election and toward Prime Minister Kishida after the election, as well as the difference in feeling thermometers toward Suga between preelection and postelection, have a positive correlation with the dependent variable, and increased feeling thermometers toward the LDP between preelection and postelection. Second, poor evaluations of the economy compared to one year ago (pocketbook evaluation) and female respondents were negatively correlated with the dependent variable and decreased feeling thermometers toward the LDP between preelection and postelection.

In addition, we decided to narrow our analysis to those who responded to both the preelection and postelection surveys and who answered they would not vote for the LDP before the election. The dependent variable is a binary variable, 1 if the respondent answered that one voted for the LDP in the postelection survey, and 0 otherwise. We estimated a logit model using the same independent and control variables as in the previous OLS model. Note that we added the difference in feeling thermometers toward the LDP between the preelection and postelection periods to the model as an independent variable.

Table 9.6 summarizes the estimated result. Only three variables have statistically significant effects at the 0.05 level and are shown in italics in the table. First, from preelection to postelection periods, people who had raised their feeling thermometers toward the LDP tended to vote for the LDP rather than other parties. Second, those who were more positive about the Tokyo Olympics and Paralympics tended to switch their vote from other parties to the LDP. Third, those who answered they were worse off than a year ago tended not to change their votes from other parties to the LDP.

The previous analysis provides the following insights. The change of government from Prime Minister Suga to Prime Minister Kishida im-

Table 9.5. Explaining the Change of Evaluation to the LDP (OLS)

Variables	*B*	*S. E.*	*Beta*	*T-Value*	*Sig.*	*95% C. I. of B*		*VIF*
						Lower	*Upper*	
Difference of the Degree at Feeling Thermometer/Kishida(Post)–Suga (Pre)	*0.259*	*0.022*	*0.344*	*11.724*	*0.000*	*0.216*	*0.303*	*1.507*
Difference of the Degree at Feeling Thermometer/Suga(Post)–Suga(Pre)	*0.126*	*0.025*	*0.129*	*4.5.5*	*0.000*	*0.071*	*0.180*	*1.444*
Tokyo Olympic Evaluation	0.019	0.059	0.008	0.315	0.753	–0.097	0.134	1.147
Change of COVID-19 Threat (Post–Pre)	0.028	0.062	0.011	0.452	0.651	–0.093	0.149	1.013
Current Economy in Japan	0.023	0.068	0.010	0.336	0.737	–0.110	0.156	1.614
Current Economy in Japan from 1 yrs. age	0.004	0.062	0.002	0.064	0.949	–0.118	0.126	1.684
Prospect to Economy in Japan	0.006	0.053	0.004	0.112	0.911	–0.098	0.110	1.738
Satisfaction to Your Household	0.005	0.058	0.003	0.080	0.936	–0.110	0.119	1.837
Current Household from 1 yrs. ago	*–0.187*	*0.093*	*–0.064*	*–2.002*	*0.046*	*–0.370*	*–0.004*	*1.796*
Prospect for Your Household	0.005	0.081	0.002	0.067	0.947	–0.153	0.163	1.950
Household Income	0.048	0.021	0.056	2.306	0.021	0.007	0.089	1.047
Age	–0.033	0.036	–0.027	–0.927	0.354	–0.104	0.037	1.472
Female (dummy)	*–0.300*	*0.104*	*–0.074*	*–2.877*	*0.004*	*–0.505*	*–0.095*	*1.159*
Vaccinated (dummy)	–0.230	0.364	–0.015	–0.632	0.527	–0.943	0.483	1.014
Job (dummy)	–0.032	0.127	–0.008	–0.251	0.802	–0.281	0.217	1.635
Permanent Employed (dummy)	–0.055	0.128	–0.013	–0.431	0.666	–0.305	0.195	1.683
Constant	0.866	0.556		1.558	0.119	–0.224	1.956	
Adjusted R-squared	0.188							
Standard Error of Regression	1.789							
Number of Observations	1421							

Table 9.6. Who Switched to Support for the LDP? (Logit)

					95% C. I. of Exp(B)	
Variables	*B*	*S. E.*	*Sig.*	*Exp(B)*	*Lower*	*Upper*
Difference of the Degree at Feeling Thermometer/ LDP (Post)–LDP (Pre)	*0.297*	*0.071*	*0.000*	*1.345*	*1.170*	*1.547*
Difference of the Degree at Feeling Thermometer/ Kishida (Post)–Suga (Pre)	0.103	0.066	0.118	1.108	0.974	1.260
Difference of the Degree at Feeling Thermometer/ Suga (Post)–Suga (Pre)	–0.044	0.074	0.553	0.957	0.827	1.107
Tokyo Olympic Evaluation	*0.490*	*0.180*	*0.007*	*1.635*	*1.147*	*2.322*
Change of COVID-19 Threat (Post–Pre)	0.046	0.172	0.788	1.047	0.748	1.466
Current Economy in Japan	–0.223	0.177	0.207	0.800	0.565	1.132
Current Economy in Japan from 1 yrs. age	0.065	0.165	0.694	1.067	0.773	1.474
Prospect to Economy in Japan	–0.183	0.155	0.235	0.832	0.615	1.127
Satisfaction to Your Household	–0.002	0.165	0.990	0.998	0.722	1.378
Current Household from 1 yrs. ago	*–0.596*	*0.259*	*0.021*	*0.551*	*0.332*	*0.915*
Prospect for Your Household	0.433	0.238	0.069	1.542	0.967	2.460
Age	–0.172	0.100	0.084	0.842	0.692	1.023
Female	0.068	0.311	0.828	1.070	0.581	1.969
Household Income	0.041	0.085	0.631	1.042	0.881	1.231
Vaccinated	0.320	1.098	0.771	1.377	0.160	11,839
Job	–0.238	0.406	0.558	0.789	0.356	1.746
Permanent Employed	0.212	0.363	0.558	1.236	0.608	2.516
Constant	–2.292	1.535	0.135	0.101		
–2LL	437.129					
Cox-Snell R-Square	0.045					
Nagelkerke R-Square	0.132					
Number of Observations	1176					

proved voters' evaluations of the LDP, while those who were worse off a year ago were dissatisfied with the LDP. Prime Minister Kishida's economic policy of a virtuous cycle of growth and distribution could appeal to those who felt worse off than a year ago. Thus, the change of government from Prime Minister Suga to Prime Minister Kishida implies a possible shift in voting behavior from retrospective voting to prospective voting.

CONCLUSION

We have explored Japanese public opinion and voting behavior under COVID-19. We began with an interesting but difficult puzzle to answer. Given that two Japanese prime ministers were forced to resign due to the policy failures against the COVID-19 pandemic, we asked why Japanese citizens reelected the LDP and placed their trust in the Kishida administration. We briefly summarize our findings here.

Our case study of the Abe and Suga administrations revealed the relationship between the infection situation and the government's response to the COVID-19 crisis and the cabinet's approval ratings during the Abe and Suga administrations. Unlike some European countries, Japanese citizens did not react emotionally to health threats from the spread of COVID-19 and did not induce a rally phenomenon. Because the government gave priority to maintaining economic activities, its response to the COVID-19 crisis was reactive and backhanded, leading to the spread of the pandemic. The Japanese public tended to perceive the rising number of infections as the government's failure to deal with COVID-19, and the cabinet's approval rating fell. Therefore, at the end of August 2021, the LDP was not able to gain sufficient support to secure a majority in the next Lower House general election.

Our analysis of the pre- and postelection surveys also revealed the factors behind the voting behavior leading to the LDP's victory in the 2021 Lower House general election. The change of government from Prime Minister Suga to Prime Minister Kishida improved voters' evaluations of the LDP, implying a sign of a possible shift in voting behavior from retrospective voting to prospective voting. Given the rapid distribution of vaccinations and the suppression of the fifth wave of infections by October, there was a certain number of people who had positive views of Suga and the LDP. Prime Minister Kishida's economic policy of a virtuous cycle of growth and distribution could appeal to those who felt worse off than a year ago. Even the controversial holding of the Tokyo Olympics encouraged voters to switch their vote from the opposition to the LDP. These are the reasons behind expectations for the LDP.

In conclusion, the rally phenomenon was not observed in Japan, where the number of infected people was overwhelmingly lower than in Europe and the United States and the logic of economic voting was fully functioning. The change in leadership within the LDP also shifted the standard of voting behavior to voting based on expectations. As a result, even the LDP, which had not been fully appreciated for its COVID-19 response, was able to secure a majority of seats in the 2021 Lower House general election.

NOTES

1. See the World Health Organization Travel Advice published on January 10, 2020, https://www.who.int/news-room/articles-detail/who-advice-for-international-travel-and-trade-in-relation-to-the-outbreak-of-pneumonia-caused-by-a-new-coronavirus-in-china (accessed February 20, 2022).
2. The cabinet approval ratings are based on opinion polls conducted by Jiji Press. For the number of infections, see the following website: https://info.vrs.digital.go.jp/dashboard/ (accessed December 1, 2021).
3. https://xn—mhlw-zj9fh02i.go.jp/stf/newpage_08906.html (accessed March 26, 2022).
4. https://www.info.gov.hk/gia/general/202002/01/P2020020100795.htm (accessed March 26, 2022).
5. https://www.bbc.com/japanese/51568233 (accessed March 26, 2022).
6. https://www.jnto.go.jp/jpn/statistics/since2003_visitor_arrivals.pdf (accessed March 26, 2022).
7. https://www.mext.go.jp/content/202002228-mxt_kouhou01-000004520_1.pdf (accessed March 27, 2022).
8. https://www.kantei.go.jp/jp/98_abe/actions/202003/05corona.html (accessed March 26, 2022).
9. https://www.kantei.go.jp/jp/singi/tokyo2020_suishin_honbu/pdf/200324pressrelease.pdf (accessed March 26, 2022).
10. https://www.kantei.go.jp/jp/98_abe/actions/202004/1corona.html (accessed March 26, 2022).
11. https://www.soumu.go.jp/menu_news/kaiken/01koho01_02000911.html (accessed April 2, 2022).
12. https://www.kantei.go.jp/jp/98_abe/statement/2020/0504kaiken.html (accessed April 2, 2022).
13. https://www.mhlw.go.jp/stf/kaiken/daijin/0000194708_00241.html (accessed April 2, 2022).
14. https://www.kantei.go.jp/jp/singi/novel_coronavirus/th_siryou/t_gaiyou_r020514.pdf (accessed April 2, 2022).
15. https://www.kantei.go.jp/jp/singi/novel_coronavirus/th_siryou/t_gaiyou_r020521.pdf (accessed April 3, 2022).

16. https://www.kantei.go.jp/jp/singi/novel_coronavirus/th_siryou/t_gaiyou_r020525.pdf (accessed April 2, 2022).
17. https://www.stat.go.jp/data/roudou/rireki/tsuki/pdf/202004.pdf (accessed April 3, 2022).
18. https://www.jiji.com/jc/article?k=2021041700410&g=soc (accessed March 26, 2022).
19. https://www.metro.tokyo.lg.jp/tosei/governor/governor/kishakaiken/2020/06/05.html (accessed April 3, 2022).
20. https://corona.go.jp/news/pdf/daijin_youshi_0613.pdf (accessed April 3, 2022).
21. https://www.mlit.go.jp/report/interview/daijin200612.html (accessed April 3, 2022).
22. https://www.kantei.go.jp/jp/98_abe/statement/2020/0618kaiken.html (accessed April 3, 2022).
23. http://www.olc.co.jp/ja/news/news_olc/20200623_02/main/0/link/20200623_03.pdf (accessed April 3, 2022).
24. https://www.mlit.go.jp/report/interview/daijin200717.html (accessed April 3, 2022).
25. https://www.reuters.com/article/emergency-declaration-japan-abe-idJPKCN252072 (accessed April 3, 2022).
26. https://www.metro.tokyo.lg.jp/tosei/governor/governor/kishakaiken/2020/08/06.html (accessed April 3, 2022).
27. https://www5.cao.go.jp/keizai1/danwa/2020/0817_danwa.pdf (accessed April 3, 2022).
28. https://www.kantei.go.jp/jp/98_abe/statement/2020/0828kaiken.html (accessed April 3, 2022).
29. https://www.kantei.go.jp/jp/99_suga/statement/2020/0916kaiken.html (accessed April 5, 2022).
30. https://www.mlit.go.jp/report/interview/daijin200929.html (accessed April 6, 2022).
31. https://corona.go.jp/news/pdf/daijin_youshi_1124.pdf (accessed April 6, 2022).
32. https://www.kantei.go.jp/jp/99_suga/statement/2020/1214kaiken02.html (accessed April 6, 2022).
33. https://www.kantei.go.jp/jp/99_suga/statement/2020/1225kaiken.html (accessed April 6, 2022).
34. https://cdp-japan.jp/news/20201228_0476 (accessed April 6, 2022).
35. https://stopcovid19.metro.tokyo.lg.jp/ (accessed April 6, 2022).
36. https://www.kantei.go.jp/jp/singi/novel_coronavirus/th_siryou/t_gaiyou_r030107.pdf (accessed April 6, 2022).

37. https://www.kantei.go.jp/jp/singi/novel_coronavirus/th_siryou/t_gaiyou_r030113.pdf (accessed April 6, 2022).

38. https://www.kantei.go.jp/jp/99_suga/statement/2021/0104kaiken.html (accessed April 5, 2022).

39. https://www.kantei.go.jp/jp/99_suga/actions/202101/22corona.html (accessed April 6, 2022).

40. https://www.jacom.or.jp/nousei/closeup/2021/210114-48828.php (accessed April 5, 2022).

41. https://www.kantei.go.jp/jp/singi/novel_coronavirus/th_siryou/t_gaiyou_r030202.pdf (accessed April 6, 2022).

42. https://www.pref.tottori.lg.jp/item/1193174.htm (accessed April 6, 2022).

43. https://www3.nhk.or.jp/news/html/20210331/k10012946781000.html (accessed April 6, 2022).

44. https://www.kantei.go.jp/jp/singi/novel_coronavirus/th_siryou/t_gaiyou_r030226.pdf (accessed April 6, 2022).

45. https://www.kantei.go.jp/jp/singi/novel_coronavirus/th_siryou/t_gaiyou_r030305.pdf (accessed April 6, 2022).

46. https://www.kantei.go.jp/jp/singi/novel_coronavirus/th_siryou/t_gaiyou_r0303018.pdf (accessed April 6, 2022).

47. "Tohoku Shinsha Fired the Prime Minister's Eldest Son over the Bribery Scandal," *Nihon Keizai Shimbun (Nikkei)*, February 26, 2021, https://www.nikkei.com/article/DGXZQODZ2672E0W1A220C2000000/ (accessed April 6, 2022).

48. https://www.kantei.go.jp/jp/singi/novel_coronavirus/th_siryou/t_gaiyou_r030423.pdf (accessed April 6, 2022).

49. https://www.kantei.go.jp/jp/singi/novel_coronavirus/th_siryou/t_gaiyou_r030507.pdf (accessed April 6, 2022).

50. https://www.kantei.go.jp/jp/singi/novel_coronavirus/th_siryou/t_gaiyou_r030514.pdf (accessed April 6, 2022).

51. https://www.kantei.go.jp/jp/singi/novel_coronavirus/th_siryou/t_gaiyou_r030521.pdf (accessed April 6, 2022).

52. https://www.kantei.go.jp/jp/singi/novel_coronavirus/th_siryou/t_gaiyou_r030528.pdf (accessed April 6, 2022).

53. https://www.kantei.go.jp/jp/singi/novel_coronavirus/th_siryou/t_gaiyou_r030617.pdf (accessed April 6, 2022).

54. https://www.kantei.go.jp/jp/singi/novel_coronavirus/th_siryou/t_gaiyou_r030708.pdf (accessed April 6, 2022).

55. https://www.kantei.go.jp/jp/singi/novel_coronavirus/th_siryou/t_gaiyou_r030730.pdf (accessed April 6, 2022).

56. https://www.kantei.go.jp/jp/singi/novel_coronavirus/th_siryou/t_gaiyou_r030817.pdf (accessed April 6, 2022).

57. https://www.kantei.go.jp/jp/singi/novel_coronavirus/th_siryou/t_gaiyou_r030825.pdf (accessed April 6, 2022).

58. https://www.kantei.go.jp/jp/singi/novel_coronavirus/th_siryou/t_gaiyou_r030928.pdf (accessed April 6, 2022).

59. https://www.kantei.go.jp/jp/singi/novel_coronavirus/th_siryou/t_gaiyou_r030928.pdf (accessed April 6, 2022).

60. https://www.kantei.go.jp/jp/99_suga/statement/2021/0903kaiken.html (accessed April 6, 2022).

61. https://info.vrs.digital.go.jp/dashboard/ (accessed April 6, 2022).

62. The respondents are provided by Rakuten Insight Inc. The preelection survey has 3,988 cases, and the postelection survey has 2,470 cases. The number of respondents who replied on both is 2,397. We designed own national representative survey sample from the view of gender, age, and area block for the proportional representation tier in the lower house election. However, our sample are biased, and we prepare and use poststratification weight using population of each generation, gender, and districts at the proportional representation tier in the lower house election.

63. On July 9, 2021, at the beginning of our preelection survey, the vaccination rate in Japan had been 31.44 percent. On October 31, the election day of the 2021 lower house election, the rate reached at 77.82 percent according to "Our World in Data" (https://github.com/owid/covid-19-data/tree/master/public/data).

64. The alternatives for each question are 1 = "regretful," 2 = "cannot say," and 3 = "good."

REFERENCES

Bækgaard, Martin, Julian Christensen, Jonas Krogh Madsen, and Kim Sass Mikkelsen. 2020. "Rallying around the Flag in Times of COVID-19: Societal Lockdown and Trust in Democratic Institutions." *Journal of Behavioral Public Administration* 3 (2): 1–12.

Erhardt, Julian, Markus Freitag, Maximilian Filsinger, and Steffen Wamsler. 2021. "The Emotional Foundations of Political Support: How Fear and Anger Affect Trust in the Government in Times of the Covid-19 Pandemic." *Swiss Political Science Review* 27 (2): 339–52.

Fiorina, Morris P. 1978. "Economic Retrospective Voting in American National Elections: A Micro-Analysis." *American Journal of Political Science* 22 (2): 426–43.

Hsieh, John Fuh-Sheng, Dean Lacy, and Emerson M. S. Niou. 1998. "Retrospective and Prospective Voting in a One-Party-Dominant Democracy: Taiwan's 1996 Presidential Election." *Public Choice* 97 (3): 383–99.

Johansson, Bengt, David Nicolas Hopmann, and Adam Shehata. 2021. "When the Rally-Around-the-Flag Effect Disappears, or: When the COVID-19 Pandemic Becomes 'Normalized.'" *Journal of Elections, Public Opinion and Parties* 31 (supl): 321–34.

Kritzinger, Sylvia, Martial Foucault, Romain Lachat, Julia Partheymüller, Carolina Plescia, and Sylvain Brouard. 2021. "'Rally Round the Flag': The COVID-19 Crisis and Trust in the National Government." *West European Politics* 44 (5–6): 1205–31.

Reed, W. Robert, and Joonmo Cho. 1998. "A Comparison of Prospective and Retrospective Voting with Heterogeneous Politicians." *Public Choice* 96 (1/2): 93–116.

10

Identity Politics and International Relations in Australia

Yu-Hua Chen

A STRATEGIC ENVIRONMENT NOT SEEN IN A CENTURY

For decades China has been a critical factor shaping U.S. global strategy. When Mao Zedong stood at the Gate of Heavenly Peace and announced the founding of the People's Republic of China (PRC) in 1949, Americans saw Communist China as an opportunity. With the tradeoff of abandoning Chiang Kai-Shek's Republic of China (ROC) on Taiwan, the Harry Truman government had the strategic goal of forming a united front with the PRC against the emerging Soviet threat. Misjudging the true intentions of Mao in the Korean War, the initial strategy Americans used to handle U.S.-China relations in the first phase of the Cold War was containment. Despite this confrontational beginning, China remained a potentially viable partner for the United States because, in the eyes of U.S. policymakers, China was more like a puppet manipulated by the Soviet Union than the main source of strategic threat. The containment strategy was less about toppling the PRC regime and more about building a *cordon sanitaire* around the Soviet Union's sphere of influence to prevent the spread of communism. China was not the United States's strategic competitor.

In the period from the 1970s to the mid-2000s, the United States and China can be viewed as informal allies tackling a wide range of global issues together. The Sino-Soviet Split in the 1960s created a mutual enemy, and therefore also created strategic momentum for the United States and China to cooperate against the Soviet Union. Henry Kissinger's secret visits to China in 1971 subsequently ushered in a new U.S. strategy toward China for the following decades—engagement. By engaging with China, the United States brought China into the Liberal International Order (LIO), which had been built by and maintained through U.S. hegemony after World War II. Although the United States and China had their share of differences, and leaders in Beijing were wary about the true intentions of the Americans, the two states dealt with a variety of global issues, such as the Soviet strategic threat, North Korean nuclear weapons, terrorism, and climate change, in a nonconfrontational manner. This informal U.S.-China alignment reached its peak when U.S. Deputy Secretary of State Robert Zoellick envisioned China taking a bigger role in world affairs as a responsible stakeholder at the National Committee on U.S.-China Relations in 2005. Based on the assumption that China was fundamentally different from the Soviet Union, he stated:

> For thirty years, our policy has been to draw out the People's Republic of China. As a result, the China of today is simply not the Soviet Union of the late 1940s: It does not seek to spread radical, anti-American ideologies; While not yet democratic, it does not see itself in a twilight conflict against democracy around the globe; While at times mercantilist, it does not see itself in a death struggle with capitalism; And most importantly, *China does not believe that its future depends on overturning the fundamental order of the international system* [emphasis added]. In fact, quite the reverse: Chinese leaders have decided that their success depends on being networked with the modern world.[1]

When the United States took the unprecedented move of making China its strategic competitor in 2017, China and the United States officially entered a competition of great powers. With material power accumulated from the era of "reform and opening up," the foreign behavior of Xi Jinping's China has fundamentally departed from Deng Xiaoping's policy of "hide your strength, bide your time," which Jiang Zemin and Hu Jintao had carefully adhered to. Aiming to restore the glorious international status China held centuries ago, China has demonstrated an aggressive, coercive approach to interacting with others. It has challenged the LIO in almost all respects, from human rights to democracy, international law to global governance, and traditional military security to 5G technology.[2] In response, the United States has officially recognized the failure of its decades-long engagement strategy in the 2017 National Security Strategy and repositioned China as a strategic competitor that is endeavoring to build a new world order antithetical to U.S. values and interests. As the scope and scale of U.S.-China competition has expanded over the years, states around the world, and particularly in East Asia, are facing the awkward and difficult strategic choice of whether to side with China or the United States. As Moon Hee-sang, the speaker of South Korea's legislature, frankly stated, "Asking whether South Korea will choose either China or the US is like asking a child whether you like your dad or your mom . . . we cannot abandon economy for the sake of security, and we cannot abandon security for the sake of economy."[3]

AUSTRALIA'S PUZZLING CHOICE

The question of what to do when a state is involved in a great power competition has constantly been asked by policymakers and scholars in both the West and East, and in the past and present. The most relevant academic discussion on this question centers around the literature on alliance theory. Essentially, there are five main strategies that the states can opt for: external balancing, internal balancing, hedging, neutrality, and bandwagoning. The way in which two states engaged in a great power competition perceive the strategic choices of smaller powers, in terms of threat perception, means that these five strategies form a strategic option spectrum for smaller states (see figure 10.1).

In a hypothetical situation where great power A and great power B are in a competition and C is involved, from A's perspective, the most threatening strategy adopted by C would be external balancing, as C's power and resources would quickly benefit A's adversary B. By contrast, A would most favor C undertaking a bandwagoning strategy for the same

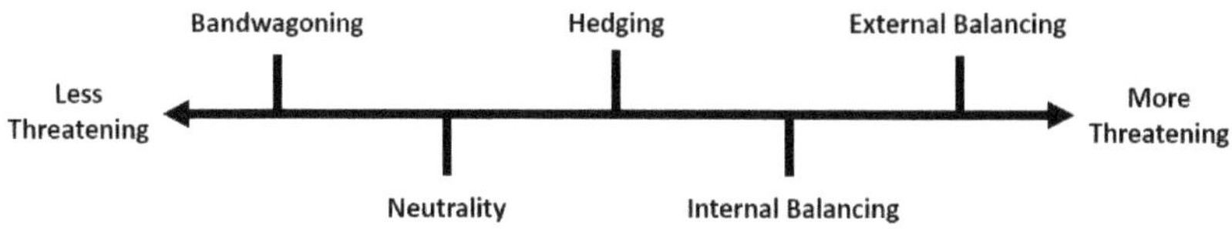

Figure 10.1. The Strategic Option Spectrum
Source: Figure created by the author.

reason. Internal balancing will be regarded by A as a less threatening strategy than external balancing because C does not formally commit to assisting B in wartime but only against A by its domestic effort. Also, training and arming the military takes a longer time and hence will not radically alter the balance of power between A and B. A hedging strategy would also be viewed favorably by A, as by hesitating to support B's invitation to collectively escalate the conflict with A, C would be demonstrating reluctance to show hostility toward A. Finally, neutrality falls somewhere between bandwagoning and hedging in this spectrum as a strategy posing no substantive threat or help to either A or B.

For many scholars, hedging is expected to be the most pervasive strategy for states in East Asia facing the U.S.-China competition for one simple reason: direct balancing against China is a costly option in a security environment full of uncertainty.[4] For small and medium-sized states in East Asia, balancing against China with the United States may not be a wise strategy because (1) they rely on China economically and (2) China, with its military and economic might, has a remarkable record of punitive behavior toward smaller players. Chinese sanctions on South Korea over the Terminal High Altitude Area Defense issue in 2016 is an illustrative example in this regard. But at the same time, those states do not want to lose their security relations with the United States either. As a result, the predictable response to this awkward strategic choice is a hedging strategy. Smaller states avoid siding with the United States by not committing to policies that aim to contain China, but keep their security relations with the United States intact in other ways. Taiwan, Malaysia, Singapore, Vietnam, Australia, and Japan are cases frequently mentioned by scholars in literature about hedging behavior.[5] Van Jackson even predicts that hedging behavior will be the most prevalent and long-term trend in the East Asian region in the era of U.S.-China competition.[6] Former prime minister of Singapore Lee Hsien Loong also warned that his country "must avoid being caught in the middle or forced into invidious choices."[7] Australia, however, is moving counter to this scholarly prediction.

Empirically, Australia is one of the states (if not the) in this region to balance against China most strongly. Australia's hardline responses to China before and during the pandemic years have surprised many China experts. It was Australia that asked for the international community to have an independent study on the origin of COVID-19 in Wuhan. It was also Australia that was most vocal among the Quadrilateral Security Dialogue (QUAD) members supporting the military integration of the member countries.[8] The most threatening move of Canberra in the eyes of Beijing recently is the formation of AUKUS, a trilateral defense partnership between Australia, the United Kingdom, and the United States. Through AUKUS, Australia will develop its nuclear submarines with the assistance of the United Kingdom and the United States to counter China's maritime ambitions in the South China Sea. Simply put, Australia is stepping up its security relations with the United States and showing obvious balancing behavior against China.

At first glance, Australia does not seem to have many incentives for leveling up its confrontations with China in this U.S.-China competition. Australia is geographically distant from China. There are more than eight thousand kilometers between Beijing and Canberra, within which they have no shared land or maritime borders. Economic relations have largely determined China-Australia relations over the decades. China is Australia's largest trading partner accounting for nearly 30 percent of Australian exports such as iron ore, coal, cotton, and various agricultural products. China is also the main source of foreign students and tourism for Australia.[9] Although China is the ninth-largest foreign investor in Australia, Chinese investment in Australia has grown remarkably in the past ten years. In a word, the economic benefits to Australia of amicable relations with China are enormous. In addition, the steadily growing Chinese community in Australia is becoming more and more politically influential. China is one main source of Australia's immigrant population. Nowadays, there are more than 1.2 million people with Chinese heritage in Australia, which is about 5 percent of the Australian population. This Chinese community exercises considerable political power at times. For example, due to his anti-Beijing stance in 2007, the former Australian prime minister John Howard was ousted by his own Sydney's Bennelong district, where 21 percent of the residents had a Chinese background.

Australia, therefore, presents a puzzling case to alliance theory literature. How can we explain Australia's balancing behavior against China in the U.S.-China competition? What drives this strategic choice? What is the impact of COVID-19 on this choice? More importantly, what lessons can Taiwan learn from Australia in the era of U.S.-China strategic competition? The remainder of this chapter will answer those questions in detail.

AUSTRALIA'S IDENTITY: FROM A PASSIVE ORDER TAKER TO PROACTIVE ORDER MAINTAINER

Identity has been one of the key approaches adopted by scholars in the field of international relations (IR) to understand state behavior from nonmainstream IR research paradigms over the past decades. The concept of identity entered social science as early as the 1950s[10] and became popular in IR along with the rise of social constructivism in the late 1980s and the early 1990s. Essentially, scholars who apply this concept in their research attempt to explain why a state is conducting behavior that makes little sense from the perspective of systemic theories of realism and liberalism by looking into the state's unique "personality"—what the state is and what it represents. For example, many leaders in Washington see the United States as the leader of the free world, so in their eyes, promoting democracy and protecting human rights worldwide is the United States's inherent responsibility. Explaining this behavior of the United States solely through material interests is not enough: it clearly involves nonmaterial interests. State identity, in other words, serves as the foundation for state behavior because it defines the values and interests that are most important in the eyes of policymakers, who collectively conceptualize the state identity.[11]

In addition, identity is relational and dynamic. What the identity a person is holding depends on who the person's significant other in discussion is. A can be a friend of B today but a foe of B tomorrow. Switching between these two identities happens when the way A and B interact with one another changed. State identity has the same logic. So, as China has seemingly begun to challenge the current international order since 2012, many states have gradually felt it necessary to recalibrate their relations with China and hence to reconsider the appropriateness of their identities in the current international order. Like all states, Australia has reexamined its identity.

For many decades, Australia had the state identity of a "passive order taker." The LIO led by the United States is embedded with values and principles that Australia identifies with and prospers from, such as democracy, human rights, free trade, freedom of navigation, and egalitarianism. Australia was happy to be complacently compliant with that order, enjoying the benefits of it, and closely followed the lead of the

United States after World War II. It is for this reason that Australia has participated in every major war that the United States has fought throughout the twentieth and twenty-first centuries: from Korea to Vietnam, then Afghanistan to Iraq. The United States has no ally more loyal than Australia. This is not to argue that, as a passive order taker, Australia had no agency in the international system or that it made no contribution to the global community. It is just that very few policymakers in Canberra seriously questioned the United States's ability to govern the order. Not to mention thinking about how to help Americans maintain the LIO. Allying with the United States has been an unquestionable component of Australia's state identity since World War II.

Being an ally of the United States does not mean that Australia sees China, with its communist ideology and authoritarian model of governance, as a natural enemy. Australia, like many states in East Asia, depends on the lucrative Chinese market to a great degree and engaged with China based on the assumption that the security and prosperity split is a false dichotomy in the post–Cold War era. Instead of viewing a powerful China as a threat to the LIO, a significant number of Australians held the view that a rising China will give Asia a better future. This optimistic view of China of Australians is reflected in a 2014 poll of the Lowy Institute, which showed most Australians regarded China as Australia's "best friend" in Asia.[12] In a scenario in which China challenges the LIO in the future, some Australian strategists even suggested Australia should keep a distance from the United States. Hugh White, a professor at Australian National University and the principal writer for Australia's 2000 Defense White Paper, is a prominent figure advocating this line of thinking. He argued that if the inevitable U.S.-China strategic rivalry arrived in Asia, Australia should not stay within the United States's orbit as it has always done but should encourage the United States to share power with China.[13]

This state identity of Australia became increasingly unsustainable after Xi's China began pushing for the Chinese International Order (CIO) in 2012. Many Chinese Communist Party (CCP) leaders are nationalists who desire China to move back to its central position in Asia and rule this region through the CIO as it did a hundred years ago. This central kingdom mentality was one important factor that drove Mao to join the Korean War to save North Korea.[14] Xi is also this type of leader. For Xi, the CIO is a hierarchical international order in which China is at the top, like an emperor governing his kingdom in whatever way he sees fit. Sinocentrism, hierarchical authority, antidemocracy and human rights, and a transactional mode of interaction are key components of this international order. China's aggressive actions in Asia since 2012 can be seen as part of a process in which China is endeavoring to replace the LIO with the CIO through its military muscle and political might. States like Taiwan, Japan, the Philippines, South Korea, Singapore, India, and Vietnam have been victims, to varying degrees, of Chinese coercion in this process. As for Australia, it has been antagonized by Chinese political influence within Australia which has attempted to break the U.S.-Australia alliance. Against this backdrop, Australian policymakers and academic circles engaged in deep reflection on Australia's state identity in relation to China, which Rory Medcalf called the Great Australian China Debate,[15] around 2016. This debate posed a series of questions reassessing two critical dimensions of Australia's order taker identity:

1. On Australia-China relations: What is the true nature of China? Is China a challenger determined to rewrite the international order? If so, will China become a threat to Australia?
2. On Australia-U.S. relations: What would be the correct position for Australia in the coming U.S.-China strategic competition? Should Australia remain in the U.S. camp and adhere to the LIO? Or should she switch to the Chinese side and support the CIO instead? Is there a third alternative?

Leaders in Canberra had few disagreements on the first dimension. Australia sees China under Xi as determined to remap the international order of East Asia. For this reason, it is quite usually to see both the Liberal-National Coalition and the Labor Party urge China to respect the rule-based international order. There is also bipartisan consensus that China is hostile to Australia and surrendering sovereignty to China is not an option. Australian policymakers, as a result, worked on three tough laws (The National Security Legislation Amendment Act 2018, Foreign Influence Transparency Scheme Act, and Electoral Legislation Amendment Act) to protect its democracy against Chinese influence in 2017 and implemented them in the following year. When asked about China's infiltration of Australian politics, former prime minister Malcolm Turnbull voiced this in Chinese:

> Modern China was founded in 1949 with these words: "中国人民站起来," "the Chinese people have stood up." It was an assertion of sovereignty; it was an assertion of pride. And we stand up, and so we say, "澳大利亚人民站起来," "the Australian people stand up."[16]

On the second dimension of redefining Australian state identity, however, it was harder to reach a consensus due to U.S. strategic retrenchment. Australia sensed that the United States's ability to govern the LIO in East Asia was in decline, mainly because the United States under the Donald Trump government had little intention to maintain its role as leader of the LIO. The United States was still the most powerful player in world affairs and will remain so for the next decade, but Trump was an isolationist. Driven by the doctrine of America first, the United States withdrew from international commitments like the Trans-Pacific Partnership and pressured many of its Asian allies, Australia included, to give Americans better treatment on a host of issues. To punish Australia for a refugee-transfer agreement, for instance, the United States sent no ambassador to Australia for nineteenth months from September 2016 to March 2019. Seeing American foreign policies like those instated one after another, some leaders in Canberra believed that the United States's security commitment to East Asia was in decline at best and U.S. leadership in world affairs was dysfunctional at worst. The United States could not be relied on as it had been in the past. Former prime minister of Australia of the Labor Party Paul Keating, for instance, asserted Australia should have its own China policy independent of the United States:

> The United States is still fundamentally pursuing the policy for the maintenance of primacy against the obvious rise of China and therefore resisting the whole idea of sharing strategic power in Asia, which I believe the United States should do with the Chinese. . . . We both need and deserved a nuanced foreign policy which does take account of these big seismic shifts in the world. . . . Strategic hegemony by the United States in the Pacific is incapable of preservation.[17]

A new state identity for Australia—a proactive order maintainer—emerged after the debate. Faced with this unprecedented strategic environment with an assertive China plus unstable U.S. commitment to East Asia, Australia ultimately determined to take a path of "self-help under anarchy," taking greater responsibility for preventing the LIO from being overthrown by China instead of simply counting on the United States. Sovereignty and values and principles that Australia has long recognized are something that money cannot buy. The new state identity of Australia is best illustrated by the 2017 Foreign Policy White Paper, which is a collaborative work by more than a hundred Australian senior diplomats across different political parties and Australia has not published a foreign policy paper of this kind for more than a decade. While recognizing the importance of U.S.-Australian alliance relations, it stresses the necessity of Australia taking a bigger responsibility for its own security and prosperity by other means such as working more closely with other major democracies in this region and increasing its defense expenditure. It believes that Australia being a more willing partner of the United States would enhance U.S. global leadership and hence a more secure strategic environment for Australia.[18]

The idea of taking more responsibility has appeared increasingly in the language used by Australian policymakers after 2017. Calling itself an "important regional leader in the global community," for instance, the Australian government has now committed a historically high amount of 270 billion (AUD) to defense spending in the newly released defense white paper to strengthen Australia's ability to shape this fragile strategic environment of Asia. Current prime minister Scott Morrison's speech introducing this defense plan is another excellent example displaying Australia's new state identity. He argues that "relations between China and the United States are fractured, at best, as they compete for political, economic and technological supremacy. But it's important to acknowledge that *they are not the only actors of consequence.*"[19] Believing middle powers in this region like Korea, Indonesia, Vietnam, and Australia are all capable of making a significant difference for the CIO, he conveyed a message to the world that Australia has determined to play its part by militarily investing its own future.

Since the Great Australian China debate, three critical and interlinked components define this new state identity of Australia for leaders in Canberra:

1. China is a potential threat to Australia: China is a challenger to the LIO and promotes the CIO, which contains principles and values antithetical to those that Australia identifies with. Joining the CIO has no appeal to Australia.
2. Australia is a supporter of the LIO centering around the United States: Allying with the United States leading the LIO remains an integrated part of Australian identity. Hedging against China is not an option.
3. Not taking the LIO for granted: Australia can no longer comfortably count on the United States for its security; it needs to proactively shoulder more responsibility for defending both itself and the LIO in this challenging time.

STATE IDENTITY STRENGTHENING

Before the outbreak of COVID-19, there was a gap between political elites and the grassroots in terms of how Australia's new state identity was perceived. As mentioned earlier, Australia, with its decades-long economic dependence on China, supposed that it could be on friendly terms with every power in the world, regardless of political systems and ideology. For most Australians, Australia's relations with China are equally important as relations with the United States, even though Australia has been an ally of the United States for many decades.[20]

Despite Chinese militarization of disputed features of the South China Sea in 2016 shocking Australian society, and despite "Power Influence," an episode of *Four Corners* of the Australian Broadcasting Corporation, which unveiled years of covert Chinese political influence operations taking advantage of the vulnerability of Australian democracy in 2017, most Australians still did not view China as a security threat to their nation. Military conflict with China was a remote possibility. Terrorism, climate change, and cyberattacks were issues Australians considered much greater threats to the safety of Australia. Voices criticizing China were frequently raised in Australian society and some scholars argued that the Australian media's reporting on China was based on "adversarial journalism,"[21] but few people asked serious questions about what actions Australia should take in a position against China before 2020. Therefore, while political leaders in Canberra knew the necessity and urgency of Australia becoming a proactive order maintainer guarding against Chinese encroachment on the LIO, most Australians lacked that awareness. This gap in the perception of Australia's new identity is evidenced in a poll by the Lowy Institute, which showed more than half of Australians surveyed saw China as more of an economic partner than a security threat before 2020.[22]

Empirically, Chinese coercive behavior at home and toward Australia during the pandemic years from 2020 to 2021 bridged this different view of Australia's new identity between leaders and the public. During the pandemic years, Australian media usually reported on how the Chinese government handled COVID-19 in quite a negative way—first that China intentionally covered up the information about the new coronavirus at Wuhan, and then that it adopted inhumane lockdowns of cities across China, sacrificing countless Chinese lives. The story of the whistleblower Dr. Li Wenliang who tried to tell the world about COVID-19 being silenced by the CCP is one infamous example of the media showcasing the authoritarian nature of China. Although the reporting adhered to the truth, the CCP's success of controlling the explosion of COVID-19 in China as well as the bureaucratic communication problems existing between the central and local governments were often ignored. Taiwan, New Zealand, and Singapore were instead referred to by the media as successful examples of containing the spread of COVID-19. China's image in the minds of Australians considerably deteriorated due to media representation.

Furthermore, Beijing's "wolverine diplomacy" toward Australia enraged many Australians. China placed massive economic sanctions on Australia after Canberra called for an independent inquiry into the origin of COVID-19 in Wuhan. It limited or slapped punitive tariffs on a wide range of Australian exports to China, including barley, beef, wine, wheat, wool, lobsters, sugar, copper, timber, grapes, iron, and coal. Although the Chinese sanctions only inflicted mild damage on Australia's trade with China overall, the sanctions themselves sent a crystal-clear political message to Australians—obey or be bullied. Then the Chinese embassy in Australia issued fourteen points of grievances to Australia, accusing Australia of poisoning bilateral relations. This sort of economic and diplomatic coercion launched by China during the pandemic years all served as a sober reminder to those who took a sanguine view of the rise of China about the true nature of China and what the world will look like if China dominates. Ultimately, political elites' and ordinary citizens' perceptions of Australia's state identity converged during the pandemic years. The Lowy Institute's polls evidence this sharp change in public perception of state identity from 2020 to 2021:[23]

1. Overall, Australians' impressions of China worsened during the pandemic years. Feelings toward China decreased seven points from 39 percent to 32 percent on the feelings thermometer of the Lowy Institute, making China the second-most disliked nation of Australians after North Korea. Regarding the tense China-Australian relations, most Australians think China is to blame.
2. In 2020, 55 percent of Australians believed that China was more of an economic partner while 41 percent saw China as a security threat. Hitting a record high, 63 percent of Australians viewed China as a security threat in 2021, while seeing China in mainly economic terms dropped to 34 percent. This sharp and substantial change of views on China is especially common in people over the age of thirty.
3. In 2020, 77 percent of Australians did not trust China to act responsibly in the world. In 2021, eight out of ten distrust China. Meanwhile, only 10 percent of Australians have confidence in Xi to do the right thing regarding world affairs in 2021, dropping from 20 percent in 2020.
4. Australians' lack of confidence in the United States has persisted during the pandemic years. 92 percent of Australians viewed the United States as handling COVID-19 badly. On confidence in the United States to act responsibly in the world, 61 percent of Australians held a positive view, significantly less than the 80 percent rate of confidence in Japan.
5. Interestingly, Australians have strongly supported the alliance with the United States before and after COVID-19, especially the older generation. Despite the vigorous Great Australian China Debate among policymakers and academic circles, most Australians saw the alliance with the United States as indispensable. 78 percent of Australians regarded alliance with the United States as very important or fairly important in 2020, and this remains consistent in 2021.
6. Although the polls did not ask what actions people in Australia wish their government to take to defend the LIO, Australians gave their

robust support to the QUAD in 2020. 88 percent recognized Australia to form the four-way security partnership with Japan, the United States, and India.

Component by component, COVID-19 has had the effect of strengthening Australia's new state identity by enlisting greater support from the public. First of all, the image of China as a dangerous challenger to the LIO and a security threat to Australia has become well established in the minds of ordinary Australians. COVID-19 put a quick end to the dwindling optimism about China in Australian society. Second, political elites and ordinary Australians are now on the same page regarding the United States as well. Although some people questioned the existing security U.S.-Australian relations during the Great Australian China Debate, abandoning the alliance relations with the United States ultimately gained no traction among leaders or the public either before or since the pandemic. This component endures the challenges of COVID-19. The final component that Australia should be more proactive is indirectly supported by the public views that the United States is incapable of managing the virus domestically and the confirmation of reaching our like-minded partners such as QUAD members. Nonetheless, it should be noted that this new Australian state identity may not be shared by Australians with Chinese heritage. In another poll conducted by the Lowy Institute, this ethnic group has developed a more favorable view of China and its system of government after COVID-19.[24]

One critical consequence of this strengthened Australian state identity is that both the Liberal-National Coalition and the Labor Party have a stronger basis for a hardline approach toward China. As happened in the United States, resisting Chinese intrusion on the LIO is one of few things that both sides of politics in Canberra agree on. There are many cases of a hardline approach against China receiving bipartisan consensus in parliament since the pandemic. For instance, the Labor Party endorsed the current Morrison government's decision to purchase nuclear submarines from the United Kingdom and the United States to better defend against Chinese military activities in the Indo-Pacific region. Though this agreement would ax a similar agreement with the French and further made China explore, Labor avoided attacking the Morrison government over this decision. The Labor Party also supported the Morrison government's criticism of China's human rights abuses in Xinjiang and Hong Kong, if not indeed being more critical. On the issue of launching an independent investigation into the origin of COVID-19 in Wuhan, the Labor leader Anthony Albanese supported the government's position and said, "It was wrong to block WHO investigators from entering . . . the fact is that it's unacceptable. . . . The whole world, not just Australia, needs to do this research, and it should be done openly and transparently, and it should be promoted by China."[25] Taking a tough approach to interacting with China is necessary for the Labor Party because "China has changed."[26]

The different sides of politics in parliament may not see eye to eye on every issue related to China, but the basic position is the same—that Australia can and should exercise its agency to do more to protect the LIO from being overthrown by China in this challenging time. The Liberal-National Coalition and the Labor Party share the same vision for the state identity of Australia, so a proactive Australia is now becoming common language for leaders of both parties. For example, Penny Wong, the shadow foreign minister, made these points clearly in her speech at the Australian National University in November 2021:

> Australia's leaders should take the world as it is, and seek to shape it for the better. . . . We need to improve our performance across the whole range of capabilities required to shape outcomes in the world.[27]

Taking more responsibility for guarding elements of the LIO, the positions of the two parties on the issue of whether Australia will defend Taiwan in a China-Taiwan military conflict are also gradually aligning. Back in 2004, the Australian foreign minister from the Liberal Party Alexander Downer once claimed Australia would not aid Taiwan if China attacked her. Now, Defense Minister Peter Dutton has unambiguously committed Australia's support to managing the stability of the Taiwan Strait by stating, "Provide a deterrence against actions . . . because the Communist party has been very clear about their intent in relation to Taiwan."[28] Wong is in line with Dutton's stance that the current status quo over the Taiwan Strait is something Australia needs to actively protect and maintain, though in terms of tactics she emphasizes the value of strategic ambiguity of Australia over the Taiwan Strait, rather than Dutton's emphasis on building deterrents against China. She said, "Labor supports AUKUS, we support ANZUS, and we are sticking to the long-held bipartisan position on Taiwan, even if Mr Dutton is walking away from it."[29]

LESSONS FOR TAIWAN

This paper argues that to make sense of Australia's puzzling balancing behavior toward China, understanding Australia's new state identity is the key. Like many states in East Asia, Australia faces an awkward strategic choice between security and prosperity, leading it to avoid taking a side in the U.S.-China rivalry. Unlike many in East Asia, however, Australia performs balancing instead of hedging against China, making it a case worthy of theoretical investigation. Faced with an unprecedented strategic environment since World War II, with a rising and more assertive China and an unstable U.S. commitment to this region, Australia has turned to self-help, and thus reshaped its state identity into that of a proactive order maintainer. Recognizing its own agency in the international system, Australia is adopting strategies to protect the LIO from being replaced by the CIO as well as defending its own sovereignty.

In hindsight, Australia has benefited from its new state identity, as it has showcased to the world during the pandemic years that security and prosperity are a false dichotomy. As the saying goes, "God helps those who help themselves." While many have assumed (Australians included) that losing the Chinese market would be an economic catastrophe and hence refuse to uphold the LIO with the United States in the U.S.-China competition, Australia has demonstrated that the economic costs are far lower than many have expected. By trade diversion, the massive economic attack China launched against Australia during the pandemic years cost Australia a net loss of just 1 billion (AUD), which is only around 0.25 of Australia's annual GDP.[30] Not only has Australia's economy ultimately become more resilient than ever before, but Australia gained improved standing in the international community for living well and standing up to China. U.S. president Joseph Biden praised Australia thus: "The United States has no closer or more reliable ally than Australia."[31]

Taiwan, though facing a structurally similar strategic environment to Australia, has not yet been through a serious state identity debate. In many ways, Taiwan faces a more ominous external environment than Australia.

For one thing, in addition to China's stronger influence over everyday life in Taiwan, Taiwan stands at the very frontline of Chinese territorial expansion. Xi has made it clear that the separation of Taiwan and China cannot last from generation to generation. Chinese aircraft circling the island of Taiwan or intruding into Taiwan's Air Defense Identification Zone has become normal in the Xi era. China's coercive diplomacy toward only increased during pandemic years. Second, although both Taiwan and Australia need to deal with the teetering U.S. commitment to East Asia, there hasn't been any formal security treaty signed between Taiwan and the United States since the 1970s, making Taiwan even more vulnerable. U.S. forces fighting for Taiwan are not obligatory under the Taiwan Relations Act. The Biden government seems to be more committed to the defense of Taiwan than the Trump government. Nevertheless, no one can be sure that there will not be another isolationist U.S. president like Trump in the future, which may be exacerbated as many in Washington see the cost of defending Taiwan as increasingly unaffordable. During the pandemic years, people of Taiwan also witnessed how the United States addressed the pandemic crisis poorly at home. Despite Taiwan's precarious situation, there is no serious state identity debate about what Taiwan is and what Taiwan stands for taking place in policy and academic circles yet.

A state identity debate is essential for the security of Taiwan for several reasons. To begin with, without a debate like this to unambiguously define friends and foes of Taiwan and unite Taiwanese political parties and people, it is difficult for the Taiwanese government to work out a long-term, sustainable China policy. A change of political power may lead to a policy *volte-face*. No one can know if the policies currently undertaken by the Tsai Ing-wen government, which were applauded by the international community, will come to an end in the next government. Because the next presidential election is just two years away, this problem is becoming increasingly urgent. Also, given that China has been conducting influence activities in Taiwan for decades, China may easily take advantage of potential political division between the Kuomintang and the Democratic Progressive Party or between the people of Taiwan and political parties whenever possible. Most importantly, Australia, Japan, and the United States now all appear to have a strategic clarity under the disguise of tactical ambiguity regarding the stability of the Taiwan Strait. Those powers are sending a message to China together that China taking over Taiwan by force is unacceptable. Having a serious debate about the position Taiwan should take in the U.S.-China competition would send a message to those security partners of Taiwan and concerned parties that Taiwan is not taking international support for granted but is very willing to defend the sovereignty of Taiwan by itself. Only by doing so can Taiwan attract more friends to help it when the central focus of world politics shifts back to the great power competition in East Asia in the postpandemic era.

NOTES

1. Please see Robert Zoellick's remark on the National Committee on U.S.-China Relations here: https://2001-2009.state.gov/s/d/former/zoellick/rem/53682.htm (accessed February 22, 2022).
2. Doshi 2021; Pillsbury 2015; Ward 2019.
3. Friedman 2019.
4. Goh 2006; Jackson 2014; Cheng-Chwee 2008; Haacke 2019; Wu 2019.
5. Wu 2019; Hiep 2013; Koga 2019; Subramanian 2020; Lee 2017.
6. Jackson 2014.
7. Lee 2020.
8. Center for Strategic and International Studies 2020.
9. Please see the figure released by the Department of Foreign Affairs and Trade of Australian Government here: https://www.dfat.gov.au/about-us/publications/trade-investment/trade-at-a-glance/Pages/trade-at-a-glance (accessed February 22, 2022).
10. Erikson 1956.
11. Jepperson, Wendt, and Katzenstein 1996.
12. Oliver 2014, 5.
13. White 2010.
14. Chen 2001.
15. Fullilove 2021; Concerned Scholars of China 2018; Open Letter Respondents 2018; Medcalf 2018.
16. Gribbin 2017.
17. Gribbin 2016.
18. Australian Government 2017.
19. Please see Scott Morrison's speech here: https://www.rev.com/blog/transcripts/scott-morrison-speech-transcript-unveiling-270bn-australian-defence-plan (accessed February 22, 2022).
20. Oliver 2017, 10.

21. Sun 2019.
22. Kassam 2021, 12.
23. Kassam 2021.
24. Kassam and Hsu n.d.
25. Hurst 2021a.
26. Hurst 2021b.
27. Wong, 2021a.
28. Hurst 2021c.
29. Wong 2021b
30. Frydenberg 2021.
31. Wintour 2021.

REFERENCES

Australian Government. 2017. The Commonwealth of Australia's 2017 Foreign Policy White Paper. November. Accessed February 22, 2022. https://www.dfat.gov.au/sites/default/files/2017-foreign-policy-white-paper.pdf.

Center for Strategic and International Studies. 2020. CSIS Briefs, March 16. Accessed February 22, 2022. https://www.csis.org/analysis/defining-diamond-past-present-and-future-quadrilateral-security-dialogue.

Cheng-Chwee, Kuik. 2008. "The Essence of Hedging: Malaysia and Singapore's Response to a Rising China." *Contemporary Southeast Asia* 30 (2): 159–85.

Chen, Jian. 2001. *Mao's China and the Cold War*. Chapel Hill and London: University of North Carolina Press.

Concerned Scholars of China. 2018. "An Open Letter from Concerned Scholars of China and the Chinese Diaspora." Policy Forum, March 26. Accessed February 22, 2022. https://www.policyforum.net/an-open-letter-from-concerned-scholars-of-china-and-the-chinese-diaspora/.

Doshi, Rush. 2021. *The Long Game: China's Grand Strategy to Displace American Order*. London: Oxford University Press.

Erikson, Erik Homburger. 1956. "The Problem of Ego Identity." *Journal of the American Psychoanalytic Association* 4 (1): 56–121.

Friedman, Rui. 2019. "How to Choose Between the U.S. and China? It's Not That Easy." *The Atlantic*, July 26. Accessed February 22, 2022. https://www.theatlantic.com/politics/archive/2019/07/south-korea-china-united-states-dilemma/594850/.

Frydenberg, Josh. 2021. "Building Resilience and the Return of Strategic Competition." Speech at Australian National University, September 6. Accessed February 22, 2022. https://ministers.treasury.gov.au/ministers/josh-frydenberg-2018/speeches/building-resilience-and-return-strategic-competition?fbclid=IwAR02Smut_Hic19OZkurRV1pEPvmVJPs0Mm5y8y3JcXnx8Z3C4fn871jQ49c.

Fullilove, Michael. 2021. "Down and Out Down Under: Australia's Uneasy American Alliance." Foreign Affairs (September/October). Accessed February 22, 2022. https://www.foreignaffairs.com/articles/2017-08-15/down-and-out-down-under.

Goh, Evelyn. 2006. "Understanding 'Hedging' in Asia-Pacific Security." *PacNet* 43.

Gribbin, Caitlyn. 2016. "Paul Keating Warns Australia to Prepare for the 'Rise of China' with Strong Foreign Policy." *ABC News*, April 30. Accessed February 22, 2022. https://www.abc.net.au/news/2016-08-31/paul-keating-warns-australia-to-prepare-for-the-rise-of-china/7800062.

Gribbin, Caitlyn. 2017. "Malcolm Turnbull Declares He Will 'Stand Up' for Australia in Response to China's Criticism." *ABC News*, December 9. Accessed February 22, 2022. https://www.abc.net.au/news/2017-12-09/malcolm-turnbull-says-he-will-stand-up-for-australia/9243274.

Haacke, Jürgen. 2019. "The Concept of Hedging and Its Application to Southeast Asia: A Critique and a Proposal for a Modified Conceptual and Methodological Framework." *International Relations of the Asia-Pacific* 19 (3): 375–417.

Hiep, Le Hong. 2013. "Vietnam's Hedging Strategy against China since Normalization." *Contemporary Southeast Asia* 35 (3): 333–68.

Hurst, Daniel. 2021a. "Australia Says China Should Allow in WHO Covid Investigators 'Without Delay.'" *The Guardian*, January 6. Accessed February 22, 2022. https://www.theguardian.com/world/2021/jan/06/australia-says-china-should-allow-in-who-covid-investigators-without-delay.

Hurst, Daniel. 2021b. "'China Has Changed': Albanese Pushes Back at Keating's Criticism of Labor and Aukus." *The Guardian*, November 11. Accessed February 22, 2022. https://www.theguardian.com/australia-news/2021/nov/11/china-has-changed-albanese-pushes-back-at-keatings-criticism-of-labor-and-aukus.

Hurst, Daniel. 2021c. "Peter Dutton Attacks Penny Wong on China Declaring He Aims to Deter 'Aggression' on Taiwan." *The Guardian*, November 23. Accessed February 22, 2022. https://www.theguardian.com/australia-news/2021/nov/23/peter-dutton-attacks-penny-wong-on-china-declaring-he-aims-to-deter-aggression-on-taiwan.

Jackson, Van. 2014. "Power, Trust, and Network Complexity: Three Logics of Hedging in Asian Security." *International Relations of the Asia-Pacific* 14 (3): 331–56.

Jepperson, Ronald L., Alexander Wendt, and Peter Katzenstein. 1996. "Norms, Identity and Culture in National Security." In *The Culture of National Security*, edited by Peter Katzenstein, 33–78. New York: Columbia University Press.

Kassam, Natasha. 2021. Lowy Institute Poll 2021. Lowy Institute. Accessed February 22, 2022. https://poll.lowyinstitute.org/files/lowyinsitutepoll-2021.pdf.

Kassam, Natasha, and Jennifer Hsu. N.d. "Being Chinese in Australia: Public Opinion in Chinese Communities." Lowy Institute. Accessed February 22, 2022. https://interactives.lowyinstitute.org/features/chinese-communities.

Koga, Kei. 2019. "Japan's 'Free and Open Indo-Pacific' Strategy: Tokyo's Tactical Hedging and the Implications for ASEAN." *Contemporary Southeast Asia* 41 (2): 286–313.

Lee, Hsien Loong. 2020. "The Endanger Asian Century: America, China, and the Perils of Confrontation." *Foreign Affairs* (July/August). Accessed February 22, 2022. https://www.foreignaffairs.com/articles/asia/2020-06-04/lee-hsien-loong-endangered-asian-century.

Lee, Ji Yun. 2017. "Hedging Strategies of the Middle Powers in East Asian Security: The Cases of South Korea and Malaysia." *East Asia: An International Quarterly* 34 (1): 23–37.

Medcalf, Rory. 2018. "The Great Australian China Debate: Issues and Implications for the United States and the World." The Sigur Center of Asian Studies of the George Washington University, September 10. Accessed February 22, 2022. https://nsc.crawford.anu.edu.au/department-news/13036/great-australian-china-debate-issues-and-implications-us-and-world.

Oliver, Alex. 2014. The Lowy Institute Poll 2014. Lowy Institute. Accessed February 22, 2022. https://www.lowyinstitute.org/sites/default/files/2014_lowy_institute_poll_0.pdf.

Oliver, Alex. 2017. The Lowy Institute Poll 2017. Lowy Institute. Accessed February 22, 2022. https://www.lowyinstitute.org/sites/default/files/documents/lowy-2017-pollreport-web.pdf.

Open Letter Respondents. 2018. "China's Influence in Australia: Maintaining the Debate." Policy Forum, March 27. Accessed February 22, 2022. http://www.policyforum.net/chinas-influence-australia-maintaining-debate/.

Pillsbury, Michael. 2015. *The Hundred-Year Marathon: China's Secret Strategy to Replace America as the Global Superpower*. New York: Henry Holt and Company.

Subramanian, Puspanathan R. M. N. 2020. "Malaysia's Hedging Strategy between United States and China." *The Journal of Defence and Security* 12 (1): 69–82.

Sun, Wanning. 2019. "Adversarial Journalism in the Coverage of China." Pearls and Irritations, December 10. Accessed February 22, 2022. https://johnmenadue.com/wanning-sun-adversarial-journalism-in-the-coverage-of-china/.

Ward, Jonathan. 2019. *China's Vision of Victory*. Fayetteville, NC: The Atlas Publishing and Media Company.

White, Hugh. 2010. "Power Shift: Australia's Future between Washington and Beijing." Quarterly essay. Collingwood, Vic.: Black Inc.

Wintour, Patrick. 2021. "US Has 'No Closer Ally than Australia,' Biden Says after AUKUS Pact." *The Guardian*, September 21. Accessed February 22, 2022. https://www.theguardian.com/world/2021/sep/21/us-has-no-closer-ally-than-australia-says-biden-after-aukus-pact.

Wong, Penny. 2021a. "Expanding Australia's Power and Influence: Speech to Australian National University." Speech at Australian National University, November 23. Accessed February 22, 2022. https://www.pennywong.com.au/media-hub/speeches/expanding-australia-s-power-and-influence-speech-to-the-national-security-college-australian-national-university-canberra-23-11-2021/.

Wong, Penny. 2021b. "Speech to Launch Peter Hartcher's 'Red Zone.'" Speech at Old Parliament House, May 19. Accessed February 22, 2022. https://www.pennywong.com.au/media-hub/speeches/speech-to-launch-peter-hartcher-s-red-zone-king-s-hall-old-parliament-house-canberra-19-05-2021/.

Wu, Charles Chong-Han. 2016. "Taiwan's Hedging against China: The Strategic Implications of Ma Ying-Jeou's Mainland Policy." *Asian Survey* 56 (3): 466–87.

Wu, Charles Chong-Han. 2019. "Why Do States Hedge in East Asia? An Empirical Study on Hedging." *Asian Perspective* 43 (3): 557–84.

11

Leadership, Public Opinion, and Party Politics in New Zealand

Alexander Tan and Neel Vanvari

INTRODUCTION

COVID-19 continues to cause disruption around the world nearly two years after it was first categorized as a "pandemic" by the World Health Organization (WHO).[1] Throughout the course of the pandemic, New Zealand's response and the leadership of the prime minister, Jacinda Ardern, have received international attention. In July 2020, the WHO praised New Zealand for its response to the pandemic and for "implementing evidence based measures."[2] In March 2021, in a study comparing how different countries responded to the pandemic, the Lowy Institute ranked New Zealand's response as being the "best performing" in its "COVID Performance Index."[3] A *New York Times* editorial called Ardern's leadership a "masterclass in how to respond."[4] Ardern has also been complemented for her effective response by "focusing on empathy" and providing "a model of compassionate leadership."[5] At the time of writing, as of February 1, 2022, New Zealand has recorded 16,620 cases and 53 deaths since the start of the pandemic in 2020.[6] As the prime minister herself stated in her opening speech to Parliament in February 2022, New Zealand's confirmed COVID-19 cases, hospitalizations, and deaths have been the lowest among OECD countries.[7] Success has also been evident in the country's vaccination drive with 93 percent of the population aged twelve years and above having been fully vaccinated with both the doses and 95 percent being vaccinated with the first dose.[8] The focus is now shifting to ensuring a quick and efficient rollout of booster doses and the vaccination of children aged five to twelve years old. At the time of writing as of February 1, 2022, 1.3 million booster doses and over 150,000 doses to children in the age group of five to twelve years have already been administered.[9] Aside from the health response, New Zealand has also been praised for its economic response measures by organizations such as the International Monetary Fund (IMF), which called it a "decisive and unprecedented fiscal and monetary policy responses."[10]

All this has been accompanied by the occasional lockdowns and with most of the past two years witnessing sporadic restrictions for most of the country. Apart from Auckland, the rest of New Zealand spent just over five weeks in complete lockdown in 2020 with restrictions on movement and gatherings being gradually lifted from June 2020 onward.[11] Following an outbreak of the delta variant, the rest of the country outside Auckland was in a complete lockdown for just three weeks after which restrictions on businesses and the movement of people were slowly lifted through the second half of 2021.[12] In the backdrop of COVID-19, New Zealand's election in October 2020 proved to be a watershed moment. Not only did Jacinda Ardern's Labour Party win the election, but it did also so resoundingly by winning 65 out of 120 parliamentary seats, which put it in a position to be able to govern alone without needing to seek coalition partners. This is significant because under New Zealand's Mixed Member Proportional (MMP) electoral system, which was adopted in 1996, this is the first time where a single political party has won an overall majority.[13]

In light of these developments, we ask the following question: What factors can account for Labour's electoral victory in 2020? We argue that Ardern's historic election victory was due to adept handling of the pandemic in the early stages, which was complemented by political leadership, government performance, and state of incumbents' vis-à-vis the opposition party.

In the next section, we examine the literature on how government performance, leadership, and voting in a crisis affects party politics and public opinion. In the third section, we focus on the prepandemic politics and issues that dominated the political landscape in New Zealand before the start of the pandemic. This will be followed by examining New Zealand's COVID-19 response and how that impacted the 2020 election. We will then discuss the result of the 2020 election and its aftermath. The final section concludes.

PUBLIC OPINION, GOVERNMENT PERFORMANCE, AND PARTY SUPPORT

New Zealand is a unique case for studying the political impact of COVID-19 for two reasons. First, whereas other Western democracies were witnessing large case numbers, significant death rates, and extreme pressure on their healthcare systems during the first wave in 2020, at the same time cases and deaths in New Zealand were very low with a lengthy period of days wherein there were no new cases recorded through the course of 2020. Second, New Zealand held an election in the same year as the COVID-19 pandemic started having a major impact on healthcare systems and economies across the world. It was an election described as "extraordinary" in which the incumbent Labour Party won an outright majority under New Zealand's MMP electoral system, a first in the country's political history.[14] There are two concepts that need to be examined when discussing elections and support for incumbents, these being public opinion and government performance.

Page and Shapiro, in their study on the relationship between these two concepts, argue that public opinion affects policy more than policy affects public opinion.[15] They observe that "policy tends to move in the same direction as public opinion most often when the opinion change is large and when it is stable, that is, not reversed by fluctuations."[16] Examining the relationship between public policy and public opinion, Wlezien and Soroka stress the role of political institutions.[17] They argue that different institutions will affect this link between public opinion and policy in different ways, such as "federalism constrains public responsiveness and that executive–legislative balance enhances policy representation."[18]

A central theme emerging in the literature on COVID-19 pandemic politics and public opinion is the observation that trust in government increased at the start of the pandemic, especially when lockdowns and other public health measures were first introduced.[19] Some scholars attribute this increase in levels of trust in government to the "rally-around-the-flag" effect.[20] Simply put, the rally-around-the-flag effect suggests that in times of crisis, the support for the incumbent government increases and public opinion tends to become more favorable toward incumbents.[21] The rally-around-the-flag effect has been previously observed during crises, predominantly conflicts, such as wars or terrorist attacks.[22] Schraff, in his study about the rise in support for incumbents, argues that due to an "anxiety effect" and the uncertainties caused by the health crisis, the public's support for political institutions and political leadership increased after the onset of the crisis.[23] In line with Hetherington and Nelson's study, Schraff states that "crises events with high levels of collective uncertainty and existential threats have the potential to activate a 'rally round the flag' dynamic."[24] In their study on the increase in levels of trust for incumbents in Austria and France, Kritzenger et al. found some evidence of a rally effect in Austria but not in France's case.[25] Cunningham's study analyzing party support in twenty-seven countries affected by COVID-19 shows some evidence of a rally effect during the first wave of COVID-19 in 2020.[26]

However, not all scholars agree that the increase in support for incumbents, as reflected in public opinion surveys, was due to the rally effect. Bol et al., in their study of fifteen European countries, argue that increasing levels of trust in government and political institutions was not due to the onset of the COVID-19 crisis but due to lockdown and other public health measures adopted by governments.[27] Johansson et al., in their study on public opinion in Sweden, argue that although support for government increased due to a rally effect, this support faded away as the crisis continued and the public opinion was determined by parameters used to measure government performance in precrisis days, such as political ideology.[28] As figure 11.1 shows, levels of trust in the incumbent Labour government also increased noticeably after the onset of the pandemic in New Zealand, in line with the global trend. Recall that the question that we are asking here pertains to the factors that account for the Labour Party's victory in the 2020 general election. So did we see a rally-around-the-flag effect in New Zealand and was this responsible for Labour's election victory in 2020 given that we saw an increase in public support for incumbents? We argue that attributing Labour's landmark election victory to the rally-around-the-flag effect is an inadequate explanation.

First, although New Zealand may have witnessed a rally-around-the-flag-effect, as some scholars note,[29] this does not always translate into election victories. As Cunningham argues, "The effect, though, is frequently ephemeral. Both Presidents Jimmy Carter and George Bush Senior benefitted from huge rallies following the Iran Hostage Crisis (up from 30% to 57%) and Operation Desert Storm (up from 59% to 89%). Yet both failed to get re-elected."[30] Second, as Johansson et al. and Kritz-

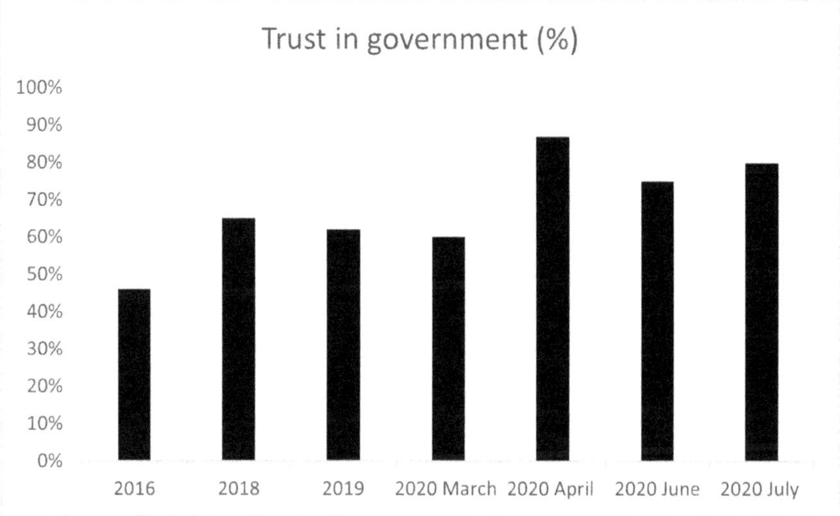

Figure 11.1. Levels of Trust in Government
Source. Chapple 2021, 212.

inger et al. found in their respective studies, the rally-around-the-flag effect in relation to COVID-19 is a short-term occurrence that fades away and there is little evidence that political leaders are able to sustain it.[31] In Sweden and Austria's case, the rally-around-the-flag effect lasted merely for a few months and started fading away as the crisis started losing salience.[32] The COVID-19 crisis began in February 2020 and the election in New Zealand was held eight months later in October. Given that the studies found the existence of a rally-around-the-flag effect to be a short-term phenomenon in relation to COVID-19, it becomes difficult to argue that the rally-around-the-flag effect led to Labour's victory in 2020.

Third, studies that argue that the COVID-19 crisis led to a rally-around-the-flag effect and the subsequent increase in public trust as a result of it associate the rally-around-the-flag effect with the numbers of cases and deaths.[33] For instance, Schraff states that higher levels of trust are witnessed due to citizens supporting political institutions and incumbents "as a lifebuoy" and this happens when the pandemic enters a phase of "exponential growth" in case numbers.[34] The onset of the health crisis followed by a steep rise in case numbers result in the anxieties and uncertainties that led to a rally-around-the-flag effect and the subsequent increase in public trust.[35] If we examine this linkage between the numbers of cases and deaths and the rally-around-the-flag effect in New Zealand's case, we can argue that the rally-around-the-flag effect was short termed and it faded away soon after the introduction of lockdown, due to the numbers of deaths and cases beginning to fall as early as April and May 2020. A rally-around-the-flag effect may have occurred in New Zealand, which resulted in the increased level of trust in government, as noted by Goldfinch et al. and Chapple.[36] However, while we agree with these scholars, we argue that attributing Labour's election victory to the rally-around-the-flag effect is an inadequate explanation. Public opinion and support for incumbents is shaped not only by evaluations of trust but also other complementary factors that can be case specific.[37]

A second concept that is important in the context of support for incumbents and elections is the concept of government performance. In a democracy, elections fulfill the functions of both representation and accountability.[38] Different institutional arrangements, including electoral systems, will fulfill both these functions differently with some systems being more representative than others and some institutions having more accountability safeguards than others.[39] In relation to incumbents and elections, the electorate will use elections to hold incumbents accountable and will judge incumbents based on their record of service while in office. Ghegrina finds that support for incumbents is based on positive evaluations of government performance.[40] When evaluating government performance, a key element of this is economic performance.[41] Scholars have argued that perceptions and evaluations about economic performance strongly influence voting preferences and affect levels of support for incumbents.[42]

The role of leadership and party leaders has become increasingly important, even in parliamentary systems. Over the years, the role of party leaders has become consequential with parliamentary politics becoming personalized and the focus on the leader has increased.[43] The traits and characteristics of political leaders have electoral consequences. For instance, Bean and Mughan argue that the effectiveness and competence of party leaders affect vote choice in Australia and the United Kingdom.[44] Leadership traits such as "competence," "responsiveness," and effectiveness improve a leader's personality traits and therefore influence election outcomes.[45] Hence, the reelection of incumbents depends not merely on government performance but also satisfactory evaluations of the party leader. As a result, parties tend to replace those leaders who may be unpopular as they may be punished electorally for keeping unpopular leaders in place.[46]

Because the 2020 election took place during an ongoing public health crisis, the impact of the crisis also needs to be considered when evaluating incumbents and elections. It is argued that crises tend to benefit incumbents. Bisbee and Honig argue that candidates who "offer to preserve the status quo will find an easier path to (re-) election."[47] De Vries et al., while examining the effect of COVD-19 on incumbent support across several European countries, argued that support for incumbents increased in countries even where COVID-19 was not a major crisis yet in that country.[48] Using the example of the Italian lockdown, "citizens in these (other) countries reacted to the Italian lockdown by increasing support for their governments, even in the absence of a similar domestic response."[49] Political parties, including opposition parties, are office seeking and one of their primary goals is to place themselves in government offices.[50] Hence, the discussion on party change will be incomplete without considering the role of the opposition, and although incumbents tend to be favored during a crisis, opposition parties will still try get into office and fulfill their goals. The strength of incumbents will be affected if the opposition parties are weaker or if they are in a stronger position compared to their incumbents. Along with leadership and government performance, we extend the analysis and also consider the role of the opposition party in a crisis to examine why the incumbent Labour government won the election in the aftermath of the COVID-19 crisis. In the next section, we analyze the most important issues and public opinion in New Zealand politics in the prepandemic phase. This allows us to examine whether any change took place after the pandemic and what is the cause of this change.

PREPANDEMIC POLITICS

Housing Market and Kiwibuild

Housing and housing reform have consistently been key policy issues in New Zealand since the 1990s.[51] Housing is often the primary asset that "makes up a substantial proportion of household wealth and retirement accumulations for many New Zealanders."[52] In the mid-2000s, debate on the issue of housing was largely focused on improving the quality of housing, especially during and after the "Leaky Building Crisis."[53] Following the election of the National Party–led government in 2008 that resulted in the adoption of "market based solutions to housing issues" and the increase in house prices as witnessed from 2008 to 2017, the debate has centered on the affordability of housing since the mid-2010s.[54] For instance, during the 2014 general election campaign, 67 percent of the respondents to Vote Compass, an online voter engagement tool, stated that the government should build "somewhat or much more affordable housing."[55]

Compared to the 2014 general election, housing, particularly rising house prices and housing affordability were regarded as even more salient issue by voters during the 2017 general election campaign.[56] A poll in June 2017 found that respondents regarded affordable housing as the second most important policy issue.[57] Another study by *Stuff*/Massey University Election Survey found that 74 percent of the respondents stated that there is a "major housing crisis in NZ right now."[58] Even political parties were focusing on housing as one of the main issues in their policy announcements during the 2017 election campaign. Housing was mentioned at least ninety-two times in the manifestos of political parties in 2017, an increase from the 2014 election campaign when it was mentioned twenty-nine times.[59]

In an attempt to address the issue of affordable housing, the Labour Party unveiled numerous policies in their 2017 manifesto. The flagship policy, however, was the Kiwbuild scheme that aimed to build affordable homes for first-time buyers.[60] Kiwibuild was launched in 2018 with the aim of building 100,000 affordable homes in ten years in order to tackle the problem of affordable housing.[61] The stated aim of the Kiwibuild scheme was to provide affordable housing primarily to those under of the age of forty as the government measured affordability against income and given that the ratio of the median house price to medium income ratio kept increasing since 2009, first home buyers under the age of forty were identifying as being the most disadvantaged.[62] However, Kiwibuild's success in delivering affordable homes was being questioned soon after its launch in 2018.[63] Problems with Kiwibuild related to the price caps at which the houses were being sold, median incomes needed to qualify for the scheme, the availability of supplementary financial help, and the ballot system.[64]

For instance, in late 2018 the then minister for housing stated that the previously specified median income of $60,000 NZD to qualify for the Kiwibuild scheme would be insufficient.[65] A similar case was the Kiwibuild project in Marfell, New Plymouth, where the median wage in the region was $23,000 NZD but only people earning a median wage of $70,000 to $90,000 NZD would be able to service a mortgage and be able quality for the scheme.[66] Other factors such as only the availability of apartments or studios instead of family homes also discouraged first-time buyers.[67]

Due to the combination of factors mentioned earlier, the Labour-led government could not meet its Kiwibuild target in the first year itself where instead of 1,000 homes, only 278 houses were completed by the July 2019 deadline.[68] In September 2019, the target of building 100,000 homes in ten years was scrapped as a "Kiwibuild reset" was launched with the aim of building as many affordable homes as possible.[69] Apart from Kiwibuild, the Labour Party also introduced other policies in order to try and address the problem of unaffordable housing. For instance, the government introduced a ban on foreigners owning houses in New Zealand in a bid to curb surging house prices in 2019.[70] Such measures had little effect in curbing house prices and received criticism for not addressing the underlying causes of increasing house prices.[71]

Toomey et. al argue that Kiwibuild failed to adequately provide for first-time buyers seeking to get into the housing market and as the scheme progressed through 2018 and 2019, the public was skeptical and not confident whether Kiwibuild would be able to deliver affordable housing.[72] Respondents to a Colmar Bruton poll believed that the government would be unable to meet its Kiwibuild targets. 69 percent of respondents said that they believed the government would miss its target of building 100,000 homes in ten years.[73] Labour's objective of trying to slow down the rate at which house prices were increasing also bears a mixed record. According to Massey University's Real Estate Analysis Unit, the median house prices kept increasing every quarter (expect from a limited period in 2019), despite the government's additional measures such as banning foreigners from owning houses.[74] Therefore, not only was the availability of affordable housing through Kiwibuild proving to be a difficult objective to attain, measures to slow down the pace of house price increases also seemed to be yielding mixed results for Labour.

Table 11.1. Top Five Issues of Concern

October 2018 (n=610)	*April 2019 (n=615)*	*November 2019 (n=615)*	*March 2020 (n=610)*
Housing/Price of Housing	Housing/Price of Housing	Housing/Price of Housing	Housing/Price of Housing
Petrol Prices/Fuel	Poverty/Inequality	Poverty/Inequality	Healthcare/ Hospitals
Inflation/Cost of Living	Inflation/Cost of Living	Inflation/Cost of Living	Poverty/Inequality
Healthcare/ Hospitals	Healthcare/ Hospitals	Healthcare/ Hospitals	Inflation/Cost of Living
Poverty/Inequality	Crime/Law	Crime/Law	Crime/Law
	After Christchurch terror attacks		Only a few COVID-19 cases in New Zealand

Source: Ipsos 2020a, 7.

In terms of public opinion, housing carried on being one of the top three issues of concern from 2018 to 2020. As table 11.1 demonstrates, respondents consistently considered housing to be the most important issue of concern from February 2018 to March 2020 before the onset of the pandemic in March 2020.[75] In addition, as figure 11.2 shows, Labour was

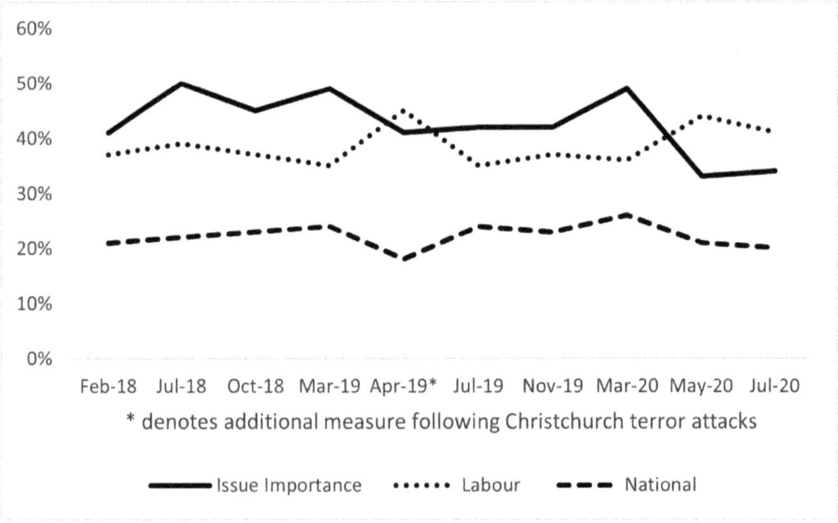

Figure 11.2. Issues of Concern and the Perceived Competence of Political Parties: Housing

Source: Ipsos 2020a, 15.

trusted more than the National Party to solve the housing issue during this period. Labour has traditionally done well and polled higher than National in relation to housing.[76] It was a Labour government who successfully built large-scale state housing after World War II, a record that the party still talks about.[77] A more recent example would be the Labour government actively looking for measures to resolve the "Leaky Building Crisis" in the mid-2000s to improve the quality of housing.[78] The Labour Party was also more willing to address housing as a "crisis" and find solutions, in stark contrast to the National Party, who refused to refer to housing as a crisis during the John Key/Bill English years.[79] Although Labour had a considerable lead over National in relation to housing, there was a slump in the polls and Labour's competence on the housing issue fell below 35 percent, following problems with Kiwibuild in July 2019.[80]

Christchurch Shootings and the Aftermath

On March 15, 2019, two consecutive mass shootings wherein a lone white supremacist gunman attacked two mosques took place in Christchurch.[81] In the aftermath of the attack, Prime Minister Ardern was praised both at home and abroad for her quick response that was unifying and emphatic.[82] Ardern's phrase, "You Are Us—Aroha Nui" was used at vigils and services across the country after the shootings, and she was applauded by world leaders for bringing the country together by providing a unifying response in the aftermath of the shootings.[83] Ardern also introduced some swift policy changes after the shootings. Following the attacks, Ardern announced that gun laws would be amended and military style semiautomatic weapons would be banned.[84] The Labour Party–led government also undertook a gun buy-back scheme to remove semiautomatic weapons from the community. In addition, a Royal Commission headed by a senior judge was set up to investigate the incident and make recommendations.[85] Other measures such as removing the livestreamed video of the massacre and the gunman's manifesto online were also undertaken by Ardern's government.[86] On the international stage, Ardern cochaired a summit of world leaders with the French president, Emmanuel Macron, with the aim of coordinating a global response to eliminate extremist content online.[87]

In terms of public opinion, data shows that the Labour Party surged ahead of the opposition National Party in the polls in the immediate

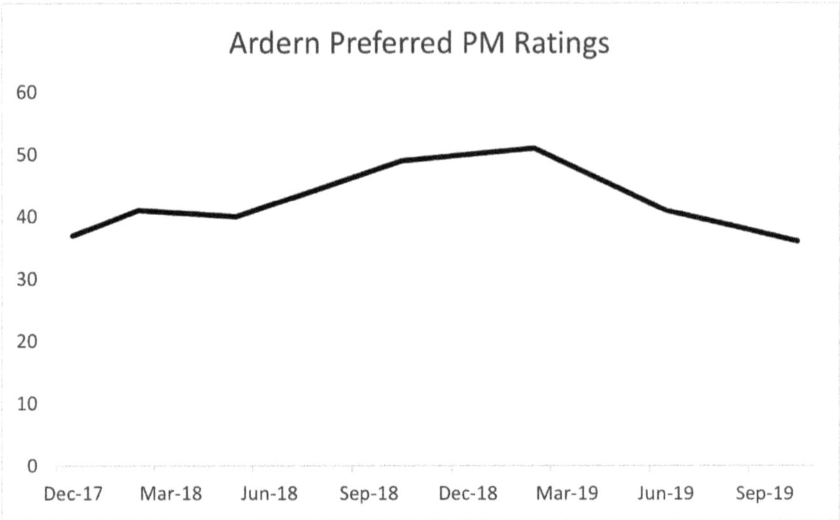

Figure 11.3. Ardern's Ratings as Preferred Prime Minister
Source: Compiled by authors using data from Colmar-Bruton and Newshub-Reid polls.

aftermath of the Christchurch massacre. In the Newshub-Reid poll immediately following the shootings, Labour had an 8.3 percent lead against National, which is the biggest lead since the Labour-led government got into office in 2017.[88] Labour's support also jumped to 48 percent from 45 percent in the Colmar Bruton poll after the shootings, and here too Labour was leading by 8 percent against National.[89] Ardern's ratings as preferred prime minister surged to 50 percent following the shootings, and until October 2019, Ardern's ratings as preferred prime minister stayed above 40 percent, as shown in figure 11.3.[90] The Labour Party also witnessed an increase in support on its handling of the other major issues such as housing from March to July 2019 in the Ipsos poll.[91] However, as shown in figure 11.4 the National Party's support started to creep back up in the polls, and from July 2019 to February 2020 National had a lead over Labour in eight out of thirteen polls conducted in this period. Although Simon Bridges's ratings as preferred prime minister saw minimal change, the party not only closed the gap of 8 percent against Labour but also reestablished a lead in the polls of its own and maintained that lead until the start of the COVID-19 pandemic in New Zealand in February 2020.

State of the Opposition

Bill English resigned in 2018 after being unable to form a coalition in the aftermath of the 2017 general election, and Simon Bridges took over as the leader of the National Party.[92] The polls show that from the outset itself, Bridges's ratings as preferred prime minister were quite low. The Colmar Bruton in May 2018 was the highest rating he ever received as preferred prime minister of 12 percent compared to Ardern at 41 percent.[93] Throughout mid-2018, Bridges's leadership was surrounded by several accusations around the misuse of expenses and wrongdoing in regard to donations.[94] There were also reports of disagreements and divisions within the National Party parliamentary caucus.[95] Despite his low ratings and the problems within caucus, the party vote polls were still favorable for National during this period. As shown in figure 11.4, the National Party was still polling between 43 percent and 47 percent between August and November 2018. Even if Labour was polling ahead of National, Labour was leading by 2 to 3 percent. Under Bridges's leadership, National was leading in the party vote in fourteen out of twenty-one polls. It even bounced back after the Christchurch shootings. One key

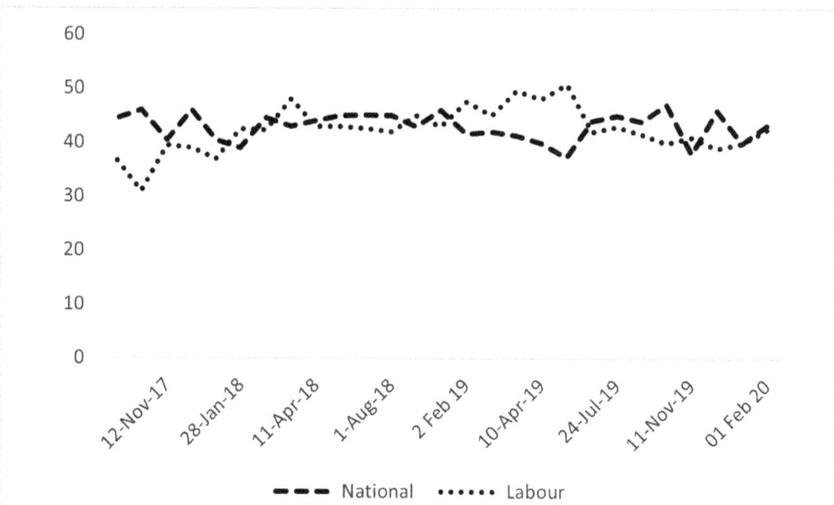

Figure 11.4. Party Vote Support for National and Labour Prepandemic
Source: Compiled by authors using data from Colmar-Bruton and Newshub-Reid polls.

observation here is that the public still perceived National to be more competent than Labour on the issue of the economy. Figure 11.5 shows this data from the Ipsos NZ Issues Monitor poll. National had an advantage over Labour when it came to the issue of the economy from February 2018 all the way until the start of the pandemic in March 2020.

What we observe in the prepandemic phase is that the party who is leading the party vote polls does not necessarily perform well in the preferred prime minister polls. While Ardern outperformed Bridges by a significant margin in the preferred prime minister polls, the National Party was performing consistently well in the party vote polls. Even when Labour had a lead in the party vote, National was able to close the gap as shown in figure 11.4. In addition, as shown in figure 11.5, National was outperforming Labour on the issue of the economy in the prepandemic phase. The gap between Ardern's strong preferred prime minister poll numbers and Labour's inability to gain an upper hand in the party vote prepandemic is explained best by Wilson who, in examining the prepandemic phase, argues that "while Ardern generally attracts positive press coverage internationally, domestically her government's popularity has never been especially strong: as recently as mid-February [2020] an influential poll showed that while Ardern then had the incumbent's advantage as 'preferred Prime Minister,' attracting 42% support, the two main oppo-

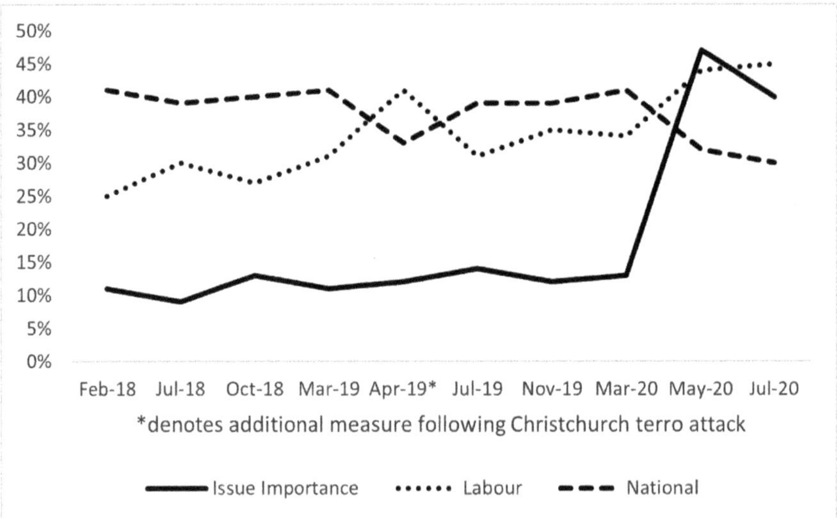

Figure 11.5. Competence of Political Parties on the Issue of the Economy
Source: Ipsos 2020a, 13.

sition parties combined had sufficient support to govern if the poll results were translated into an actual election."[96]

PANDEMIC AND PUBLIC OPINION

In the previous section, we observed that in the prepandemic phase, even though Simon Bridges's personal ratings in the preferred prime minister polls were never above 14 percent, under his leadership the National Party, while in opposition, was still performing well in the polls in terms of the party vote. Even after the boost in the polls for Ardern and Labour following significant events like the Christchurch terror attacks, the National Party was able to close the gap in the polls in the prepandemic phase. Two Colmar Bruton polls, one in late November 2019 and the second in early February 2020, placed National's party vote ahead of Labour's and predicted that the center-right block, consisting of the National Party and the ACT Party, would have enough seats to form a government.[97] However, once the pandemic began and case numbers started to increase in New Zealand, there was a change in the trend noticed in the polls. Figure 11.6 tracks the party vote support for Labour and National

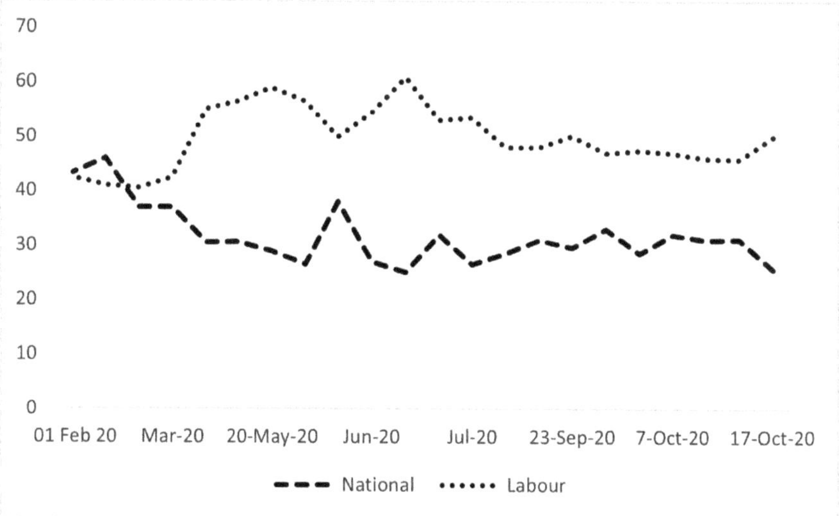

Figure 11.6. Party Vote Support in the Pandemic Phase—Labour and National
Source: Compiled by authors using data from Colmar-Bruton and Newshub-Reid polls.

using data from Colmar Bruton and Newshub-Reid opinion polls. We can observe that as the pandemic continued to progress from February 2020 up until the election in October 2020, the gap in the party vote support widened between Labour and National. This is different from the prepandemic phase as shown in figure 11.4, wherein National was able to regain support in the polls and there was no consequential divergence in party vote support between the two major parties. As the pandemic rolled on, Labour was not only able to lead by a significant margin in the polls but also widen its lead as the election drew closer in October 2020.

So what was the cause of this change in the polls and why did Labour win the 2020 election? We argue that Labour's favorable poll numbers and subsequent victory was due to a convergence of the following factors: adept handling of the pandemic by introducing measures early on in the outbreak, the role of leadership during the crisis, government performance in both the health and economic spheres, and finally, the role of incumbents and opposition during a crisis. We begin by looking at the measures that the Labour-led government adopted to deal with the pandemic as it unfolded from early 2020.

On February 28, 2020, New Zealand reported its first case of COVID-19.[98] However, the government had already put some measures in place to try to mitigate the impact of COVID-19 even before the first case was detected in the community. Table 11.2 contains a timeline of New Zealand's COVID response in 2020. The government's initial response consisted of evacuating citizens from severely affected areas like Wuhan in China and monitoring the spread of the virus abroad.[99] The Ministry of Health set up an incident monitoring and response group as early as January 2020. In early February, the government put in place self-isolation requirements for some travelers arriving from China. Just after the first case was detected in New Zealand, by early March restrictions were also put in place for travelers coming in from Iran, Italy, and South Korea, as these countries were also experiencing high case numbers. Border measures were further strengthened in mid-March where self-isolation was made mandatory for all arrivals and on March 19, the government announced that New Zealand's borders would be closed to everybody except New Zealand citizens and permanent residents. Thus, even before New Zealand reported its first one hundred cases of COVID-19 and before a complete lockdown was implemented, the government had put in place several border measures to try and delay the spread of the virus in the community by slowly tightening border measures in early 2020.[100] Some have argued that delaying the entry of the virus into the community and containing it at the border allowed New Zealand to put public health measures in place and prepare its healthcare systems.[101] The prime minister, while outlining these preemptive border measures on March 14, 2020, stated that "we must go hard, and go early, and do everything we can to protect New Zealanders health."[102]

Table 11.2. Timeline of COVID-19 Measures in New Zealand

Date	*Policy Measure*
January 24, 2020	New Zealand Ministry of Health establishes an Incident Management Team
January 30, 2020	New Zealand evacuates citizens from Wuhan, China
February 3, 2020	Entry restrictions on foreign nationals entering from China Self-isolation implemented for some incoming passengers
February 28, 2020	First case of COVID-19 reported in New Zealand More travel restrictions placed on incoming passengers from Iran
March 2, 2020	Entry restrictions on incoming travelers from Italy and South Korea
March 5, 2020	First person-to-person transmission confirmed in New Zealand
March 14, 2020	Self-isolation made mandatory for all incoming travelers
March 17, 2020	The government assigns $12.1 billion NZD to help the healthcare sector along with businesses and workers
March 19, 2020	Border closed to all except New Zealand citizens and permanent residents
March 21, 2020	New Zealand introduced a four-tiered alert level system with all of New Zealand immediately put into Alert Level 2 with some restrictions
March 23, 2020	New Zealand put into Alert Level 3 with more restrictions put in place for businesses and citizens
March 25, 2020	State of emergency declared due to detected community transmission of COVID-19
March 26, 2020	New Zealand moved to Alert Level 4 with a complete lockdown for at least four weeks
April 20, 2020	Alert Level 4 extended for at least another week
April 27, 2020	New Zealand moves to Alert Level 3, lockdown is lifted and restrictions eased
May 14, 2020	New Zealand enters Alert Level 2 with further easing of restrictions Government announces a $50 billion NZD COVID Rescue package
June 9, 2020	No active cases of COVID-19 in the community New Zealand enters Alert Level 1; all restrictions are lifted

Source: Compiled by authors. Data from Jamieson 2020, 599; Levine 2021, 34–37; Ministry of Health 2020.

However, border restrictions were just one aspect of New Zealand's COVID response. With community transmission of COVID-19 and the steady increase of case numbers, New Zealand adopted the "elimination strategy" to "stamp out" the virus and adopted a four-tiered alert level system in mid-March.[103] With just over one hundred cases reported in the country, Ardern moved the country to "Alert Level 4" and announced a complete lockdown for at least four weeks. Thus, within a month of the first case being reported, the government moved swiftly to put in place measures to mitigate the spread of the virus with the aim of protecting "lives and livelihoods" and to protect the healthcare system from being overburdened by a surge in cases.[104] In April 2020, just over a month after New Zealand was placed in complete lockdown, recovered cases were exceeding new cases and in June 2020, the country recorded zero cases in the community and restrictions were slowly lifted before a phased return to Alert Level 1.[105] Decisive and swift policy measures were instrumental in ensuring that New Zealand succeeded in its elimination strategy of no community transmission of the virus.[106] Polls show that the public did support the government and the lockdown measures. Two Colmar Bruton polls, one conducted in early April 2020 and the second at the end of April 2020, found that 88 percent and 87 percent of respondents supported the government's measures to tackle the virus showing that there was considerable public support for the government's actions in the early stages of the pandemic.[107]

The second factor that we look at us is the role of leadership. As discussed earlier, the role of political leaders is becoming increasingly important, even in parliamentary systems. Ardern's leadership during a crisis has been analyzed before, she was praised for her response and "empathic" leadership in the aftermath of the Christchurch terror attacks.[108] COVID-19 posed a serious challenge to leaders around the world, as restricting the movement of citizens to protect healthcare systems, through lockdowns and other public health measures such as social distancing, would invariably harm the economy and bring economic activity to a standstill.[109] The nature of this health emergency was even more acute in New Zealand, as there has been underinvestment in its healthcare system over the years and the country has the lowest number of ICU beds in the OECD at 4 per 100,000 people.[110] A disease modeling report in March 2020 estimated that the impact of COVID-19 on New

Zealand's healthcare system would be "severe" and estimated the number of fatalities to be over 12,500 if the spread of the virus was not curtailed.[111] Given the nature of the crisis and the measures being proposed, collective action and a "buy-in" from the public in favor of these restrictions was imperative in order to slow the spread of the virus.[112] As Tan states, "challenge of the public-health response has been how to bring 'everyone' along to observe and abide by the guidelines established for the elimination of the virus and for the control strategy to be effective."[113] Political leadership was a key component of New Zealand's COVID-19 response as it sought to address this "collective action" problem through her "pandemic leadership" approach.[114]

Central to New Zealand's pandemic response was ensuring that advice from public health experts, epidemiologists, and specialists was followed and incorporated in the policy formulation process.[115] As Wilson argues, "New Zealand government's approach has been guided by scientific advice, facts, evidence and a willingness to listen to those with relevant expertise to help inform its decision making."[116] According to Tan, "In New Zealand, political leadership decided early on that the crisis at hand was primarily a public-health, public-safety, medical, and epidemiological concern."[117]

Although the public health response has been led primarily by specialists, technocrats, and health experts such as Dr. Ashley Bloomfield, director-general of the Ministry of Health, these experts have constantly been supported publicly by the prime minister and her cabinet. Effective political communication has been vital, complementing the science-led and evidence-based approach that New Zealand has adopted. This primarily was achieved through daily press conferences during the first outbreak in 2020, wherein the prime minister and the director-general of health would appear together and provide an update on case numbers, hospitalizations, the latest criteria being considered before the cabinet decided on a move between "Alert Levels" and other public health advice such as the distribution of personal protective equipment (PPE) and mask wearing.[118] Direct communication by the prime minister and other ministers through alternative methods, such as "Facebook Live," where Ardern spoke directly to the public providing public health information such as the importance of handwashing also played an important part.[119] Tan argues that defining the COVID-19 emergency as a public health crisis and by introducing technical terminologies such as "flattening the curve," "bubbles," and "social distancing," the number of participants has been limited through "issue contraction."[120] According to Tan, "the political leadership's ability to navigate issue definition through issue contraction provided the much-needed space, time, and flexibility for . . . government to map an appropriate and effective pandemic response."[121] Underpinning this leadership and communication strategy is the "Unite Against COVID-19" campaign actively promoted as the central theme of New Zealand's pandemic response.[122] Phrases such as "team of five million," "be safe and be kind," and "we are all in this together" have been used to foster a sense of collective belonging and a shared purpose, along with "mobilising collective effort."[123]

Through the daily press conferences and her Facebook Live sessions, Ardern personally led the pandemic response, through clear and effective communication, emphasizing the need to follow public health guidelines but also fostering a sense of collective belonging by being empathic and relatable.[124] Figure 11.7 shows Ardern's ratings in the preferred prime minister during the pandemic phase. Since the start of the pandemic and after leading the pandemic response, Ardern's ratings as preferred prime minister increased significantly. Data from a UMR postelection poll in

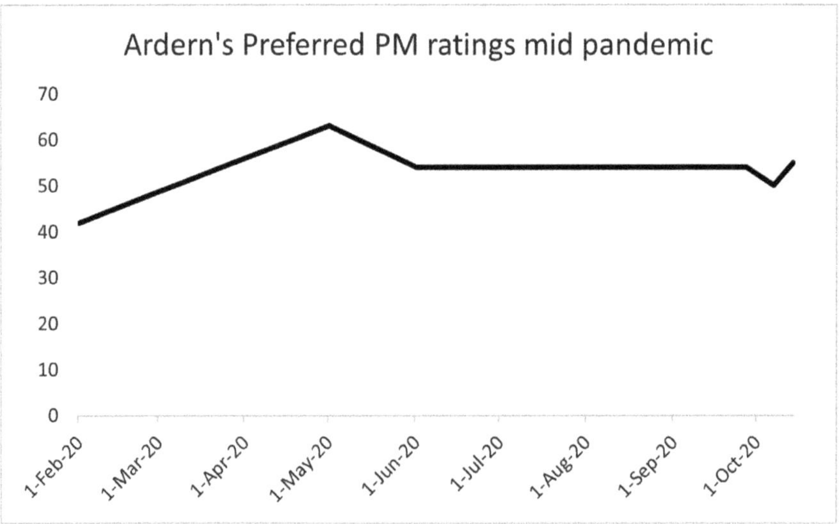

Figure 11.7. Ardern's Support as Preferred Prime Minister Mid-Pandemic
Source: Compiled by authors using data from Colmar-Bruton and Newshub-Reid polls.

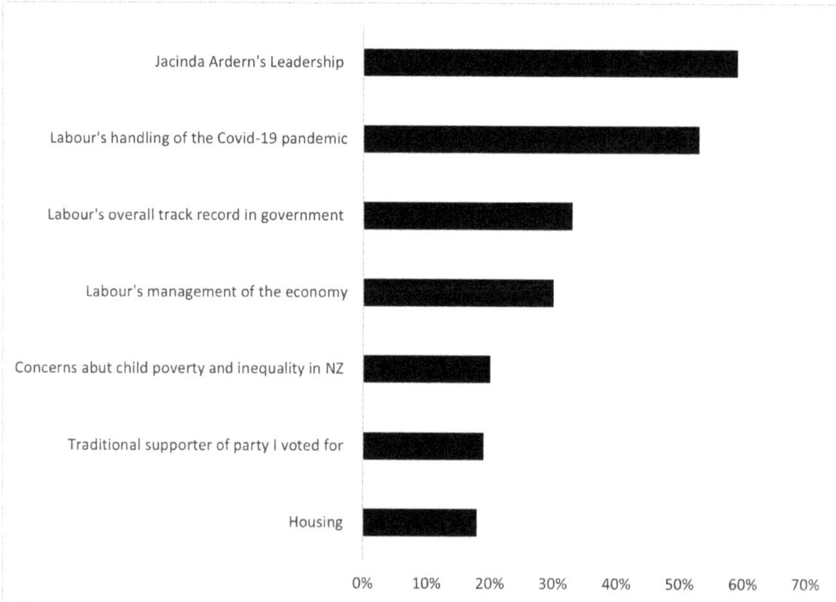

Figure 11.8. Labour Vote Deciders—Prompted: In terms of finally deciding which party you were going to vote for in the recent general election, would you say the following factors were (%critically important, Labour voters top ten)
Source: UMR postelection poll, in Mills, Downs, and Butt 2021, 300.

figure 11.8 shows that Ardern's leadership was considered "critically important" by 59 percent of the public who voted for Labour and 53 percent of voters who backed Labour considered Labour's handling of the pandemic to be a critical factor.

The third factor that we consider is government performance. As discussed earlier, voters will hold incumbents accountable at the ballot box based on their performance during their time in office. As noted by scholars, economic performance and the state of the economy is a key element in the evaluation of government performance. COVID-19 was not merely a health emergency, it also significantly endangered to the economic prospects of countries. Numerous countries, which were hit hard by COVID-19, were already reeling from the uncertainties prevalent in the global economy since 2008. For many governments, COVID-19 posed a challenge as closing borders, instituting lockdowns, restricting the movement of people, and curbing the operation of businesses would bring significant economic consequences, even though those measures would help to flatten the curve and safeguard the healthcare systems. The Labour-led

Table 11.3. Issues that the Public Are Most Concerned about Postpandemic

November 19 (n=615)	*March 20 (n=610)*	*May 20 (n=1,000)*	*July 20 (n=1,000)*	*September 20 (n=1,000)*	*November 20 (n=1,001)*
Housing/Price of Housing	Housing/Price of Housing	The Economy	The Economy	The Economy	Housing/Price of Housing
Poverty/Inequality	Healthcare/ Hospitals	Unemployment	Housing/Price of Housing	Housing/Price of Housing	The Economy
Inflation/Cost of living	Poverty/Inequality	Housing/Price of Housing	Unemployment	Unemployment	Poverty/Inequality
Healthcare/ Hospitals	Inflation/Cost of Living	Healthcare/ Hospitals	Healthcare/ Hospitals	Healthcare/ Hospitals	Healthcare/ Hospitals
Crime/Law	Crime/Law	Poverty/Inequality	Poverty/Inequality	Poverty/Inequality	Inflation/Cost of Living
	Only a few COVID-19 cases in New Zealand	New Zealand moves out of Alert Level 4	Alert Level 1	Alert Level 2 (second wave)	Alert Level 1/first wave postelection

Source: Ipsos 2020c, 8.

government's performance in protecting the country's health system by effectively controlling the spread of the virus has already been examined in the preceding discussion. We now turn to the economic response and measures introduced as a result of COVID-19.

COVID-19 presented a significant challenge for New Zealand's economy, as tourism and international students studying in New Zealand tertiary institutions were significant sectors of the economy that were immediately impacted due to border closures.[125] As noted before, even though the government addressed the COVID-19 crisis as being primarily a public health and epidemiological issue,[126] the government also took actions in the economic sphere during the crisis. Business leaders were consulted and their help seeking essential supplies like PPE was enlisted by Ardern and her finance minister before the implementation of the first Alert Level 4 lockdown in March 2020.[127] In the same month, the government announced a NZ$12.1 billion (approximately US$8.47 billion) economic rescue package to help those businesses and workers who were adversely affected due to restrictions put in place such as a limit on gatherings in hospitality venues.[128] This figure was further increased to NZ$52 billion (approximately US$36.4 billion) in May 2020 to address the economic consequences of COVID-19.[129] A range of initiatives to support workers and businesses such as the Wage Subsidy scheme, Business Finance Guarantee scheme, the essential workers leave scheme, and other measures targeted to support small and medium-sized enterprises were put in place.[130] Economic initiatives and the 2020 budget in general was framed as being part of and complementing the healthcare response with phrases such as "Recover and Rebuild from COVID-19 Together" being put into action.[131]

After the beginning of the pandemic, the economy and unemployment became critical issues for the public. According to an Ipsos poll, shown in table 11.3, the economy and unemployment were in the top three issues that the public were most concerned about.[132] This is a noticeable difference from the prepandemic phase wherein the neither the economy nor unemployment feature as being the top three most concerning issues to the public as prominently as they did after the pandemic. There is another observation from this poll that must be noted. As shown in figure 11.9, not only was the economy as an issue of concern more prominent, but the public also perceived Labour as being more capable to deal with the

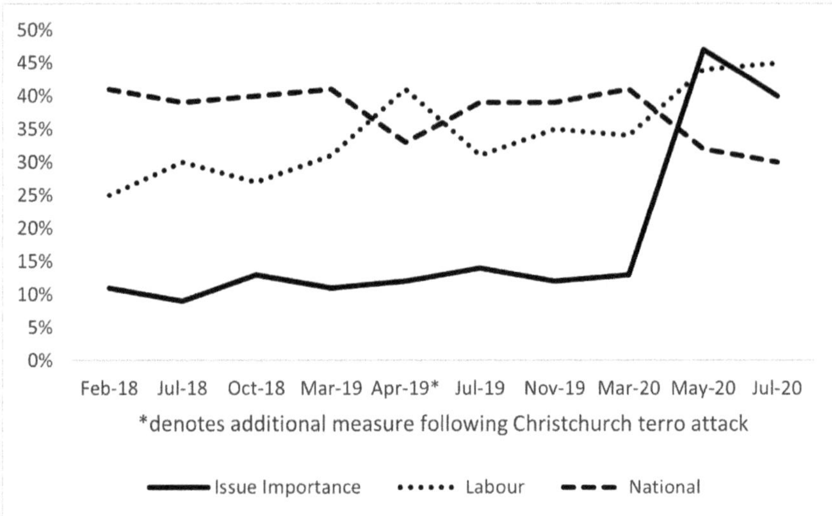

Figure 11.9. Important Issues and Perceived Competence of Political Parties: The Economy
Source: Ipsos November 2020b, 17.

economy over National.[133] This is also a marked difference from the pre-pandemic phase because the economy was the only issue that the public perceived National to handle better than Labour. After the pandemic and in the lead up the election, based on data from the Ipsos poll, Labour took over National on the issue of the economy. There is another set of data with which we can gaze the public's perception about the government's performance. As represented in figure 11.10, data from UMR and Roy Morgan Research examines whether respondents thought that New Zealand was heading in the right direction or whether the country was on the wrong track. The data shows that there was a noticeable increase in those who believed that New Zealand was on the right track. After the pandemic began, the percentage of respondents who thought that the country was on the right track jumped from 52 percent to 73 percent in February 2020 and it stayed at those levels, hovering between 68 percent and 73 percent through the course of the pandemic until after the election in 2020.

The last factor that we examine is state of the incumbent and the opposition parties during the crisis. As discussed previously, crises benefit incumbents as voters become risk averse and tend to lean toward maintaining the status quo. However, we cannot fully examine the concept

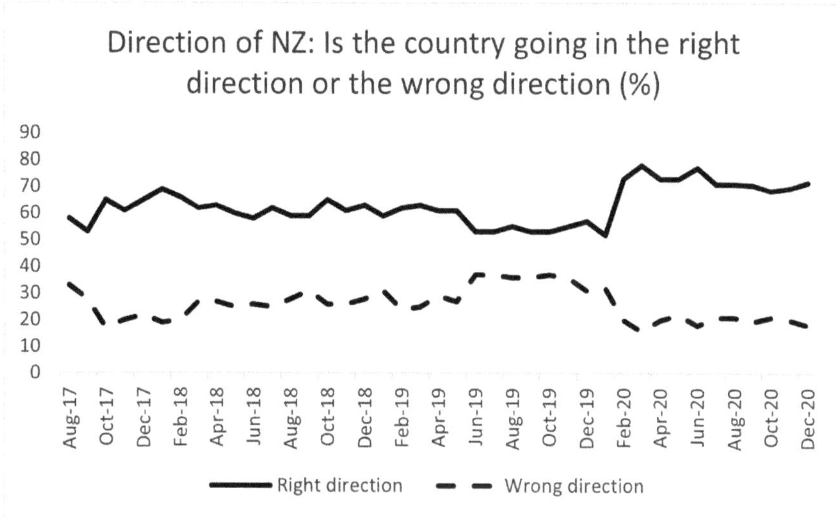

Figure 11.10. New Zealand Heading in the "Right" Direction or the "Wrong" Direction
Source: Compiled by authors. Data from Mills, Downs, and Butt 2021, 300; Roy Morgan Research 2017.

of party change by focusing solely on incumbents and without analyzing the opposition party. After the 2017 election, National won 55 of the 120 seats and was the largest party in Parliament. In the prepandemic phase, even though Simon Bridges was not performing well in the preferred prime minister polls, the National party was doing well in terms of the party vote. Even after crisis events such as the Christchurch terror attacks, when Labour gained an upper hand against National in the party vote, National was able to close the gap and gain some momentum in the party vote polls again. Thus, from the 2017 election to the start of the pandemic, National had a strong position in the polls as far as the party vote is concerned.

In May 2020, while New Zealand was still in the midst of dealing with its community outbreak of COVID-19, Simon Bridges was voted out by caucus as the Leader of the National Party and replaced by Todd Muller.[134] Although the election of Todd Muller gives National a small boost in the party vote polls, Labour still had a 12 percent lead against National in the party vote.[135] However, Muller's time as leader of the opposition was mired in allegations of intraparty disputes especially considering the political fate of his predecessor Simon Bridges and allegations of misconduct such as the leaking of confidential information by one of his MPs.[136] After just fifty-nine days, Todd Muller resigned as the leader of the National Party in July 2020 and was replaced by former cabinet minister Judith Collins.[137] In just five months, the National Party had seen three new leaders at the helm. In addition, under all three leaders, the party saw intraparty disputes and allegations of misconduct against both MPs and organizational members of the party. Changing party leaders and divisions within the party can be costly for political parties.

Florence So notes that "leadership contests can send conflicting signals on what its [party's] future directions should be, even when the party eventual settles on a winner."[138] Leadership contests can prove to be detrimental to a party's electoral prospects.[139] Furthermore, Greene and Haber argue that intraparty divisions influence how voters perceive the competency of a political party.[140] According to Greene and Haber, "public intra-party divisions fuel negative evaluations of parties' cohesiveness and that these perceptions influence elections in two ways. Voters perceive intra-party disagreement as an inability to coordinate and develop rigorous policies."[141] In figure 11.11, we find some evidence that National's leaderships contests and other problems were taken into account by the voters. At least 16 percent of Labour voters rated National's leaderships problems and other issues as being "critically important" when casting their vote.

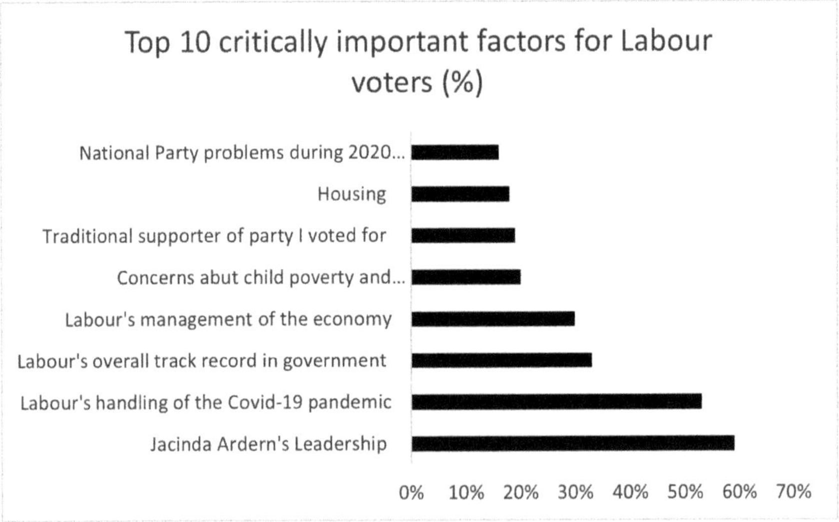

Figure 11.11. Labour Vote Deciders—Prompted: In terms of finally deciding which party you were going to vote for in the recent general election, would you say the following factors were (%critically important, Labour voters top ten)

Source: UMR postelection poll, in Mills, Downs, and Butt 2021, 300.

In a crisis, opposition parties often face the dilemma of either cooperating with the government or criticizing the government for its response to the crisis.[142] This also entails a tradeoff for parties as either they can have some sway in the policymaking process by adopting a consensual approach and cooperating with the government during a crisis, or they can adopt an adversarial approach by criticizing the government, thereby distinguishing themselves from the government's crisis response in the hope of a future electoral gain.[143] As a strategy to attract voters in a crisis, parties may shift their attention to claim "ownership" of salient issues, particularly an area in which they have a "track record" on the issue in question.[144] The National Party was generally supportive of the government's COVID-19 response, adopting a more consensual approach when the pandemic first began.[145] However, the National Party slowly began to oppose the government as the pandemic rolled on. For instance, National voted against an emergency bill in Parliament that would grant the government powers to enforce Alert Level 2 restrictions in May 2020.[146] There is some evidence to suggest that National was unable to claim ownership of any issue during the crisis. Figure 11.4 shows a poll from the Ipsos NZ Issues Monitor poll taken in September 2020 representing the political party the voters think is most capable of addressing the top twenty "most concerning" issues. As Figure 11.4 shows, the public perceived Labour, or in the instance of environment issues, the Green Party to be more capable than National at addressing the most concerning issues. On the contrary, as discussed earlier, during the pandemic National lost ownership of the only issue on which it was performing better than Labour prepandemic: the economy.

Table 11.4. Political Party Most Capable of Managing Issues

Issue	*Political Party*	*Issue*	*Political Party*
1. The Economy	Labour	11. Household Debt/Personal Debt	Labour
2 Housing/Price of Housing	Labour	12. Immigration	Labour
3. Poverty/Inequality	Labour	13. Education	Labour
4. Healthcare/Hospitals	Labour	14. Race Relations/Racism	Labour
5. Unemployment	Labour	15. Transport/Public Transport/ Infrastructure	Labour
6. Inflation/Cost of Living	Labour	16. Taxation	Labour
7. Climate Change	Green	17. Petrol Prices/Fuel	Labour
8. Crime/Law and Order	Labour	18. Issues facing Māori	Labour
9. Drug/Alcohol Abuse	Labour	19. Population/Overpopulation	Labour
10 Environmental Pollution/ Water Concerns	Green	20. Defense/Foreign Affairs	Labour

Source: Ipsos 2020b, 13.

The last point of distinction between the incumbent and opposition parties is the impact of party leaders and leadership image. We noted earlier that party leader image is a key indicator of voting intention and party leaders have an effect on electoral prospects. Figure 11.7 shows that Ardern's support in the preferred prime minister poll was significantly high during the pandemic phase. Figure 11.12 shows the poll ratings of Judith Collins and the other two National leaders in the Colmar Bruton preferred prime minister polls. Although Judith Collins had higher poll numbers as preferred prime minister than either Simon Bridges or Todd Muller, there was still a significant gap between Ardern's numbers and Collin's support and Ardern had a considerable lead. In relation to the party leader image, Mills et al. observe that while Ardern's strengths were centered on empathy and there were very few and small negatives for the opposition to work on, Judith Collins, while having a certain set of positives, also had significant negatives such as being too aggressive and arrogant.[147] It is vital to note that in the pandemic phase, Labour was able to lead both in the preferred prime minister polls and the party vote and this is different from the prepandemic phase. In addition, in the pandemic phase, Labour was also perceived to be more competent than National by the public in relation to the economy, something that was not observed before the pandemic.

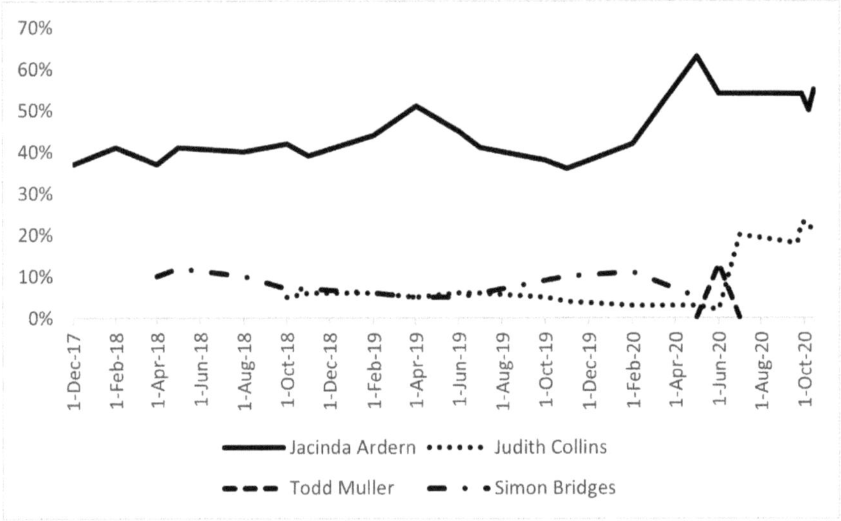

Figure 11.12. Preferred Prime Minister Poll
Source: Colmar Bruton 2020b, 9.

ELECTION IN A PANDEMIC

In order to examine the election results of 2020, it is vital to first discuss New Zealand's electoral system. In 1996, New Zealand adopted the MMP system.[148] Since then, no single party has been able to gain a majority of the seats in Parliament and coalition governments have become the norm since 1996.[149] Under MMP, the total number of seats that a party wins is ultimately determined by the percentage of the party vote.[150] Thus, if out of 100 seats, Party A wins 10 electorate seats and has won 20 percent of the party vote, Party A gets 10 members of Parliament from the list allocation to bring its total number of seats to 20, which will theoretically reflect 20 percent of seats in line with the 20 percent of the party vote won by Party A.[151] Scholars argue that MMP, being more proportional than a majoritarian electoral system such as First Past the Post (FPP), is more advantageous to smaller parties.[152] As Shugart and Tan argue, since the adoption of MMP, the number of parties being represented in the legislature has increased since the days of FPP prior to 1996.[153] Although MMP is advantageous to small parties, it is vital to note that the two large parties in New Zealand have survived "better than expected."[154] This, coupled with the existence of several "micro parties" that do not tend to last beyond a few electoral cycles, makes New Zealand's MMP system distinct from other countries where MMP is also in use.[155]

New Zealand recorded zero community cases for 102 days until COVID-19 was detected in the community again when a family in South Auckland tested positive for the virus in August 2020.[156] The government acted quickly and moved Auckland into Alert Level 3 and the rest of the country was moved to Alert Level 2.[157] As a result, due to restrictions in movement and gatherings, the election was postponed by a month and was held in October 2020 instead.[158] By the end of September, all of New Zealand was moved back down to Alert Level 1and for the remainder of the campaign, there no more restrictions.[159] Until the Auckland delta outbreak in August 2021, New Zealand witnessed no more restrictions for the better part of a year.[160] The 2020 election witnessed a record number people either voting by mail or voting in advance.[161] The election result of 2020 was consequential in many ways and it resulted in a very different composition in Parliament compared to 2017. Labour performed well in both in terms of the electorate seats and the seats allotted via party lists. In terms of the party vote, Labour was leading in the party vote in seventy-one out of seventy-two constituencies.[162] In addition, only one Labour member of Parliament lost their electorate seat, that too to the Maori Party, not National.[163] UMR's postelection poll, as represented in figure 11.13, showed that 19 percent of National's 2017 vote went to Labour in 2020. The Labour party won sixty-five seats, an overall majority and hence was put in a position where Labour was able to form a government by itself without needing coalition partners, if it chose to do so.[164]

Using Laakso and Taagapera's Effective Number of Parties Index, the effective number of electoral parties in New Zealand after the 2020 election was 2.6.[165] This was down from 3.6 in the 2017 election, further lending credence to Vowles's argument about the two large parties surviving better than expected under MMP.[166] Since the introduction of MMP in 1996, no party has ever been able to win an outright majority alone. It is vital to note that the mechanical effect of MMP is such that small parties benefit from MMP as it is a proportional system and consequently, the large parties do not have the same advantages as they would in a majoritarian system like FPP.[167] The result of the 2020 election is significant not only because one party won an overall majority for the first time but also because the result of the election did not correspond with the theoretical mechanical effect of the electoral system.

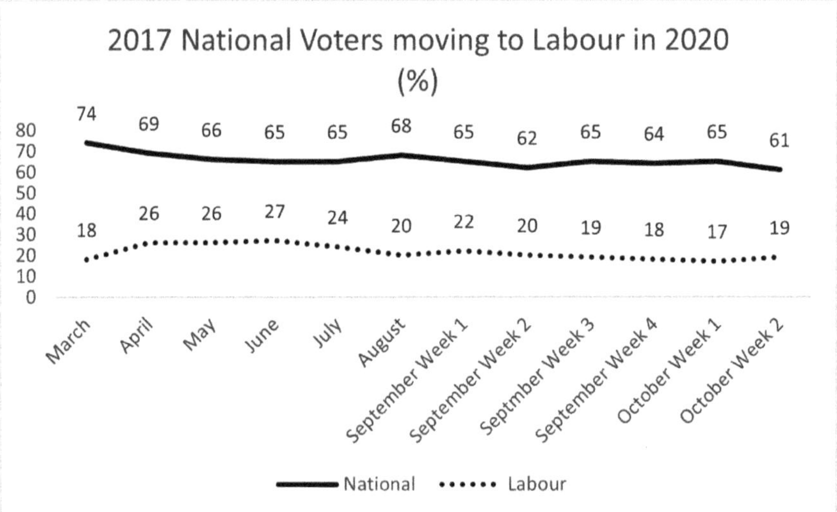

Figure 11.13. 2017 National Party Voters Moving to Labour in 2020 (%)
Source: UMR postelection poll, in Mills, Downs, and Butt 2021, 300.

CONCLUDING OBSERVATIONS

As the pandemic progressed and the nature of the crisis changed with new variants such as delta and omicron emerging, so did New Zealand's pandemic response. There were long stretches of no community spread of the virus for most of 2020 and 2021. In August 2021, an outbreak of the Delta variant resulted in a complete lockdown for two weeks across the country, with restrictions for Auckland being in place for the remainder of the year. The government launched an aggressive vaccination campaign in light of the delta variant, and although mass vaccination for the general public began only in April 2021, New Zealand was able to achieve very high vaccination rates of close to 90 percent at the end of year. By August 12 only 21.6 percent of the eligible population were fully vaccinated. By October 31, it had reached 75 percent. By December 17, 2021, 90 percent were fully vaccinated and 94 percent had first dose.[168] After the onset of the delta outbreak, the government announced that the elimination strategy, which had been the linchpin of the government's pandemic response, would be "phased out" and three-tier traffic light system as part of the "living with COVID" strategy.[169] In 2022, after omicron was detected in New Zealand, the government also kick started a booster campaign and made vaccine doses available for children and young adults. As figure 11.14 and 11.15 show, Labour and Ardern have continued to enjoy strong support in the polls after the election. Labour would still be the leading party in government if the election was held today.

In conclusion, we argue that Labour's historic election victory under MMP in 2020 was due to a combination of factors. Labour and Ardern's performance before the pandemic were achieving mixed results at best. Despite strong support after crises, in the prepandemic phase Labour was not able to sustain this support and National was able to regain its lead in the party vote. However, we see a marked change in the numbers once the pandemic began. The government benefitted from strong support of its pandemic response and lockdown measures early in the crisis that was complemented by effective leadership and Ardern's personal involvement and leadership in the pandemic response. Effective communication was a key part of this leadership approach. The government's initial economic measures during the pandemic also enabled Labour to take the lead over National on the issue of the economy. Although economic problems such

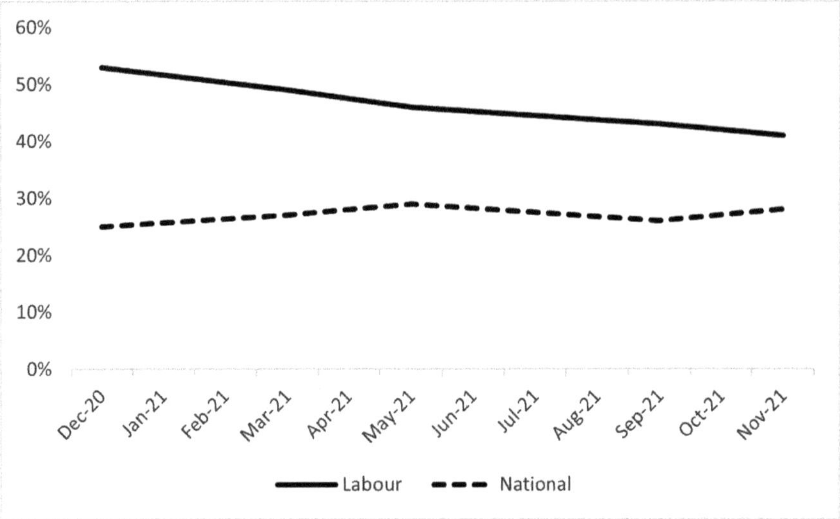

Figure 11.14. Postelection Polls—Party Vote
Source: Compiled by authors using data from Colmar Bruton and Newshub-Reid.

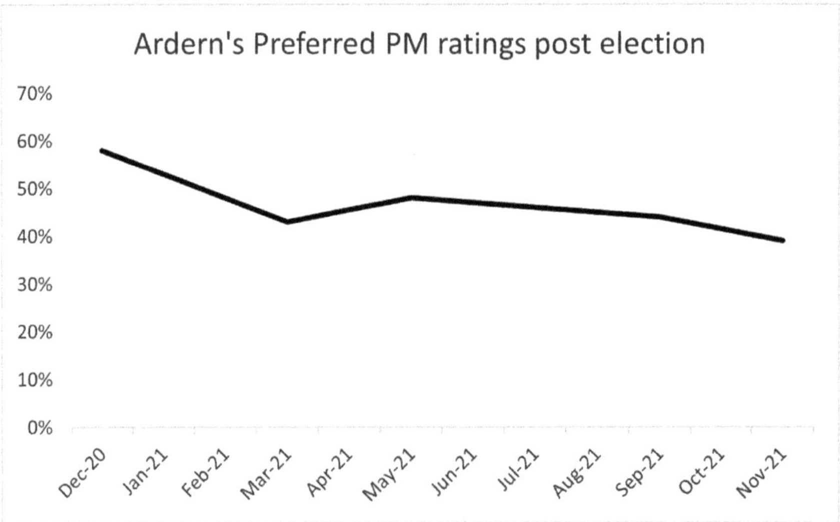

Figure 11.15. Ardern's Preferred Prime Minister Ratings: Postelection
Source: Compiled by authors using data from Colmar Bruton and Newshub-Reid.

as house prices and inflation have become serious issues in New Zealand in the postelection phase, from the perspective of assessing government performance as a factor in the preelection phase, data shows us that Labour was doing well on this issue throughout 2020. Finally, a weak opposition party also gave Labour a considerable advantage. Neither was the National Party able to claim ownership of salient issues during the pandemic, it was also riddled with intraparty divisions and frequent leadership changes that harmed the party electorally. In summary, Labour's historic and triumphal election victory was due to a deft early response, leadership particularly that of the party leaders, a satisfactory evaluation of the government's performance and a weak opposition party during the crisis.

NOTES

1. *BBC* 2020a.
2. Deguara 2020.
3. Lowy Institute 2021.
4. Manhire 2020.
5. *1News* 2020; Clark 2020.
6. Ministry of Health n.d.a.
7. Malpass 2022.
8. Ministry of Health n.d.b.
9. Ibid.
10. International Monetary Fund 2021.
11. *RNZ* 2021.
12. Brockett 2021.
13. *BBC* 2020c.
14. Levine 2021, 33–67.
15. Page and Shapiro 1983.
16. Ibid., 181
17. Wlezien and Soroka 2012, 1425.
18. Ibid.
19. Bol et al. 2021, 497–505; *The Economist* 2020.
20. Cunningham 2020; Schraff 2021, 1007–17.
21. Mueller 1970, 18–34; Mueller 1973.
22. Hetherington and Nelson 2003, 37–42; Gaines 2002, 531–36.
23. Schraff 2021, 1007.
24. Ibid., 1008; Hetherington and Nelson 2003, 37–42.

25. Kritzinger et al. 2021, 1205–31.
26. Cunningham 2020.
27. Bol et al. 2021, 497–505.
28. Johansson, Hopmann, and Shehata 2021, 321–34.
29. Goldfinch, Taplin, and Gauld 2021, 3–11; Chapple 2021, 214.
30. Cunningham 2020.
31. Johansson, Hopmann, and Shehata 2021, 321–34; Kritzinger et al. 2021, 1205–31.
32. Johansson, Hopmann, and Shehata 2021, 321–34; Kritzinger et al. 2021, 1205–31.
33. Schraff 2021, 1007–17; Johansson, Hopmann, and Shehata 2021, 321–34.
34. Schraff 2021, 1007.
35. Ibid .
36. Goldfinch, Taplin, and Gauld 2021, 3–11; Chapple 2021, 214.
37. Kritzinger et al. 2021, 1223.
38. Manin, Przeworski, and Stokes 1999, 29–55.
39. Lijphart 1984; Powell 2000.
40. Manin, Przeworski, and Stokes 1999, 29–55.
41. Gherghina 2011.
42. Lewis-Beck and Stegmaier 2000, 183–219; Roper 2003, 85–100; Anderson 2000, 151–70.
43. Bittner 2011; Mughan 2000, 6.
44. Bean and Mughan 1989.
45. Bittner 2011; Stewart and Clarke 1992, 447–70.
46. Mughan 2015, 28–39.
47. Bisbee and Honig 2021, 70.
48. De Vries et al. 2021, 452.
49. Ibid.
50. Janda 1980.
51. Murphy 2014, 893–909.
52. Law and Meehan 2013.
53. Bierre and Howden-Chapman 2020, 29–49.
54. Murphy 2014, 899; White and Nandedkar 2021, 219.
55. Lees-Marshment et al. 2015, 103.
56. Mills, Berti, and Rupar 2018, 164.
57. Roy Morgan Research 2017.
58. Duncan 2018, 120.
59. Mills, Berti, and Rupar 2018, 165.
60. *RNZ* 2017.

61. Ministry of Housing and Urban Development n.d.
62. Ibid.
63. Toomey, Collins, and Jenkins 2021, 93–117.
64. Ibid.
65. Toomey, Collins, and Jenkins 2021, 96; *New Zealand Parliament* 2018.
66. Martin 2018; Edmunds 2018.
67. Toomey, Collins, and Jenkins 2021, 100.
68. Toomey, Collins, and Jenkins 2021, 102; Cooke 2019.
69. McCullough 2019.
70. Furley 2018.
71. Corlett 2018.
72. Toomey, Collins, and Jenkins 2021, 102.
73. *1News* 2019.
74. Real Estate Analysis Unit, *Home Affordability Report (December 2019)*.
75. Ipsos 2020a.
76. Bierre and Howden-Chapman 2020, 29–49; White and Nandedkar 2021, 213–34.
77. Hall 2021.
78. White and Nandedkar 2021, 213–34.
79. Ibid.
80. Toomey, Collins, and Jenkins 2021, 93-117.
81. *BBC* 2019.
82. Satherly and Prendergast, "Jacinda Ardern's Response"; Malik 2019.
83. Ellis and Muller 2020, 332–48; Crothers and O'Brien 2020, 247–59.
84. *Reuters* 2020.
85. Crothers and O'Brien 2020, 247–59.
86. *RNZ* 2019.
87. *New Zealand Herald* 2019.
88. Trevett 2019.
89. Colmar Bruton 2019.
90. Ibid.
91. Ipsos 2020a, 8.
92. *RNZ* 2018.
93. Colmar Bruton 2019, 10.
94. Walters 2020.
95. Small and Burrows 2020.
96. Wilson 2020, 283.
97. Colmar Bruton 2019, 13; Colmar Bruton 2020, 16.
98. *RNZ* 2021.

99. Jamieson 2020, 599.
100. Ibid.
101. Baker, Kvalsvig, and Verrall 2020.
102. Ardern 2020.
103. Baker 2021, 193.
104. Wilson 2020, 279–93.
105. Jamieson 2020, 599.
106. Cousins 2020.
107. Cooke 2020; Coughlan 2020.
108. Nagesh 2019.
109. Kritzinger et al. 2021, 1206.
110. Young, Psirides, and Streat 2021, 8–10.
111. Wilson et al. 2020, 9.
112. Wilson 2020, 279–93.
113. Tan 2020, 93.
114. Ibid., 79–99; Wilson 2020, 279–93.
115. Tan 2020; Wilson 2020.
116. Wilson 2020, 285.
117. Tan 2020, 94.
118. Hunt 2021.
119. Wilson 2020, 286.
120. Tan 2020, 95.
121. Ibid., 99.
122. Tan 2020, 79–99; Wilson 2020, 279–93.
123. Tan 2020, 79–99; Wilson 2020, 279–93.
124. Wilson 2020, 287.
125. Martin 2021.
126. Tan 2020, 94.
127. Stock 2020.
128. Jamieson 2020, 599.
129. Ibid.
130. New Zealand Government 2020, 7.
131. Ibid.
132. Ipsos 2020c, 8.
133. Ibid., 17.
134. *RNZ* 2020b.
135. Levine 2021, 38.
136. RNZ 2020c.
137. Graham-McLay 2020.
138. So 2021, 4.

139. Ibid.
140. Greene and Haber 2015, 16.
141. Ibid.
142. Moury and De Giorgi 2015, 1–13.
143. Ibid.
144. Walgrave and Swert 2007, 37; Greene and Haber 2015, 16.
145. Tan 2000, 94.
146. Molyneux 2020.
147. Mills, Downs, and Butt 2021, 299–300.
148. Boston 2011, 79–105; Shugart and Tan 2016, 247–77; Vowels 2018, 147–60.
149. Boston 2011, 79–105; Shugart and Tan 2016, 247–77; Curtin and Miller 2010, 120–36.
150. Shugart and Tan 2016, 249.
151. Ibid.
152. Boston 2011, 79–105; Shugart and Tan 2016, 247–77.
153. Shugart and Tan 2016, 247–77.
154. Vowels 2017, 805–24.
155. Shugart and Tan 2016, 247–77.
156. *RNZ* 2021.
157. Ibid.
158. *BBC* 2020b.
159. *RNZ* 2021.
160. Ibid.
161. *RNZ* 2020a.
162. Levine 2021, 57.
163. Ibid., 58.
164. *BBC* 2020c.
165. Laakso and Taagepera 1979, 3–27.
166. Vowels 2018, 147–60.
167. Shugart and Tan 2016, 247–77.
168. Ministry of Health n.d.b; *RNZ* 2021.
169. Corlett 2021.

REFERENCES

1News. 2019. "1 NEWS Poll: Public Faith Fades in Government's 100,000 KiwiBuild Target." February 25. https://www.1news.co.nz/2019/02/25/1-news-poll-public-faith-fades-in-governments-100000-kiwibuild-target/.

1News. 2020. "'Empathy in a Crisis'—Jacinda Ardern's Covid-19 Leadership Praised by International Media." April 20. https://www.1news.co.nz/2020/04/19/empathy-in-a-crisis-jacinda-arderns-covid-19-leadership-praised-by-international-media/.

Anderson, Christopher J. 2000. "Economic Voting and Political Context: A Comparative Perspective." *Electoral Studies* 19 (2): 151–70.

Ardern, Jacinda. 2020. "Major Steps Taken to Protect New Zealanders from COVID-19." The Beehive, March 14. https://www.beehive.govt.nz/release/major-steps-taken-protect-new-zealanders-covid-19.

Baker, Michael. 2021. "The 2020 Election, the COVID-19 Emergency, and the Need to Improve Our Response Capacity for Even More Serious Threats." In *Politics in a Pandemic: Jacinda Ardern and New Zealand's 2020 Election*, edited by Stephen Levine, 193–202. Wellington: Victoria University of Wellington Press.

Baker, Michael G., Amanda Kvalsvig, and Ayesha J. Verrall. 2020. "New Zealand's COVID-19 Elimination Strategy." *Medical Journal of Australia* 213 (5): 198–200.e1.

BBC. 2019. "Christchurch Shootings: 49 Dead in New Zealand Mosque Attacks." March 15. https://www.bbc.com/news/world-asia-47578798.

BBC. 2020a. "Coronavirus Confirmed as Pandemic by World Health Organization." March 11. https://www.bbc.com/news/world-51839944.

BBC. 2020b. "New Zealand: Jacinda Ardern Delays Election over Coronavirus Fears." August 17. https://www.bbc.com/news/world-asia-53796434.

BBC. 2020c. "New Zealand Election: Jacinda Ardern's Labour Party Scores Landslide Win." October 17. https://www.bbc.com/news/world-asia-54519628.

Bean, Clive, and Anthony Mughan. 1989. "Leadership Effects in Parliamentary Elections in Australia and Britain." *The American Political Science Review* 83 (4): 1165–79.

Bierre, Sarah, and Philippa Howden-Chapman. 2020. "Telling Stories: The Role of Narratives in Rental Housing Policy Change in New Zealand." *Housing Studies* 35 (1): 29–49.

Bisbee, James, and Dan Honig. 2021. "Flight to Safety: COVID-Induced Changes in the Intensity of Status Quo Preference and Voting Behavior." *The American Political Science Review*: 1–17.

Bittner, Amanda. 2011. *Platform or Personality?: The Role of Party Leaders in Elections*. New York and Oxford: Oxford University Press.

Bol, Damien, Marco Giani, Andre Blais, and Peter John Loewen. 2021. "The Effect of COVID-19 Lockdowns on Political Support: Some Good News for Democracy?" *European Journal of Political Research* 60 (2): 497–505.

Boston, Jonathan. 2011. "Government Formation in New Zealand Under MMP: Theory and Practice." *Political Science* 63 (1): 79–105.

Brockett, Matthew. 2021. "New Zealand Lifts Lockdown Outside Auckland as Outbreak Wanes." *Bloomberg*, September 6. https://www.bloomberg.com/news/articles/2021-09-06/ardern-lifts-lockdown-outside-auckland-as-delta-cases-dwindle.

Clark, Pilita. 2020. "Arise Saint Jacinda, a Leader for Our Troubled Times." *The Financial Times*, April 19. https://www.ft.com/content/d26564b4-80ba-11ea-82f6-150830b3b99a.

Chapple, Simon. 2021. "Well-Being and the Covid Crunch: The Economy and the 2020 Election." In *Politics in a Pandemic: Jacinda Ardern and New Zealand's 2020 Election*, edited by Stephen Levine, 203–14. Wellington: Victoria University of Wellington Press.

Colmar Bruton. 2019. *1 News Colmar Bruton Poll November 27–29, 2019*. December 2. https://static.colmarbrunton.co.nz/wp-content/uploads/2019/05/Prelim_23-27-Nov-2019_1-NEWS-Colmar-Brunton-Poll-report-.pdf.

Colmar Bruton. 2020a. *1 News Colmar Bruton Poll February 8–12, 2020*. February 13. https://static.colmarbrunton.co.nz/wp-content/uploads/2019/05/8-12-Feb-2020_1-NEWS-Colmar-Brunton-Poll-report-.pdf.

Colmar Bruton. 2020b. *1 News Colmar Bruton Poll October 10–14, 2020*. October 15. https://static.colmarbrunton.co.nz/wp-content/uploads/2019/05/10-14-October-2020_1-NEWS-Colmar-Brunton-Poll-report-1.pdf.

Cooke, Henry. 2019. "KiwiBuild Failure Is More than a Broken Promise, It's a Betrayal." *Stuff*, May 12. https://www.stuff.co.nz/national/politics/112627636/kiwibuild-failure-is-more-than-a-broken-promise-its-a-betrayal.

Cooke, Henry. 2020. "Coronavirus: Public Surge in Trust of Government during Covid-19 Crisis." *Stuff*, April 8. https://www.stuff.co.nz/national/health/coronavirus/120911320/coronavirus-public-surge-in-trust-of-government-and-national-pride.

Corlett, Eva. 2018. "Foreign House Buyer Problem 'Was Never Real.'" *RNZ*, June 20. https://www.rnz.co.nz/news/national/359991/foreign-house-buyer-problem-was-never-real.

Corlett, Eva. 2021. "New Zealand Covid Elimination Strategy to Be Phased Out, Ardern Says." *The Guardian*, October 4. https://www.theguardian.com/world/2021/oct/04/new-zealand-covid-strategy-in-transition-ardern-says-as-auckland-awaits-lockdown-decision.

Coughlan, Thomas. 2020. "Coronavirus: The Government's Covid-19 Lockdown Measures Have Overwhelming Public Support, According to a Poll." *Stuff*, April 23. https://www.stuff.co.nz/national/121231591/coronavirus-the-governments-covid19-lockdown-measures-have-overwhelming-public-support-according-to-a-poll.

Cousins, Sophie. 2020. "New Zealand Eliminates COVID-19." *The Lancet (British Edition)* 395 (235): 1474–74.

Crothers, Charles, and Thomas O'Brien. 2020. "The Contexts of the Christchurch Terror Attacks: Social Science Perspectives." *Kōtuitui New Zealand Journal of Social Sciences* 15 (2): 247–59.

Cunningham, Kevin. 2020. "The Rally-Round-the-Flag-Effect and Covid-19." UK in a Changing Europe, King's College London, May 28. https://ukandeu.ac.uk/the-rally-round-the-flag-effect-and-covid-19/.

Curtin, Jennifer, and Raymond Miller. 2010. "New Zealand's Future Party System: A Multi-Party Mirage?" In *Key to Victory: The New Zealand General Election of 2008*, edited by Stephen Levine and Nigel S. Roberts, 120–36. Wellington: Victoria University Press.

Deguara, Brittney. 2020. "Coronavirus: WHO Showcases, Praises New Zealand's Effective Covid-19 Response with Documentary." *Stuff*, July 24. https://www.stuff.co.nz/national/health/coronavirus/122247181/coronavirus-who-showcases-praises-new-zealands-effective-covid19-response-with-documentary.

De Vries, C. E., B. N. Bakker, S. B. Hobolt, and K. Arceneaux. 2021. "Crisis Signaling: How Italy's Coronavirus Lockdown Affected Incumbent Support in Other European Countries." *Political Science Research and Methods* 9 (3): 451–67.

Duncan, Grant. 2018. "Trust, Distrust, and the End of Politics-as-We-Knew-it: The Mood of the Nation Prior to Election 2017." *Kōtuitui New Zealand Journal of Social Sciences* 13 (2): 114–31.

Edmunds, Susan. 2018. "New Plymouth KiwiBuild Houses Set to Sell for $100k More than Suburb's Median Price." *Stuff*, November 21. https://www.stuff.co.nz/business/108755451/new-plymouth-kiwibuild-houses-set-to-sell-for-100k-more-than-suburbs-median-price.

Ellis, Gavin, and Denis Muller. 2020. "The Proximity Filter: The Effect of Distance on Media Coverage of the Christchurch Mosque Attacks." *Kōtuitui New Zealand Journal of Social Sciences* 15 (2): 332–48.

Furley, Tom. 2018. "One Year On: How Has the Govt Performed on Housing?" *RNZ*, October 23. https://www.rnz.co.nz/news/political/369208/one-year-on-how-has-the-govt-performed-on-housing.

Gaines, Brian J. 2002. "Where's the Rally? Approval and Trust of the President, Cabinet, Congress, and Government since September 11." *PS: Political Science & Politics* 35 (3): 531–36.

Gherghina, Sergiu. 2011. "Does Government Performance Matter? Electoral Support for Incumbents in Six Post-Communist Countries." *Contemporary Politics* 17 (3): 257–77.

Goldfinch, Shaun, Ross Taplin, and Robin Gauld. 2021. "Trust in Government Increased during the Covid-19 Pandemic in Australia and New Zealand." *Australian Journal of Public Administration* 80 (1): 3–11.

Graham-McLay, Charlotte. 2020. "Judith Collins Named New Zealand National Party's New Leader." *The Guardian*, July 14. https://www.theguardian.com/world/2020/jul/14/judith-collins-named-new-zealand-national-party-new-leader.

Greene, Zachary David, and Matthias Haber. 2015. "The Consequences of Appearing Divided: An Analysis of Party Evaluations and Vote Choice." *Electoral Studies* 37: 15–27.

Hall, Michael. 2021. "Can Labour Tackle the Housing Crisis like Its Lauded Party Predecessors? What You Need to Know." *RNZ*, August 14. https://www.rnz.co.nz/news/what-you-need-to-know/449159/can-labour-tackle-the-housing-crisis-like-its-lauded-party-predecessors-what-you-need-to-know.

Hetherington, Marc J., and Michael Nelson. 2003. "Anatomy of a Rally Effect: George W. Bush and the War on Terrorism." *PS: Political Science & Politics* 36 (1): 37–42.

Hunt, Elle. 2021. "Words Matter: How New Zealand's Clear Messaging Helped Beat Covid." *The Guardian*, February 26. https://www.theguardian.com/world/2021/feb/26/words-matter-how-new-zealands-clear-messaging-helped-beat-covid.

International Monetary Fund. 2021. *New Zealand: Staff Concluding Statement of the 2021 Article IV Discussions*. 2021. Accessed February 1, 2022. https://www.imf.org/en/News/Articles/2021/03/11/mcs031121-new-zealand-staff-concluding-statement-of-the-2021-article-iv-discussions.

Ipsos. 2020a. *The Ipsos New Zealand Issues Monitor*. July. Accessed January 24, 2022. https://www.ipsos.com/sites/default/files/9th-ipsos-new-zealand-issues-monitor-090720.pdf.

Ipsos. 2020b. *The Ipsos New Zealand Issues Monitor*. September. Accessed January 30, 2020. https://www.ipsos.com/sites/default/files/ct/news/documents/2020-09/11th_ipsos_new_zealand_issues_monitor_sept_2020.pdf.

Ipsos. 2020c. *The Ipsos New Zealand Issues Monitor*. November. Accessed January 28, 2022. https://www.ipsos.com/sites/default/files/ct/news/documents/2020-11/12th_ipsos_new_zealand_issues_monitor_nov_2020.pdf.

Jamieson, Thomas. 2020. "'Go Hard, Go Early': Preliminary Lessons from New Zealand's Response to COVID-19." *American Review of Public Administration* 50 (6–7): 598–605.

Janda, Kenneth. 1980. *Political Parties: A Cross-National Survey*. New York: Free Press; London: Collier Macmillan.

Johansson, Bengt, David Nicolas Hopmann, and Adam Shehata. 2021. "When the Rally-Around-the-Flag Effect Disappears, Or: When the COVID-19 Pandemic Becomes 'Normalized.'" *Journal of Elections, Public Opinion and Parties* 31 (S1): 321–34.

Kritzinger, Sylvia, Martial Foucault, Romain Lachat, Julia Partheymüller, Carolina Plescia, and Sylvain Brouard. 2021. "'Rally Round the Flag': The COVID-19 Crisis and Trust in the National Government." *West European Politics* 44 (5–6): 1205–31.

Laakso, Markku, and Rein Taagepera. 1979. "'Effective' Number of Parties: A Measure with Application to West Europe." *Comparative Political Studies* 12 (1): 3–27.

Law, David, and Lisa Meehan. 2013. *Housing Affordability in New Zealand: Evidence from Household Surveys (WP 13/14).* New Zealand Productivity Commission, July 16. https://www.productivity.govt.nz/assets/Documents/do-nz-firms-catch-up-to-the-domestic-productivity-frontierhistory-of-tertiary-educaion-5/4da073556f/Housing-Affordability-in-New-Zealand_-Evidence-from-Household-Surveys-WP-13_14.pdf.

Lees-Marshment, Jennifer, Yannick Dufresne, Gregory Eady, Danny Osborne, Cliff van der Linden, and Jack Vowles. 2015. "Vote Compass in the 2014 New Zealand Election: Hearing the Voice of New Zealand Voters." *Political Science* 67 (2): 94–124.

Levine, Stephen. 2021. "Politics in a Pandemic: New Zealand's 2020 Election." In *Politics in a Pandemic: Jacinda Ardern and New Zealand's 2020 Election,* edited by Stephen Levine, 33–67. Wellington: Victoria University of Wellington Press.

Lewis-Beck, Michael S., and Mary Stegmaier. 2000. "Economic Determinants of Electoral Outcomes." *Annual Review of Political Science* 3 (1): 183–219.

Lijphart, Arend. 1984. *Democracies: Patterns of Majoritarian and Consensus Government in Twenty-One Countries.* New Haven, CT: Yale University Press.

Lowy Institute. 2021. *COVID Performance Index.* Accessed February 1, 2022. https://interactives.lowyinstitute.org/features/covid-performance/.

Malik, Nesrine. 2019. "With Respect: How Jacinda Ardern Showed the World What a Leader Should Be." *The Guardian,* March 28. https://www.theguardian.com/world/2019/mar/28/with-respect-how-jacinda-ardern-showed-the-world-what-a-leader-should-be.

Malpass, Luke. 2022. "The Political Lines Have Been Drawn for a Traditional Left-Right Battle." *Stuff,* February 8. https://www.stuff.co.nz/national/politics/opinion/127712758/the-political-lines-have-been-drawn-for-a-traditional-leftright-battle?fbclid=IwAR0iD74y77scRGIqEm8JrseYNUm1J9klbufMdkXm7qdDdFlLBRLw_3lrKfM.

Manhire, Toby. 2020. "NZ Ranked First in World for Covid-19 Response Communications." *The Spinoff,* May 6. https://thespinoff.co.nz/politics/06-05-2020/nz-ranked-first-in-world-for-covid-19-response-communications.

Manin, Bernard, Adam Przeworski, and Susan Carol Stokes. 1999. *Democracy, Accountability, and Representation.* New York: Cambridge University Press.

Martin, Hannah. 2021. "Covid-19: One Year on from NZ Closing Its Border, What Will Happen Next?" *Stuff*, March 14. https://www.stuff.co.nz/national/health/300247817/covid19-one-year-on-from-nz-closing-its-border-what-will-happen-next.

Martin, Robbin. 2018. "Price Point Casts Doubt Over KiwiBuild Homes in New Plymouth." *RNZ*, November 20. https://www.rnz.co.nz/news/national/376417/price-point-casts-doubt-over-kiwibuild-homes-in-new-plymouth.

McCullough, Yvonne. 2019. "KiwiBuild Reset: Government Drops 100,000-Home Target, Adds $400m Fund." *RNZ*, September 4. https://www.rnz.co.nz/news/political/398097/kiwibuild-reset-government-drops-100-000-home-target-adds-400m-fund.

Mills, Keri, Carlo Berti, and Verica Rupar. 2018. "What Kind of Country We Want for Our Children: An Analysis of Media Coverage of the 2017 New Zealand General Election." *Kōtuitui New Zealand Journal of Social Sciences* 13 (2): 161–76.

Mills, Stephen, Marcus Downs, and Thomas Butt. 2021. "Why Labour Won—Survey Findings and the 2020 Election." In *Politics in a Pandemic: Jacinda Ardern and New Zealand's 2020 Election*, edited by Stephen Levine, 298–305. Wellington: Victoria University of Wellington Press.

Ministry of Health. 2020. *Novel Coronavirus Update—24th January 2020*. January 24. https://www.health.govt.nz/news-media/news-items/novel-coronavirus-update-24th-january-2020.

Ministry of Health. N.d.a. *COVID-19: Current Cases*. Accessed February 1, 2022. https://www.health.govt.nz/our-work/diseases-and-conditions/covid-19-novel-coronavirus/covid-19-data-and-statistics/covid-19-current-cases

Ministry of Health. N.d.b. *COVID-19: Vaccine Data*. Accessed February 1, 2022. https://www.health.govt.nz/covid-19-novel-coronavirus/covid-19-data-and-statistics/covid-19-vaccine-data.

Ministry of Housing and Urban Development. N.d. *Kiwibuild Eligibility Criteria.* Accessed January 30, 2022. https://www.hud.govt.nz/assets/Residential-Housing/Housing-Affordability/KiwiBuild/37d9374b24/Cabinet-paper-KiwiBuild-eligibility-criteria.pdf.

Molyneux, Vita. 2020. "National Votes against Government's Alert Level 2 Enforcement Bill." *Newshub*, May 12. https://www.newshub.co.nz/home/politics/2020/05/national-votes-against-government-s-alert-level-2-enforcement-bill.html.

Moury, Catherine, and Elisabetta De Giorgi. 2015. "Introduction: Conflict and Consensus in Parliament during the Economic Crisis." *Journal of Legislative Studies* 21 (1): 1–13.

Mueller, John E. 1970. "Presidential Popularity from Truman to Johnson." *The American Political Science Review* 64 (1): 18–34.

Mueller, John E. 1973. *War, Presidents, and Public Opinion*. New York: Wiley.

Mughan, Anthony. 2000. *Media and the Presidentialization of Parliamentary Elections*. New York; Houndmills, Basingstoke, Hampshire: Palgrave.

Mughan, Anthony. 2015. "Parties, Conditionality and Leader Effects in Parliamentary Elections." *Party Politics* 21 (1): 28–39.

Murphy, Laurence. 2014. "'Houston, We've Got a Problem': The Political Construction of a Housing Affordability Metric in New Zealand." *Housing Studies* 29 (7): 893–909.

Nagesh, Ashitha. 2019. "Jacinda Ardern: 'A Leader with Love on Full Display.'" *BBC*, March 21. https://www.bbc.com/news/world-asia-47630129.

Newshub. 2019. "Jacinda Ardern's Response to the Christchurch Terror Attack, 'They Are Us,' Named Quote of the Year." December 12. https://www.newshub.co.nz/home/new-zealand/2019/12/jacinda-ardern-s-response-to-the-christchurch-terror-attack-they-are-us-named-quote-of-the-year.html.

New Zealand Government. 2020. *Budget Speech Hon. Grant Robertson*. May 14. https://www.treasury.govt.nz/sites/default/files/2020-05/b20-speech.pdf.

New Zealand Herald. 2019. "Core Group of World Leaders to Attend Jacinda Ardern-Led Paris Summit." April 29. https://www.nzherald.co.nz/nz/core-group-of-world-leaders-to-attend-jacinda-ardern-led-paris-summit/ICFA7SVF5Q3PVC6GXIXCN7ZKEQ/?c_id=1&objectid=12226274.

New Zealand Parliament. 2018. *11863 (2018). Hon Judith Collins to the Minister of Housing and Urban Development*. June 12. https://www.parliament.nz/en/pb/order-paper-questions/written-questions/document/WQ_11863_2018/11863-2018-hon-judith-collins-to-the-minister-of-housing.

Page, Benjamin I., and Robert Y. Shapiro. 1983. "Effects of Public Opinion on Policy." The *American Political Science Review* 77 (1): 175–90.

Powell, G. Bingham. 2000. *Elections as Instruments of Democracy: Majoritarian and Proportional Visions*. New Haven, CT: Yale University Press.

Reuters. 2020. "New Zealand Tightens Gun Laws Further in Response to Mass Shooting." June 18. https://www.reuters.com/article/us-newzealand-shooting-idUSKBN23P0TE.

RNZ. 2017. "Know Your Policy: Housing." August 30. https://www.rnz.co.nz/programmes/policy-comparisons/story/201856645/know-your-policy-housing.

RNZ. 2018. "Bill English Delivers Emotional Resignation Speech." February 13. https://www.rnz.co.nz/news/political/350294/bill-english-delivers-emotional-resignation-speech.

RNZ. 2019. "Christchurch Mosque Shootings: 'Manifesto' Deemed Objectionable." March 23. https://www.rnz.co.nz/news/national/385399/christchurch-mosque-shootings-manifesto-deemed-objectionable.

RNZ. 2020a. "Election 2020: Advance Votes Surpass Total in 2017." October 13. https://www.rnz.co.nz/news/political/428240/election-2020-advance-votes-surpass-total-in-2017.

RNZ. 2020b. "Simon Bridges on Losing National Party Leadership: 'It's Been a Heck of a Ride.'" May 22. https://www.rnz.co.nz/news/political/417279/simon-bridges-on-losing-national-party-leadership-it-s-been-a-heck-of-a-ride.

RNZ. 2020c. "What Did Todd Muller Achieve in His 53 Days as National Leader?" July 14. https://www.rnz.co.nz/news/political/421163/what-did-todd-muller-achieve-in-his-53-days-as-national-leader.

RNZ. 2021. "Timeline: The Year of Covid-19 in New Zealand." March 24. https://www.rnz.co.nz/news/national/437359/timeline-the-year-of-covid-19-in-new-zealand.

Roper, Steven D. 2003. "Is There an Economic Basis for Post-Communist Voting? Evidence from Romanian Elections, 1992–2000." *East European Quarterly* 37 (1): 85–100.

Roy Morgan Research. 2017. "New Zealanders' Concerns Highlighted in Run to Election: Poverty and the Gap between Rich and Poor Is the Single Biggest Issue Facing New Zealand and the World According to New Zealanders." June 30. http://www.roymorgan.com/findings/7254-new-zealand-most-important-problems-may-2017-201706301533.

Roy Morgan Research. N.d. "NZ Government Confidence (2007–2022)." Accessed January 24, 2022. http://www.roymorgan.com/morganpoll/new-zealand/nz-government-confidence.

Schraff, Dominik. 2021. "Political Trust during the Covid-19 Pandemic: Rally Around the Flag or Lockdown Effects?" *European Journal of Political Research* 60 (4): 1007–17.

Shugart, Matthew S., and Alexander C. Tan. 2016. "Political Consequences of New Zealand's MMP System in Comparative Perspective." In *Mixed-Member Electoral Systems in Constitutional Context*, edited by Nathan F. Batto, Chi Huang, Alexander C. Tan, and Gary W. Cox, 247–77. Ann Arbor: University of Michigan.

Small, Zane, and Matt Burrows. 2020. "The Rise and Demise of Simon Bridges: A Timeline of His Key Moments as National Leader." *Newshub*, May 22.

https://www.newshub.co.nz/home/politics/2020/05/the-rise-and-demise-of-simon-bridges-a-timeline-of-his-key-moments-as-national-leader.html.

So, Florence. 2021. "Don't Air Your Dirty Laundry: Party Leadership Contests and Parliamentary Election Outcomes." *European Journal of Political Research* 60 (1): 3–24.

Stewart, Marianne C., and Harold D. Clarke. 1992. "The (Un)Importance of Party Leaders: Leader Images and Party Choice in the 1987 British Election." *The Journal of Politics* 54 (2): 447–70.

Stock, Rob. 2020. "Coronavirus: How Tindall, Morgan and Fyfe Worked to Ready Country for Covid-19 Fight." *Stuff*, April 9. https://www.stuff.co.nz/business/120912415/coronavirus-how-tindall-morgan-and-fyfe-worked-to-ready-country-for-covid19-fight.

Tan, Alexander C. 2020. "Solving the Collective Action Problem Taiwan, New Zealand, and the COVID-19 Battle." *Taiwan Journal of Democracy* 16 (2): 79–99.

The Economist. 2020. "Covid-19 Has Given Most World Leaders a Temporary rise in Popularity." May 9. https://www.economist.com/graphic-detail/2020/05/09/covid-19-has-given-most-world-leaders-a-temporary-rise-in-popularity.

Toomey, Elizabeth, Toni Collins, and Kate Jenkins. 2021. "The New Zealand Experiment: KiwiBuild for First-Homebuyers." *Australian Property Law Journal* 29 (1): 93–117.

Trevett, Claire. 2019. "Claire Trevett: Poll Puts Labour Support Up After Mosque Attacks but Tax Is Back in Debate." *New Zealand Herald*, April 11. https://www.nzherald.co.nz/nz/claire-trevett-poll-puts-labour-support-up-after-mosque-attacks-but-tax-is-back-in-debate/AA2JYNQVNFWD6ZHOB4V4CQAI7I/?c_id=1&objectid=12221107.

Vowels, Jack. 2017. "Electoral Systems in Context: New Zealand." In *The Oxford Handbook of Electoral Systems*, edited by Erik S. Herron, Robert Pekkanen, and Matthew Søberg Shugart, 805–24. Oxford: Oxford University Press.

Vowels, Jack. 2018. "Surprise, Surprise: The New Zealand General Election of 2017." *Kōtuitui New Zealand Journal of Social Sciences* 13 (2): 147–60.

Walgrave, Stefaan, and Knut De Swert. 2007. "Where Does Issue Ownership Come From? From the Party or from the Media? Issue-Party Identifications in Belgium, 1991–2005." *Harvard International Journal of Press/Politics* 12 (1): 37–67.

Walters, Laura. 2020. "Jami-Lee Ross Leaves More Questions than Answers." *Newsroom*, October 23. https://www.newsroom.co.nz/jami-lee-ross-leaves-more-questions-than-answers.

White, Iain, and Gauri Nandedkar. 2021. "The Housing Crisis as an Ideological Artefact: Analysing how Political Discourse Defines, Diagnoses, and Responds." *Housing Studies* 36 (2): 213–34.

Wilson, Nicholas, Lucy Telfar Barnard, Amanda Kvalsvig, Michael Baker, New Zealand Ministry of Health, and University of Otago. 2020. *Potential Health Impacts from the COVID-19 Pandemic for New Zealand If Eradication Fails: Report to the NZ Ministry of Health.* Wellington: Ministry of Health.

Wilson, Suze. 2020. "Pandemic Leadership: Lessons from New Zealand's Approach to COVID-19." *Leadership (London, England)* 16 (3): 279–93.

Wlezien, Christopher, and Stuart N. Soroka. 2012. "Political Institutions and the Opinion-Policy Link." *West European Politics* 35 (6): 1407–32.

Young, Paul J., Alex Psirides, and Stephen Streat. 2021. "New Zealand's Staffed ICU Bed Capacity and COVID-19 Surge Capacity." *New Zealand Medical Journal* 134 (1545): 8–10.

Index

Page References for illustrations and tables are *italicized*

About the Contributors

Chia-hung Tsai is a research fellow at the Election Study Center, National Chengchi University, and holds a joint appointment with the Graduate Institute of East Asian Studies. His fields of specialization include public opinion, methodology, and comparative politics. He has published research in peer-reviewed journals such as *Electoral Studies*, *Social Science Quarterly*, *Asian Journal of Communication*, *Political Science*, *Party Politics*, *International Political Science Review*, *Journal of Asian and African Studies*, and *PLoS ONE*. Dr. Tsai holds a doctorate degree in political science from the Ohio State University. He was also a commissioner of the Central Election Commission (2017–2021), recipient of visiting scholarship of Top University Alliance (2012–2013), and recipient of Taiwan's 2022–2023 senior Fulbright Research Grants.

Yao-Yuan Yeh is Fayez Sarofim–Cullen Trust for Higher Education endowed chair and professor in international studies, department chair of international studies and modern languages, department chair of political science, director of the Master of Diplomacy & Strategic Affairs Program, director of the Taiwan & East Asia Studies Program, and director of the Mandarin Center of the Universities of St. Thomas and Wenzao Ursuline at the University of St. Thomas, Houston. He received his PhD in political science from Texas A&M University. His research focuses on public opinion, foreign policy, international security, U.S.-China-Taiwan relations, East Asian politics, terrorism and political violence, and quantitative methods. Dr. Yeh's academic and policy work has been published in various prestigious platforms, including but not limited to *British Journal of Political Science*, *Terrorism and Political Violence*, *The China Quarterly*, *Social Science Quarterly*, *Scientific Data*, *International Relations of the Asia-Pacific*, *The Defense Post*, *THE DIPLOMAT*, *East Asia Forum*, and *The National Interest*. He has coedited a volume titled *Taiwan: The Development of an Asian Tiger* (Lynne Rienner Publishers, 2019) and coauthored in *Presidentialism, Violence, and the Prospect of Democracy* (Lexington Book, 2021).

Nathan F. Batto is associate research fellow at the Institute of Political Science, Academia Sinica, and the Election Study Center, National Chengchi University. He studies electoral, legislative, and party politics in Taiwan. He is coeditor of *Mixed-Member Electoral Systems in Constitutional Context*, and recent research has appeared in the *Journal of Politics*, *International Journal of Taiwan Studies*, *Journal of Women, Politics, & Policy*, and *Asian Survey*. His blog is Frozen Garlic.

Fang-Yu Chen is assistant professor in the Department of Political Science at Soochow University, Taipei, Taiwan. He received his PhD in political science from Michigan State University. He specializes in East Asian politics, democratization, and foreign policy.

Yi-Ning Katherine Chen (PhD, The University of Texas at Austin) is distinguished professor of communication at National Chengchi University (NCCU), Taiwan. Between 2014 and 2018, she was on secondment as commissioner at the National Communications Commission, Taiwan. Professor Chen has spoken at various regulatory forums and international academic conferences in Europe, the United States, and Asia, in which topics focus on the internet users' behavior and pay TV vs. OTT TV regulation. She is also a board member of the Oversight Board for Meta.

Yu-Hua Chen is an assistant professor in China studies at Global Studies Program of Akita International University (AIU), Japan. He graduated from the Australian National University (ANU). His research interests include China's foreign and security policy, history of modern China, international relations theory, foreign policy of Taiwan, and geopolitics. Prior to teaching at AIU, he was a visiting fellow at George Washington University and a lecturer at the ANU.

Chi Huang is a university chair professor of political science, director of the Taiwan Institute for Governance and Communication Research (TIGCR), and research fellow of the Election Study Center at National Chengchi University, Taiwan. His research interests focus on survey research, quantitative methodology, electoral systems, and voting behavior. He has coauthored or coedited seven books and published articles in leading international and Taiwanese journals, including *APSR*, *AJPS*, *JOP*, *Comparative Political Studies*, *Electoral Studies*, *Party Politics*, *Political Research Quarterly*, *Asian Survey*, *Asian Journal of Communication*, and *Taiwanese Political Science Review*. He cofounded the Conference Group on Taiwan Studies (CGOTS) in the American Political Science Association in 1991, cofounded the Institute for Political Methodology (IPM, Taiwan) program in 2001, served as president of the Taiwanese Political Science Association (2003–2005), and founded the Taiwan's Election and Democratization Study (TEDS) interuniversity survey project in 2000, and served as the TEDS Coordinator until 2020.

Iain Johnston is the Gov. James Albert Noe and Linda Noe Laine Professor of China in World Affairs in the Government Department at Harvard University. He has written on socialization theory, identity and political behavior, and strategic culture, mostly with application to the study of East Asian international relations and Chinese foreign policy. Johnston is the author of *Cultural Realism: Strategic Culture and Grand Strategy in Chinese History* (Princeton, 1995) and *Social States: China in International Institutions, 1980–2000* (Princeton University Press, 2008), and is coeditor of *Engaging China: The Management of an Emerging Power* (Routledge, 1999), *New Directions in the Study of China's Foreign Policy* (Stanford, 2006), *Crafting Cooperation: Regional Institutions in Comparative Perspective* (Cambridge, 2007), *Measuring Identity: A Guide for Social Scientists* (Cambridge, 2009), and *Perception and Misperception in American and Chinese Views of the Other* (Carnegie Endowment for International Peace, 2015).

Koji Kagotani is an assistant professor in the Faculty of Policy Studies at Chuo University. He received a PhD in political science from the University of California, Los Angeles, in 2010. His specialization is international relations, formal theory, and political methodology. His works appeared in *International Relations of the Asia-Pacific*, *International Studies Quarterly*, *Japanese Journal of Political Science*, and *PS: Political Science and Politics*.

Chiung-Chu Lin is currently an associate professor in the Department of Political Science, National Chung Cheng University, Taiwan. Her research interests focus on voting behavior, electoral politics, opinion polls, and party politics. Her articles have appeared in *Journal of Electoral Studies*, *The Soochow Journal of Political Science*, *Issues & Studies*, *The Taiwanese Political Science Review*, *Survey Research—Method and Application*, and *Taiwan Democracy Quarterly*.

Hsuan-Yu Shane Lin is a postdoctoral research fellow at the Institute of Political Science at Academia Sinica (Taiwan) and a nonresident associate in research at the Fairbank Center for Chinese Studies at Harvard University. His research is focused on how social media impacts international security, especially the escalation of crises. His research can advance our understanding of the validity of the democratic peace theory in the social media era. His research has been supported by the Fairbank Center at Harvard, the Democratic Statecraft Lab at the University of Virginia, and the Fulbright Foundation. He was a predoctoral research fellow at the Fairbank Center. He received his PhD from the Department of Politics at the University of Virginia and his MA and BA from the Department of Political Science at National Taiwan University.

Alexander Tan is professor of political science and international relations at the University of Canterbury in Christchurch, New Zealand, and university chair professor of political science at National Chengchi University in Taipei, Taiwan. He has published widely contemporary democracies, party politics, Taiwan politics, and political economy with a focus on East and Southeast Asia.

Neel Vanvari is a PhD candidate in the Department of Political Science and International Relations at the University of Canterbury, New Zealand. His research interests include political economy, political parties, and party systems.

Austin Wang is assistant professor of political science at the University of Nevada, Las Vegas. Dr. Wang received his PhD in political science from Duke University. He specializes in survey research, electoral politics, political methodology, and East Asian politics.

Ching-Hsing Wang is an associate professor in the Department of Political Science at National Cheng Kung University in Taiwan. His research interests include research methods, political behavior, political psychology, public opinion, and Asian politics. He has published articles in such scholarly journals as *Democratization*, *Electoral Studies*, *International Political Science Review*, *Japanese Journal of Political Science*, *Party Politics*, *Political Science*, *Social Science Quarterly*, *The Social Science Journal*, *Taiwanese Political Science Review*, and other journals.

Dennis Lu-Chung Weng is an associate professor of political science at Sam Houston State University. Currently, he serves as an international research fellow for democracy studies at Stellenbosch University in South Africa and the Center of Southeast Asia Studies at the National Chengchi University in Taiwan. Dr. Weng's research and teaching interests are in the fields of comparative politics, East and Southeast Asia politics, political behavior, and survey research. Dr. Weng has published various scholarly articles in edited volumes and peer-reviewed journals. His op-eds have appeared in many Asian News media.

Charles K. S. Wu is an assistant professor in the Department of Political Science and Criminal Justice at the University of South Alabama. He received his PhD in political science from Purdue University. His primary research interests fall into the intersection between international relations and American politics, and his research agenda focuses on the factors that influence public opinion on military operations overseas. Dr. Wu's academic and policy work has been published in *Social Politics*, *Scientific Data*, *Journal of East Asian Studies*, *Journal of Asian and African Studies*, *International Relations of the Asia-Pacific*, *The National Interest*, *The Diplomat*, and *The Pacific Forum*. His latest coauthored book is *Presidentialism, Violence, and the Prospect of Democracy* (Lexington Book, 2021).

Masahiro Yamada is a professor at the School of Law and Politics, Kwansei Gakuin University. He received a PhD in law from University of Tsukuba. His specialization is political participation, voting behavior, and electoral politics. His works appeared in the *Journal of Politics*, and *Political Science Research and Methods*.

George Yin is a national service postdoctoral fellow at the National Taiwan University Department of Political Science. He is also a research fellow at National Taiwan University and a research associate at the Harvard Fairbank Center for Chinese Studies. Previously, he taught at Swarthmore College and was a nonresident senior fellow at the Atlantic Council.

Eric Chen-hua Yu is a research fellow of the Election Study Center and jointly appointed as a professor of political science at National Chengchi University in Taipei, Taiwan. Before he returned to Taiwan to teach in his alma mater, he was a research fellow and program manager of the Center on Democracy, Development, and the Rule of Law (CDDRL) at Stanford's Freeman Spogli Institute for International Studies (FSI) for three years. His research interests and recent publications have focused on electoral politics, public opinion, and public policy analysis. Yu received an MS in public policy analysis from the University of Rochester and a PhD in political science from Columbia University.

www.ingramcontent.com/pod-product-compliance
Ingram Content Group UK Ltd.
Pitfield, Milton Keynes, MK11 3LW, UK
UKHW020904190926
475560UK00011B/338

9 781666 940978